Clinical Acupunct

Springer

Berlin
Heidelberg
New York
Barcelona
Hong Kong
London
Milan
Paris
Singapore
Tokyo

Gabriel Stux
Richard Hammerschlag
(Editors)

Clinical Acupuncture

Scientific Basis

With Contributions by
B. M. Berman, S. Birch, C. M. Cassidy, Z. H. Cho,
J. Ezzo, R. Hammerschlag, J. S. Han, L. Lao, T. Oleson,
B. Pomeranz, C. Shang, G. Stux, C. Takeshige

With 40 Illustrations, some in Color
and 27 Tables

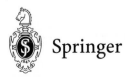 Springer

Gabriel Stux, M.D.
Akupunktur Centrum
Goltsteinstrasse 26
40211 Düsseldorf
Germany
106657.3550@compuserve.com

Richard Hammerschlag, Ph. D.
Oregon College of Oriental Medicine
10525 S. E. Cherry Blossom Drive
Portland, Oregon 97216, USA
rzhammer@compuserve.com

ISBN 3-540-64054-1 Springer-Verlag Berlin Heidelberg New York

Library of Congress Cataloging-in-Publication Data
Clinical acupuncture : scientific basis / G. Stux, R. Hammerschlag (eds.).
p. ; cm.
Includes bibliographical references and index.
ISBN 3-540-64054-1 (softcover : alk. paper)
1. Acupunctur.   I. Stux, Gabriel. II. Hammerschlag, R. (Richard)
[DNLM: 1. Acupuncture. 2. Research. 3. Treatment Outcome.
WB 369 C641 2001]   RM184.C635 2001   615.8'92--dc21

Springer-Verlag Berlin Heidelberg New York
a member of BertelsmannSpringer Science + Business Media GmbH

© Springer-Verlag Berlin Heidelberg 2001
Printed in Germany

The use of general descriptive names, registered names, trademarks, etc. in this publication does not imply, even in the absence of a specific statement, that such names are
exempt from the relevant protective laws and regulations and therefore free for general use.

Product liability: The publisher cannot guarantee the accuracy of any information
about dosage and application contained in this book. In every individual case the user
check such information by consulting the relevant literature.

Production: PRO EDIT GmbH, 69126 Heidelberg, Germany
Cover design: design & production, 69121 Heidelberg, Germany
Typesetting: Mitterweger & Partner, 68723 Plankstadt, Germany
Printed on acid-free paper   SPIN: 10653473   22/3130   5 4 3 2 1 0

Preface

In 1988, when "Scientific Bases of Acupuncture" was published, its editors noted that 12 years had passed since the acupuncture endorphin hypothesis was first postulated, an event that marked the start of serious basic research on acupuncture. The editors also suggested that more was known about the mechanisms of acupuncture analgesia than many procedures of conventional medicine and, in consequence, it was time to stop referring to acupuncture as an "experimental procedure."

Now another 12 years have passed. Acupuncture research, both basic and clinical, has greatly expanded. Modern biomedical techniques, including those of molecular biology and medical imaging, have revealed increasingly detailed physiological correlates of acupuncture action. Clinical researchers from Europe, North America, and Asia have devised a variety of protocols to test acupuncture efficacy according to generally accepted standards for randomized controlled trials. A critical review of acupuncture research by the United States Food and Drug Administration resulted in the label "experimental" being legally removed from the packaging of acupuncture needles in 1996, just as the editors of "Scientific Bases of Acupuncture" had proposed. A year later, again in large part a result of increased and improved acupuncture research, a consensus conference on acupuncture convened by the U. S. National Institutes of Health concluded its panel report with the endorsement "... *there is sufficient evidence of acupuncture's value to expand its use into conventional medicine and to encourage further studies of its physiology and clinical value*" (JAMA 280:1518–24).

The present book is nothing less than a celebration of the coming of age of acupuncture research. Reflecting the broad spectrum of modern-day acupuncture research, its chapters include an assessment of systematic reviews of acupuncture trials, proposed standards of acupuncture treatment in clinical research, qualitative methods to gauge patient satisfaction with Oriental medicine treatment, and physiological models of auricular acupuncture, meridians, and homeostatic responses to acupuncture. Our hope is that the state-of-the-art reviews presented in these pages will encourage consideration of the millennia-old practice of acupuncture as a contemporary, evidence-based treatment option.

July, 2000   Gabriel Stux
                                               Richard Hammerschlag

Contents

Contributors

Brian M. Berman (bberman@compmed.ummc.umaryland.edu)
Complementary Medicine Program, University of Maryland School
of Medicine, James L. Kernan Hospital Mansion, 2200 Kernan Drive,
Baltimore, MD 21207–6697, USA

Stephen Birch (71524.3461@compuserve.com)
Foundation for the Study of Traditional East Asian Medicine
W.G. Plein 330, 1054 SG Amsterdam, The Netherlands

Claire M. Cassidy (honeeum@aol.com)
Paradigms Found Consulting, 6201 Winnebago Road, Bethesda,
MD 20816, USA

Zang Hee Cho (zcho@uci.edu)
Department of Radiological Sciences, University of California,
Irvine, CA 92697, USA

Jeanette Ezzo (jeanetteezzo@prodigy.net)
Epidemiology Faculty, Project LEAD, 1905 W. Rogers Avenue,
Baltimore, MD 21209, USA

Richard Hammerschlag (rzhammer@compuserve.com)
Oregon College of Oriental Medicine, 10525 S.E. Cherry Blossom
Drive, Portland, OR 97216, USA

Ji-Sheng Han (jshh@public.bta.net.cn)
Neuroscience Research Center, Beijing Medical University, Beijing,
China 100083

I.-K. Hong
Dept. of Information Engineering, Kwangju Institute of Science
and Technology, Kwanju, Korea

Lixing Lao (LLao@compmed.ummc.umaryland.edu)
Complementary Medicine Program, University of Maryland School
of Medicine, James L. Kernan Hospital Mansion, 2200 Kernan Drive,
Baltimore, MD 21207–6697, USA

S.-H. Lee
Dept. of Acupuncture, South Baylo University, Anaheim, CA 92801,
USA

C.-S. Na
  Dept. of Meridianology, Oriental Medical College, Dong Shin
  University, Naju, Korea

Terry Oleson (terryoleson@earthlink.net)
  Health Care Alternatives, PMB 2657, 8033 Sunset Boulevard,
  Los Angeles, CA 90046–2427, USA

Bruce Pomeranz (varadi9180@home.com)
  Departments of Zoology and Physiology, University of Toronto,
  25 Harbor Street, Toronto, Ontario M5S 1A1, Canada

Charles Shang (cshang@emory.edu)
  Department of Medicine, Emory University School of Medicine,
  69 Butler Street, S.E., Atlanta, GA 30303, USA

Gabriel Stux (106657.3550@compuserve.com)
  Acupuncture Center Düsseldorf, Goltsteinstraße 26,
  40211 Düsseldorf, Germany

Chifuyu Takeshige (Makoton@cc.showa-u.ac.jp)
  Department of Medicine, Showa University, 1–5-8 Hatanodai,
  Shinagawa-ku, Tokyo 142, Japan

E. K. Wang (ekwong@uci.edu)
  Dept. of Ophthalmology, University of California, Irvine, CA 92697,
  USA

CHAPTER 1

Acupuncture Analgesia – Basic Research

B. Pomeranz

1.1
Introduction

In recent years, acupuncture analgesia (AA) in the west has been restricted mainly to the treatment of chronic pain and not used for surgical procedures, except for demonstration purposes. In some Western countries, however, AA is used in combination with nitrous oxide, sufficient N_2O being given to render the patient unconscious but not for analgesia [80], or with fentanyl [89]. How could a needle inserted in the hand possibly relieve a toothache? Because such phenomena do not conform to accepted physiological concepts, scientists were puzzled and skeptical. Many explained it by the well-known placebo effect, which works through suggestion, distraction, or even hypnosis [201, 202]. In 1945, Beecher [9] showed that morphine relieved pain in 70% of patients, while sugar injections (placebo) reduced pain in 35% of patients who believed they were receiving morphine. Thus, many medical scientists in the early 1970s assumed that AA worked by this placebo (psychological) effect. However, there were several problems with this idea. How does one explain the use of AA in veterinary medicine over the past 1000 years in China and approximately 100 years in Europe and its growing use on animals in America? Animals are not suggestible and only a very few species are capable of the still reaction (so-called animal hypnosis). Similarly, small children also respond to AA. Moreover, several studies in which patients were given psychological tests for suggestibility did not show a good correlation between AA and suggestibility [101]. Hypnosis has also been ruled out as an explanation, as two studies [6, 58] have shown that hypnosis and AA respond to naloxone differently, AA being blocked and hypnosis being unaffected by this endorphin antagonist.

Until 1973, the evidence for AA was mainly anecdotal, with a huge collection of case histories drawn from one quarter of the world's population. Unfortunately, there were few scientifically controlled experiments to convince the skeptics. In the past 25 years, however, this situation has changed considerably. Scientists have been asking two important questions: does AA really work by a physiological rather than a placebo/psychological effect and, if so, by what mechanism?

The first question had to be approached via controlled experiments to rule out placebo effects, spontaneous remissions, etc. These experiments have been carried out in clinical practice on patients with chronic pain, in the laboratory on humans, studying acute laboratory-induced pain (see Sect. 1.6), and on animals (see Sect. 1.6). From these numerous studies, it can be concluded that AA works much better than placebo.

Hence, AA must have some physiological basis. But what are the possible mechanisms? Only the answer to the second question (how does AA work?) could possibly dispel the deep skepticism toward acupuncture.

1.2
Neural Mechanisms of Acupuncture Analgesia

Twenty years of research in my laboratory coupled with over 100 papers from the western scientific literature led to a compelling hypothesis: AA is initiated by the stimulation of small diameter nerves in muscles which send impulses to the spinal cord. Then, three neural centers (spinal cord, midbrain, and pituitary) are activated to release transmitter chemicals (endorphins and monoamines) which block "pain" messages. Figures 1 and 2 summarize various aspects of the hypothesis of the neural mechanism of AA.

We explain the figures and present some of the evidence for this hypothesis. Fig. 1 shows how pain messages are transmitted from the skin to the cerebral cortex. On the left is skin, with a muscle beneath it in the lower left corner. An acupuncture needle penetrates the muscle. The next rectangle is the spinal cord, and to the right are rectangles depicting various brain structures: midbrain, thalamus, pituitary-hypothalamus, and cerebral cortex. As shown in the legend to Fig. 1, open triangles represent excitatory terminals (acting at the synapse) and closed triangles inhibitory terminals. Large arrows indicate the direction of impulse flow in the axons and small arrows the painful stimulus.

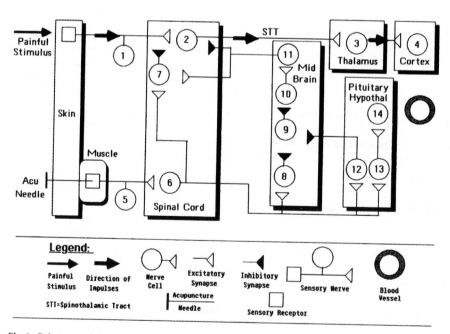

Fig. 1. Pain transmission

To understand the pain transmission as shown in Fig. 1, follow the thick arrows at the top. An injury to the skin activates the sensory receptors of small afferent nerve fibers (labeled 1) of A delta and C axon size. (Nerve fibers are classified by size and according to whether they originate in skin or muscle: large diameter myelinated nerves A beta (skin) or type I (muscle) carry "touch" and proprioception, respectively. Small diameter myelinated A delta (skin) or types II and III (muscle) carry "pain" messages, as do the smallest unmyelinated C (skin) and type IV (muscle). Types II, III, IV, and C also carry nonpainful messages.) Cell 1 synapses onto the spinothalamic tract (STT) cell in the spinal cord (labeled 2). The STT (cell 2) projects its axon to the thalamus to synapse onto cell 3, which sends impulses to the cortex to activate cell 4 (probably in the primary somatosensory cortex). I must point out that this diagram is oversimplified, since there are at least six possible pathways carrying pain messages from the spinal cord to the cortex but, for the sake of clarity, only the STT is shown.

It is best to go to Fig. 2 to see how the other cells operate (cells 5–14). In Fig. 2, the acupuncture needle is shown activating a sensory receptor (square) inside the muscle, and this sends impulses to the spinal cord via the cell labeled 5, which represents type II and III muscle afferent nerves (small diameter myelinated afferents). Type II afferents are thought to signal the numbness of De Qi needling sensations and type III the fullness (heaviness and mild aching) sensation [203]. Any soreness felt is carried by unmyelinated type IV afferents from the muscle, although soreness is not

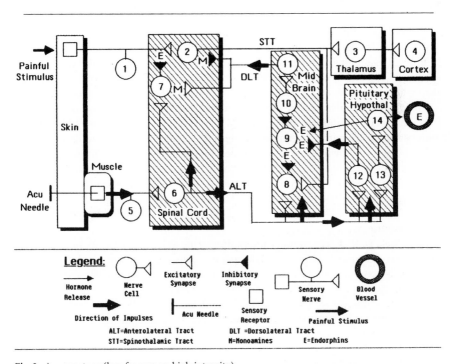

Fig. 2. Acupuncture (low frequency, high intensity)

usually part of the De Qi sensations. In some acupuncture points, e. g., at the fingertips or over major nerve trunks, there are no muscles and here different fibers are
involved. If cutaneous nerves are activated, A delta fibers are the relevant ones. Cell
number 5 synapses in the spinal cord onto an anterolateral tract (ALT) cell (labeled 6)
which projects to three centers, the spinal cord, the midbrain, and the pituitary-
hypothalamic complex.

Within the spinal cord, cell 6 sends a short segmental branch to cell 7, which is an
endorphinergic cell. This cell releases either enkephalin or dynorphin, but not beta-
endorphin. (There are three families of endorphins: enkephalin, β-endorphin, and
dynorphin, and in Fig. 2 these are all labeled E.) The spinal cord endorphins cause
presynaptic inhibition of cell 1, preventing transmission of the painful message from
cell 1 to cell 2.

As there are very few axo-axonal synapses between cell 7 and cell 1, it is thought
that the endorphin peptides merely diffuse to the receptors located on the terminals
of cell 1. There are also postsynaptic endorphin synapses acting directly on cell 2
from cell 7, although these are not shown. Thus, enkephalins and dynorphins block
pain transmission at the spinal cord level. The presynaptic inhibition probably works
by reducing calcium current inflow during the action potential in the terminals of cell
1, resulting in reduced release of the pain transmitter.

What Fig. 2 does not show are the numerous peptides present in the cell 1 terminals, including cholecystokinin, somatostatin, neurotensin, bombesin, calcitonin
gene-related peptide, angiotensin, substance P, and vasoactive intestinal peptide. So
far, only cholecystokinin (CCK) has been shown to play a role in AA [72], acting like
the opiate antagonist naloxone to block endorphin-mediated AA. Perhaps the ratio of
CCK and endorphins is the important variable in producing analgesia.

As shown in Fig. 2, cell 6 also projects to the midbrain, ascending the spinal cord
in the ALT. Here, it excites cells 8 and 9 in the periaqueducal gray (PAG), which
release enkephalin to disinhibit cell 10, which is thus excited) and in turn activates
the raphe nucleus, located in the caudal end of the medulla oblongata (cell 11), causing it to send impulses down the dorsolateral tract (DLT) to release monoamines
(serotonin and norepinephrine, labeled M) onto the spinal cord cells [66]. Cell 2 is
inhibited by postsynaptic inhibition, while cell 1 is presynaptically inhibited via cell
7. (Cell 7 is excited while cell 2 is inhibited by the monoamines.) Either of the two
monoamine mechanisms can suppress the pain transmission. In addition to the
raphe magnus, which releases serotonin onto the cord, there is the adjacent reticularis paragigantocellularis (not shown), which may release norepinephrine via the DLT
onto the spinal cord. Norepinephrine binds to an alpha receptor in the cord to block
pain transmission.

Some believe that serotonin and norepinephrine act synergistically in this regard
[64]. There is some evidence that the peptide neurotensin may be the excitatory
transmitter between cells 10 and 11 [7]. The precise relationship of these descending
monoamine effects to AA is not clear at present, and results suggest that some of the
raphe serotonin effect in AA may be mediated by ascending fibers from the raphe to
the forebrain (not shown). More work is needed on the role of the monoamine system
in AA.

Even less well understood is the action of cell 6 onto cells 12 and 13, the pituitary
hypothalamic complex. Cell 12 in the arcuate nucleus may activate the raphe via

β-endorphin, and cell 13 in the hypothalamus may release β-endorphin from the pituitary gland from cell 14 (Fig. 2). While there is some agreement that AA is accompanied by elevated beta-endorphin in the CSF [169] and blood and that pituitary lesions suppress AA [42], there is no agreement on how the β-endorphin from the pituitary reaches the brain to cause analgesia. Too little of it reaches the blood to cross the blood-brain barrier in sufficient quantities. Some evidence suggests that the pituitary-portal venous system can carry hormones in a retrograde direction directly to the brain [13]. Perhaps cell 14 can influence cell 9, as shown by the thin arrows in Fig. 2, without having to cross the blood-brain barrier. If so, the role of circulating endorphins in the blood is unclear. However, there is an important correlate of pituitary β-endorphin release: adrenocorticotrophic hormone (ACTH) and β-endorphin are coreleased into the circulation on an equimolar basis [19, 158]. (They stem from a common precursor).

The ACTH travels to the adrenal cortex, where cortisol is released into the blood [43], which may explain why acupuncture is helpful in blocking the inflammation of arthritis and the bronchospasms of asthma (the doses of cortisol released by acupuncture are small and finely regulated, thus avoiding the side effects of cortisol drug therapy). Because of insufficient data, other centers implicated in the AA-endorphin effects have been left out of our description. These include the nucleus accumbens, amygdala, habenula, and anterior caudate [77, 224]. In Fig. 2, the axon from the STT cell (cell 2) has a collateral fiber dropping down to excite cell 8 in the midbrain to cause analgesia. This is because of a phenomenon discovered in 1979 by Le Bars et al. [95] called DNIC (diffuse noxious inhibitory control), in which one pain inhibits another. Its role in AA has been suggested but never clearly established [14].

In summary, acupuncture stimulates nerve fibers in the muscle which send impulses to the spinal cord and activate three centers (spinal cord, midbrain, and hypothalamus/pituitary) to cause analgesia. The spinal site uses enkephalin and dynorphin to block incoming messages with stimulation at low frequency and other transmitters (perhaps gamma-aminobutyric acid, or GABA) with stimulation at high frequency. The midbrain uses enkephalin to activate the raphe descending system, which inhibits spinal cord pain transmission by a synergistic effect of the monoamines, serotonin, and norepinephrine. The midbrain also has a circuit which bypasses the endorphinergic links at high frequency stimulation. Finally, at the third, or hypothalamus/pituitary center, the pituitary releases β-endorphin into the blood and CSF to cause analgesia at a distance. Also, the hypothalamus sends long axons to the midbrain and activates the descending analgesia system via β-endorphin. This third center is not activated at high frequency stimulation but only at low frequency.

What is the practical significance of this three-level system? When needles are placed close to the site of pain or in the tender (trigger, or Ah Shi) points, they are maximizing the segmental circuits operating at cell 7 within the spinal cord while also bringing in cells 11 and 14 in the other two centers (Fig. 2). When needles are placed in distal points far from the painful region, they activate the midbrain and hypothalamus-pituitary (cells 11 and 14) without the benefit of local segmental effects at cell 7. Moreover, cells 11 and 14 produce analgesia throughout the body, while cell 7 produces analgesia only locally.

Local segmental needling usually gives a more intensive analgesia than distal non-segmental needling because it uses all three centers. Generally, the two kinds of needling (local and distal) are used together on each patient to enhance one another. Another important practical consequence of this system is the frequency/intensity effect. As shown in Fig. 2, low frequency (2–4 Hz), high intensity needling works through the endorphin system and acts in all three centers, while high frequency (50–200 Hz), low intensity needling only activates cells 7 and 11, bypassing the endorphin system. Numerous studies have shown that the types of analgesia produced by these two approaches are quite different [2]: the low frequency method produces an analgesia of slower onset and, more importantly, of long duration, outlasting the 20-minute stimulation session by 30 minutes to many hours. Also, its effects are cumulative, improving increasingly after several treatments. In contrast, the high frequency, low intensity analgesia is rapid in onset but of very short duration and with no cumulative effects. Many authors have arbitrarily described the low frequency, high intensity type of analgesia as "acupuncture-like" transcutaneous electrical nerve stimulation (TENS) and the high frequency, low intensity type as "conventional" TENS.

Because low frequency, high intensity analgesia produces a cumulative effect, repeated treatment produces more and more benefit for the patient [109, 154, 200] or laboratory animal [151]. This could be due to long-lasting effects of endorphins in the low frequency system. Most conventional TENS (high frequency) devices must be worn continuously by the patients, as the effect is of short duration, and in over 70 % of cases the effectiveness wears off after some months of continuous use because tolerance develops [209]. In contrast, low frequency acupuncture need only be given daily or twice a week because of its long-term cumulative effects [154]. Indeed, too frequent application of low frequency acupuncture produces tolerance. For example, if applied continuously for 6 h, the analgesia weakens and finally disappears [71]. This effect is cross-tolerant with morphine tolerance [71], and the mechanisms involved may be similar to those of addiction to endorphins. Hence, spacing the acupuncture treatments with long enough intervals may prevent tolerance while promoting the cumulative effects.

Perhaps the failure of some Western clinics to achieve success is due to the use of very infrequent treatments (e.g., one per week) and the termination of treatment after only five to ten sessions. In some clinics in Asia, patients are treated daily for a month, then weekly for 6 months, and the results reported anecdotally are excellent. Of course, some patients will never respond to acupuncture for various reasons; nonresponders may be genetically deficient in opiate receptors. We have shown that mice genetically lacking endorphin receptors respond poorly to acupuncture [135]. Other failures may be due to deficiency in endorphin molecules; rats lacking endorphin compounds respond poorly to acupuncture [123]. Some nonresponders can be converted to responders by treatment with the safe drug jd-phenylalanine, which potentiates endorphins [39, 51, 183]. In clinical practice, a strategy must be developed to allow nonresponders to be recognized while not aborting therapy too soon for potential responders who might show delayed cumulative effects. (One way is to decide after five treatments: if there is no benefit whatsoever, abort; if mild to moderate effects occur, continue and reassess after 10–15 treatments.) Often, the cost of repeated office visits is prohibitive. Hence, our group developed a home acupuncture-like TENS device which gives De Qi sensations and can be used by the patient over acupuncture points for 30 min/day for several months [41].

Most books might have ended the discussion of AA right here. However, because acupuncture is relatively new to Western medicine and so controversial, more data are needed to convince students that the acupuncture mechanisms outlined in Figs. 1 and 2 are well-established. Those who are in a hurry can skim or skip the next few pages but should nonetheless scrutinize the reference list (this omits the huge literature from China which, if included, would double the number of citations). It should be apparent that we know more about AA than about many chemical drugs in routine use. For example, we know very little about the mechanisms of most anesthetic gases but still use them regularly. The reader is also referred to the reviews [3, 66, 68, 76, 86, 100, 117, 139, 142, 143, 150, 168, 173, 215, 223, 226].

1.3
Evidence for Endorphins and Acupuncture Analgesia

Perhaps the most exciting experiments which opened up the field of AA to scientific research were those in which endorphin antagonists (e.g., naloxone and naltrexone) were used. That naloxone could antagonize AA was reported initially by two groups [113, 147]. Studying acute laboratory-induced tooth pain in human volunteers, Mayer et al. [113] produced AA by manual twirling of needles in LI.4 (first dorsal interosseous muscle of the hand). In a double-blind design, they gave one group of subjects IV naloxone while another group received IV saline. The saline group achieved AA with a time course typical for clinical reports (30 min to onset of analgesia and effects lasting for over 1 h). The naloxone group showed no AA. As no controls received naloxone alone, one might argue that naloxone hyperalgesia simply subtracted from the analgesia of AA. However, this is probably not the case, since numerous studies on acute laboratory-induced pain have shown that naloxone alone rarely produces hyperalgesia [57]. This suggests that endorphins do not have a basal tone during acute pain. Mayer et al. [113] studied a control group receiving placebo injections. The placebo subjects were told to expect a strong analgesic effect and none was observed, as predicted from Beecher's work on acute pain, where only 3 % of subjects reported placebo analgesia [9].

The other early naloxone study was by Pomeranz and Chiu [147] in awake mice; they used the mouse squeak latency paradigm and gave electroacupuncture (EA) at LI.4. Numerous control groups were used in this latter experiment in an attempt to determine some of the possible artifacts. Each group received one of the following treatments: EA alone, EA plus saline, EA plus IV naloxone, sham EA in a nonacupuncture point, naloxone alone, saline alone, and no treatment at all (just handling, restraint, and repeated pain testing). The results were unequivocal: naloxone completely blocked AA, sham EA produced no effect, and naloxone alone produced very little hyperalgesia (not enough to explain reduction of AA by subtraction). Moreover, the results in mice and in humans indicated firstly that AA was not a psychological effect and secondly that AA truly was blocked by naloxone. In a later study, Cheng and Pomeranz [36, 37] produced a dose-response curve for naloxone and found that increasing doses produced increasing blockade. In a third study in anesthetized cats [146] recording from layer-5 cells in the spinal cord (cell 2 in Fig. 1), the same researchers completely prevented the EA effects with IV naloxone.

Since these early papers, there have been numerous studies in which systemically administered endorphin antagonists have been used to test the endorphin-AA hypothesis. Although most researchers reported naloxone antagonism [25, 28, 32,

34–39, 46, 53, 62, 78, 93, 97, 98, 133, 135, 146, 147, 151, 160, 164, 165, 170, 171, 174, 175, 187, 193, 208, 210, 224, 225], some found no effects of naloxone [1, 30, 31, 137, 185, 200, 211]. Three of these seven failures were obtained with high frequency, low intensity stimulation, which is probably not endorphinergic [1, 200, 211]. In one of the failures [31] low intensity stimulation was used which did not lead to De Qi sensations. In spite of this, four of seven subjects in that study showed naloxone antagonism.

While the reasons for the other three negative papers [30, 137, 185] are not entirely clear, a possible explanation has emerged. Antagonists work best when given before the treatment [144, 206] and fail to reverse analgesia that has already been initiated. Thus, naloxone can prevent AA but often cannot reverse it. (In the three failed experiments, researchers tried to reverse AA, giving the endorphin antagonist after, not before the acupuncture treatments.) Taken together, the overwhelming weight of evidence shows that naloxone antagonizes AA and that the few negative results may be due to poor timing of the naloxone administration. In biology, negative results are often less valid than positive ones.

A few weeks after the first naloxone results were announced in the research news section of Science [110], a letter to the editor in the same journal justifiably criticized the use of naloxone as the sole proof of the AA-endorphin hypothesis [75]. This criticism is based mainly on the argument that naloxone might possess unknown side effects unrelated to opiate receptor blocking. Small doses which were effective in preventing AA in man ($5 \cdot 10^{-8}$ M) and in mice and cats (10^{-6} M) would tend to implicate receptor effects, but the effectiveness of small doses of naloxone is clearly not enough evidence to prove specificity [162]. However, since that letter was written, 17 different lines of experimentation have emerged which have independently provided support for the AA-endorphin hypothesis:

1. Many different opiate antagonists block AA [33–37].
2. Naloxone has a stereospecific effect [36, 37].
3. Microinjection of naloxone or antibodies to endorphins blocks AA only if given into analgesic sites in the central nervous system [15, 45, 67, 72, 73, 133, 144, 151, 216, 221, 224].
4. Mice genetically deficient in opiate receptors show poor AA [135, 159].
5. Rats deficient in endorphin show poor AA [123, 175].
6. Endorphin levels rise in blood and CSF during AA and fall in specific brain regions during AA [5, 45, 52, 74, 77, 83, 90, 108, 111, 125, 136, 169, 195, 225].
7. AA is enhanced by protecting endorphins from enzyme degradation [39, 45, 51, 54, 63, 82, 91, 123, 175, 225].
8. AA can be transmitted to a second animal by CSF transfer or by cross-circulation and this effect is blocked by naloxone [98, 105, 157].
9. Reduction of pituitary endorphins suppresses AA [42, 111, 152, 177, 179, 180, 181].
10. There was a rise in messenger RNA for proenkephalin in brain and pituitary. This lasted 24–48 h after 30 min of EA, indicating a prolonged increased rate of enkephalin synthesis. This could explain the enduring effects of EA and the potentiation of repeated daily treatments [60, 220].
11. There is cross-tolerance between AA and morphine analgesia, implicating endorphins in AA [33, 34, 71].

12. AA is more effective against emotional aspects of pain. This is typical of endorphins [218].

13. Lesions of the arcuate nucleus of the hypothalamus (the site of β-endorphins) abolishes AA; this is cell 12 in Fig. 2 [177, 178, 204].

14. Lesions of the periaqueductal gray (site of endorphins) abolishes AA [205].

15. The level of c-Fos gene protein (which measures increased neural activity) is elevated in endorphin-related areas of the brain during AA [59, 96, 132].

16. Evidence suggests that, in addition to monoamines mediating 100 Hz EA effects, dynorphin (one of the three endorphins) may also be involved. Thus, at 100 Hz there is an elevation of dynorphin levels in the dorsal horn of rat spinal cord [217] and there is an elevation of dynorphin A in lumbar punctures in humans receiving 100 Hz EA [69, 70]. Moreover, rats given EA at 100 Hz show AA, which is blocked by the dynorphin kappa antagonist (norbinaltorphimine), while the EA at 2 Hz is blocked by mu and delta antagonists, suggesting involvement of enkephalins and β-endorphin at these lower frequencies [34, 35].

17. Electroacupuncture in rats elevated precursors of the three endorphins, preproenkephalin, preprodynorphin, and preproendorphin mRNA. Moreover, antisense nucleotides for c-fos or c-jun successfully blocked the EA-induced preprodynorphin mRNA [60].

In summary, 17 different lines of research strongly support the AA-endorphin hypothesis. Despite so much convergent evidence for this hypothesis, skepticism persists:

1. Some cite the few failures of naloxone to reverse AA [31]. It has already been suggested above that naloxone reversal experiments are prone to difficulty because naloxone prevents but does not reverse AA. Moreover, the number of successful naloxone antagonisms of AA far exceeds the number of failures (28 successes versus 7 failures). In general, negative results in biomedical research are less reliable than positive results.

2. Some state that naloxone antagonism is necessary but not sufficient evidence [75]. That is why we have presented 17 different lines of evidence (only one line of evidence depends on naloxone).

3. Some attack the animal studies of AA as being unrelated to AA in humans [31]. Firstly, there have been numerous experiments in humans with the same AA-endorphin outcome as in lower animals. Secondly, the similarity of results across many species proves the generality of the phenomenon. Thirdly, there is no proper objective measure of pain in man. Fourthly, if skeptics are correct, then the entire animal "pain" literature should be discarded, a literature which provided our initial insights into endorphins, brain stimulation analgesia, TENS, and other results that have been highly applicable to human pain.

4. Some are concerned that AA in animals may be merely stress-induced analgesia (which also releases endorphins) and hence has nothing to do with acupuncture in humans [31]. At a conference on stress-induced analgesia at the New York Academy of Sciences, we gave a lecture entitled "Relation of stress-induced analgesia to acupuncture analgesia." Some of the points made in that paper [140] were:

   A. Sham EA on nearby nonacupuncture points in animals induces no AA, thus controlling for stress [27, 43, 55, 56, 102, 147, 176, 186].

B. AA elicited in anesthetized rats and cats or decerebrate cats does not involve psychological stress [27, 55, 56, 134, 144, 146, 148, 151, 152, 186].
C. AA at one frequency is endorphin-mediated while, at another, it is serotonin-mediated. Yet both give similar levels of stress [38, 170].
D. Many mechanisms of stress analgesia are very different from those of AA.
E. Results in mice and rats were obtained with mild stimulation activating A beta nerve fibers, a nonpainful procedure no more stressful than sham point stimulation [133, 149, 186].

In conclusion, the objections raised by a few skeptics are easily refuted. The overwhelming evidence supports the AA-endorphin hypothesis. Zhang [223] reviewed other differences between AA and stress analgesia:

1. AA is reversible with naloxone but stress analgesia is only partly antagonized by large doses of naloxone (20 times higher than that for reversing AA).
2. Plasma cyclic adenosine monophosphate (cAMP) levels decrease during AA but rise during stress analgesia.
3. The periaqueductal gray is essential for AA but not for stress analgesia.
4. Dorsolateral spinal cord lesions eliminate AA but not stress analgesia.

Nevertheless, a note of caution is needed here. Some animal models of AA are indeed stressful to the animals, especially those done in the awake conscious state using strong stimulation of the needles. One such experiment involves the rat model used by Professor Han of Beijing Medical University which has been challenged by Professor Mayer of the University of Virginia [20–22].

1.4
Evidence for Midbrain Monoamines and Acupuncture Analgesia

There are numerous papers implicating the midbrain monoamines in AA, especially serotonin and norepinephrine. As the raphe magnus in the brainstem contains most of the serotonin cells in the brain, lesions which destroy these cells or their axons in the DLT would presumably impair AA if serotonin were involved. Such lesions also abolish morphine analgesia, which is mediated by descending inhibition via the raphe-DLT-serotonin system [7]. Numerous experiments show that lesions to this system in animals block AA [40, 48, 87, 116, 163, 212]. Moreover, antagonistic drugs which block serotonin receptors also block AA in mice [40, 165]. In the above tests of the serotonin-AA hypothesis, the drugs were given systemically (usually IP). However, local microinjection studies produced surprising results, suggesting that the descending serotonin-DLT inhibitory system may not be as important as the raphe projections to the forebrain: intrathecal injections of serotonin antagonists over the spinal cord produced no blockade of AA in rats [133], while lesions of the ascending raphe tracts caused a selective decrease in cerebral serotonin and a correlated decrease in AA in the rat [65].

Microinjection of serotonin antagonists into the various brain regions confirmed the importance of ascending serotonin pathways; AA was blocked by injections into the limbic system and the midbrain PAG [65]. Enhancement of AA was observed in mice [40] and rats [65] when serotonin was increased by giving 5-HTP (a precursor of 5-HT) systemically or intracerebroventricularly [65, 219], the latter route being more effective than the intrathecal route. Measurement of 5-HT and its metabolite 5-hydroxyindoleacetic acid (5-HIAA) in the brain and spinal cord of rats during AA showed increased synthesis and utilization of 5-HT [190, 222]. The importance of serotonin in AA has also been confirmed clinically in patients using the serotonin uptake blocker clomipramine, where AA was potentiated in a double-blind study [221].

All this leaves us with the questions of why a lesion of the DLT in the spinal cord inhibits AA [163] if spinal cord serotonin does not mediate AA effects and whether the DLT contains other transmitters that mediate AA. Mayer and Watkins suggest that a synergism between descending serotonin and norepinephrine is the possible answer [112]. Indeed, Hammond [64] showed that combined intrathecal antagonists (for serotonin and norepinephrine) produced the best antagonism of descending analgesia produced by brainstem stimulation. Perhaps this should be tried for AA, since combined intrathecal antagonists should block AA more effectively than single antagonists.

There have been studies on the effects of norepinephrine (alone, without serotonin) on AA. Intrathecal injection of a norepinephrine antagonist blocked AA, showing the importance of descending norepinephrine pathways [66]. Clearly, the monoamine story needs more work. If synergism of descending serotonin and norepinephrine is important, then combined intrathecal blockers should be used in all future studies of monoamines in AA. The relative roles of the ascending and descending tracts need to be clarified.

In conclusion, there is no doubt that the monoamines (serotonin and norepinephrine) play a role in AA. Serotonin projections from the raphe to higher centers may mediate AA. Descending projections to the spinal cord via the DLT may work synergically with descending norepinephrine effects to block pain transmission in the spinal cord.

1.5
Evidence for Pituitary Hypothalamic System and Acupuncture Analgesia

The third possible center mediating low frequency endorphin analgesia is the pituitary-hypothalamic system. The arcuate nucleus of the ventromedial hypothalamus and the pituitary gland contain all the β-endorphin cells in the brain [16]. As the arcuate cells have long axons, β-endorphin is found in other brain loci, but it all originates from the hypothalamic cells [207]. The arcuate cells can produce analgesia via these long axons (stimulating the midbrain PAG, for example). Lesions of the arcuate nucleus abolish AA in rats [161].

There is a good deal of confusion regarding the possible relationship of the pituitary (hormonal) β-endorphins to pain modulation. We have already mentioned the evidence (lesion and blood biochemistry studies) implicating pituitary endorphins in AA. Involvement of the pituitary in other forms of analgesia has also been studied. For example, stress-produced analgesia is at least partly mediated by pituitary β-endorphins [158]. Here problems arise, because pituitary ablation is a very unreliable technique. Moreover, injection of the drug naloxone could have side effects. To make matters worse, in some species (e.g., rat) the blood-brain barrier for β-endorphin is very tight [158], although mice, rabbits, and man have a weaker barrier [192]. A new route for pituitary endorphins to reach the brain while bypassing the barrier has been discovered [13, 121] in the hypothalamic pituitary portal system (reverse flow occurs). Perhaps the endorphins can reach the third ventricles and, via the CSF, influence such structures as the PAG. Perhaps more important than the pituitary release of endorphins is the corelease of adrenocorticotropic hormone (ACTH) which occurs during AA [108, 111, 125], because this stimulates the adrenals to raise blood cortisol levels after AA [18, 43, 99, 102]. Sham acupuncture does not raise blood cortisol levels [43, 99], thus ruling out stress as the cause of cortisol release. It is tempting to speculate that this cortisol mediates the treatment effects of acupuncture in arthritis, effects which seem to go beyond analgesia [41]. Similarly, asthma might be helped by cortisol release [12, 182, 184].

Conclusions

In conclusion, the evidence for the mediation of AA by endorphins is very strong, while that for the involvement of monoamines needs more work to verify the possible synergism of serotonin and norepinephrine. Moreover, the circuits depicted in Figs. 1 and 2 are quite well established, although there is some uncertainty about the role of the pituitary.

1.6
Acupuncture Points – Do They Really Exist?

The question of the existence of acupuncture points, or acupoints, has been explored in several ways:
1. By comparing the effects of needling at true points versus sham points
2. By studying the unique anatomical structures at acupoints
3. By studying the electrical properties of skin at acupoints
4. By studying the nerves being activated by acupuncture at acupoints

1.6.1
Does Needling Work Better at True Points Than at Sham Points?

Several experimenters have shown that, for acute laboratory-induced pain in human subjects, needling of true points produces marked analgesia while needling of sham points produces very weak effects [23, 29, 172]. These results were clear-cut, because effects of sham point stimulation are nonexistent in acute laboratory pain. Placebo pills also have poor efficacy in acute pain, causing analgesia in only 3 % of cases.

In contrast to those clear-cut results, the work on chronic pain patients has been less convincing. Placebo analgesia in chronic pain has a strong effect, working in 30 %–35 % of patients. Moreover, needling in sham points seems to work in about 33 %–50 % of patients, while true points are effective in about 55 %–85 % of cases [197]. Therefore, to show statistical significance in the differences between sham point needling and true point needling requires huge numbers of patients (at least 122 per study); and experiments that would allow definitive conclusions have not yet been done [197]. It is puzzling that sham acupuncture works in 33 %–50 % of patients with chronic pain but not at all in acute laboratory-induced pain. Because of these problems, the specificity of acupoints in humans has been shown only in acute pain studies but has yet to be properly studied in patients with chronic pain, where the number of patients studied has never exceeded the required statistical minimum of 122 [199].

In animal studies in mouse [147], cat [27, 56], horse [43], rat [176, 186], and rabbit [55, 102], many researchers have shown that true acupuncture works better than sham needling in acute pain studies. These results are consistent with the research on acute pain in humans. In such studies, it is important to use mild stimulation in awake animals to avoid inducing stress: strong stimulation of sham sites could cause stress-induced analgesia [140]. Stress analgesia is a well-documented phenomenon [107] that is often mediated by endorphins. If the stimulation used is very strong, animals are highly stressed by both true and sham point needling.

Hence, numerous studies on acute pain in animals and humans clearly demonstrate that AA from needling true points is far superior to AA from needling sham points. However, more studies are needed to make the comparison in chronic pain.

1.6.2
Are There Unique Anatomical Structures at Acupuncture Points?

Despite several histological studies of the skin and subcutaneous structures under acupoints, no unique structures have been found. However, several authors [61, 119, 120] have made the astute observation that the majority of acupuncture points coincide with trigger points. For example, Melzack et al. found that 71 % of acupuncture points do so [119, 120]. This suggests that needles activate the sensory nerves which arise in muscles. This agrees with findings that stimulation of muscle afferents is important for producing analgesia [44, 104, 203].

The work of Travell on trigger points, begun in 1952 [188] and culminating in a large book published in 1983 [189], shows that there are small hypersensitive loci in the myofascial structures which, when touched or probed, give rise to a larger area of pain in an adjacent or distant (referred) area. She observed that "dry needling" (with needles containing no drugs) of these trigger points produced pain relief. When sites are tender, the Chinese call them Ah Shi points, and needling of them is recommended. Trigger points can often be found outside muscle bellies, in skin, scars, tendons, joint capsules, ligaments, and periosteum [189]. Travell stresses the importance of precise needling of trigger points, as missing the tense knotted muscle fiber could aggravate the problem by causing spasms. Similarly, strong electrical stimulation should be avoided. Thus, mild stimulation with needles inserted directly into trigger points is recommended [189]. The majority of trigger points are located on or near the following acupoints: SI.10–13, 15; SJ.13, 14; UB.12–17, 28, 29, 36–41, 48, 49; and GB.27–30. Although the cause of trigger point tenderness is unknown, one possibility is that poor inactivation of calcium by muscle sarcoplasmic reticulum causes calcium to cross-link the actin and myosin, with ensuing permanent contracture. How needling rectifies this problem, however, is unclear [189].

In a review on the subject of the anatomy of acupuncture points, Dung [50] listed ten structures which are found in the vicinity of acupoints (see especially numbers 5, 6, and 9 regarding trigger points). In decreasing order of importance, he found:

1. Large peripheral nerves. The larger the nerve, the more effective.
2. Nerves emerging from a deep to a more superficial location.
3. Cutaneous nerves emerging from deep fascia.
4. Nerves emerging from bone foramina.
5. Motor points of neuromuscular attachments. A neuromuscular attachment is the site where a nerve enters the muscle mass. This is not always the actual neuromuscular synapse, which may lie a few centimeters further along the nerve, after it has divided into smaller branches. The pathophysiological significance of this neuromuscular attachment is unknown. Travell emphasizes that many authors have used the term "motor point" interchangeably with "trigger point," but in most cases these are not at the same locations [189].
6. Blood vessels in the vicinity of neuromuscular attachments.
7. Nerves composed of fibers of varying sizes (diameters). This is more likely on muscular nerves than on cutaneous nerves.
8. Bifurcation points of peripheral nerves.
9. Ligaments (muscle tendons, joint capsules, fascial sheets, collateral ligaments), as these are rich in nerve endings.
10. Suture lines of the skull.

It is obvious from this list that no particular structure dominates at acupuncture points. Perhaps the major correlate is the presence of nerves, be they in large nerve bundles (items 1–8) or nerve endings (items 9 and 10). A report by Heine revealed that 80 % of acupoints correlate with perforations in the superficial fascia of cadavers. Through these holes, a cutaneous nerve vessel bundle penetrates to the skin. If replicated, this finding could be the morphological basis for acupoints [79].

The abolition of AA by injection of local anesthetics into an acupoint before stimulation begins [44, 149] strongly suggests that nerves are important for this phenomenon (Sect. 1.6.4). However, we should not rule out other mechanisms to explain the effects of acupuncture in immunological, allergic, and other non-AA phenomena. One can speculate on the possible release of arachidonic acid from lesioned membranes during needling, giving rise to leukotrienes and prostaglandins, which could affect immunity. Also, currents of injury (electric currents generated from a hole in the skin) might be important for nerve regeneration (Sect. 1.6.3).

It would be easy to find out if local anesthetics prevent all acupuncture effects as they do for AA, but few experiments have been done on nonanalgesic effects. Evidence suggests the existence of channels which may correlate with meridians. Vernejoul et al. [196] injected to a depth of 4 mm a radioactive isotope into 130 humans subcutaneously, using technetium-99 in sodium pertechnetate in a volume of 0.05 ml. They compared migration of the isotope (using a gamma camera) after injection into acupoints with injection into nonacupoints. They claimed that vertical lines of migration were seen only from acupoints. These extended as far as 30 cm within 5 min and resembled meridian lines in their distribution. Moreover the migration velocity was altered under pathological conditions. From the photographs in the papers, however, it was difficult to draw conclusions. Also, one must rule out lymphatic drainage. Several reports have favored venous drainage as the explanation for this isotope migration, raising serious doubts about this method for studying meridians [94, 167, 213, 215]. Replications by other laboratories are definitely needed before conclusions can be drawn from this controversial research.

1.6.3
Do Acupuncture Points Have Unique Physiological Features?

There have been a number of reports that the skin resistance (impedance) over acupuncture points is lower than that of surrounding skin [8, 26], but this result has been attributed to pressure artifacts from electrodes [114, 127, 191]. Normally, dry skin has a DC resistance in the order of 200 000–2 million ohms. At acupuncture points, this is down to 50 000 ohms in the studies claiming unique properties of acupoints. These observations have led to the marketing of "point finders," pencil-shaped metal-tipped probes attached by wires to an ohmmeter. The circuit is completed by a second electrode in a hand-held metal cylinder (with large skin contact on the sweaty palm and hence with a low resistance in the order of 1000 ohms). The point finder generally measures DC resistance based on Ohm's law (E = IR): a constant voltage is applied to the wires and the resultant current (I) is measured, from which resistance (R) is instantly computed. This can be read out on a Wheatstone bridge or directly on a meter. Most devices produce a beeping tone whose frequency or intensity is proportional to the resistance being measured. This allows the clinician to move the roving pencil probe around the body surface while listening to the tones. Anecdotal reports suggest that these devices work best in certain regions (e.g., hands, face, or ears) in which acupuncture points and low resistance often coincide (but see [118] for negative results on the ear). It is further claimed that, during disease of particular organs, the resistances at acupoints are abnormally low, even lower than the usual low resistance at acupoints (but see [118]). Indeed, the Japanese (Ryodoraku) method of measuring the acupoint skin resistance on the body has been in widespread use in Japan since its introduction by Nakatani in 1950 [124], while Nogier and the French school [126] have made observations at ear acupoints (see also [118]). In Germany, the Voll machine has concentrated on another skin electrical phenomenon, whereby the initial peak resistance reading is ignored while the capacitive "fall-back" of the reading to a steady-state (higher resistance) value is considered diagnostic. In the USSR, Gaikin developed the toboscope as a point finder, which was shown at the Montreal World Fair in 1967. This was further developed by Nechushkin in the 1970s.

There have been two careful experiments performed to validate the claims of ear "point finders" [118, 129]. Oleson et al. [129] took 40 patients and, in a "blind" design, compared diagnoses made with a point finder (9 V DC, 50 mA) on the ear with diagnoses made on the same patients by means of a Western medical workup. The researchers were blind to the Western diagnosis to ensure that no clues were available to them. Amazingly, the correlation between ear diagnosis and Western diagnosis was 72.5 %, which was highly significant [129]. Melzack and Katz [118] could find no difference in conductance between acupuncture points and nearby control points in patients with chronic pain [118] when they measured skin resistance in the ear. Unfortunately, neither Ryodoraku nor the Voll machine has been validated by similar controlled studies. Moreover, further claims for the Voll machine that homeopathic remedies placed in parallel with the measuring wires can modify the readings and thereby indicate appropriate treatments for the diagnosed ailment have never been scientifically tested [88].

Until recently, we were quite skeptical of the entire skin resistance phenomenon. This was because the measurements were not made in accordance with established

biophysical practice. Neither the published reports [8, 26, 155, 156] nor clinical anecdotal observations were based on properly conducted studies, as pointed out by
others [26, 114, 127, 191]. We improved the methodology. Ag/AgCl electrodes were
used with a salt bridge to avoid electrochemical potentials, biphasic pulses were used
to avoid polarization from DC currents, small (microampere) currents were applied
to avoid electrical damage to skin, spring-loaded probes were used to avoid mechanical injury of the skin, and very small amounts of saline were supplied from the salt
bridge through a Millipore filter to overcome skin moisture variations. When these
precautions were taken, a highly reliable technique developed [166]. Preliminary
results to date suggest that acupuncture points do sometimes have lower impedance
than surrounding skin. Whether or not this is true, the point finders commercially
available are very unreliable [166].

We have no idea what the physiological significance could be, if any, of low resistance at acupoints. It is known that sweating has a profound effect on skin resistance;
this forms the basis of lie detector tests. Stress, which activates the sympathetics,
causes sweating and a drop in skin resistance. In a preliminary study, we determined
that sweating occurs uniformly over the skin surface, equally at acupoints and over the
surrounding skin. Moreover, the earlobe is practically devoid of sweat glands, yet
resistance phenomena are claimed to occur there as well [129] (but see [118]). We have
not yet validated the claims of a drop in resistance during disease; if this phenomenon
proves to be true, the pathophysiological mechanism is unclear. Can sympathetics
affect local sweating during disease? Why should this be localized to acupoints when
sweating normally appears to be diffusely organized? It is also unclear why, acupoints
in normal people should have a low resistance. Could the presence of a large nerve,
emerging from deep tissues to more superficial layers, induce skin changes?

Another finding at acupuncture points is the presence of a voltage source [8] (i.e.,
a potential difference is reported to exist between acupoints and the neighboring
skin), with the points being measured at 5 mV higher than the nonpoints. Unfortunately, as mentioned above for resistance, most of these voltage measurements did
not use state of the art biophysical methodology. This is particularly unfortunate, as
electrochemical potential artifacts produced at the electrode-skin interface are large
compared with the millivolts being generated by the body. An outstanding study was
published by Jaffe et al. [85], showing that the human skin has a resting potential
across its epidermal layer of 20–90 mV (outside negative, inside positive). This paper
paid no attention to acupuncture points. Nevertheless, one can speculate that acupuncture points, having low resistance, tend to short-circuit this battery across the
skin and hence give rise to a source of current in a source-sink map of the skin. In
other words, acupuncture points provide a path of least resistance for currents driven
by the 20–90 mV resting potential which exists across the entire skin, which is consistent with the 5 mV readings mentioned above [8].

An important measurement in the same paper by Jaffe et al. [85] showed that a
lesion (a cut) in the skin produces a current of injury which is due to short-circuiting
of the skin battery. Preliminary results [166] indicate that insertion of acupuncture
needles into the skin might also produce a current of injury which has biological
influences on the underlying tissues. Indeed, our team has reported that weak currents (only 1–10 mA) promote nerve growth in the leg of an adult rat when applied
through acupuncture needles [115, 141, 145, 153]. In China, over 100 000 patients

with Bell's palsy of the seventh nerve have been reported anecdotally to benefit from EA and plain needling [214]. Perhaps the current of injury caused by needling and generated by the 20--90 mV resting potential across the intact skin promotes nerve regeneration in these cases. It is important to note that in a weak DC electric field, nerves grown in cell cultures will grow branches toward the electrodes [131]. Moreover, this growth is maximal in the direction of the negative pole [131]. The papers from our laboratory also show enhanced nerve growth toward the negative pole of the applied DC field [115, 141, 145, 153]. Holes made by needles would also cause a negativity at the site of injury due to the current of injury.

Regeneration of amputated amphibian limbs has been shown to be enhanced by applied electric fields and currents in the direction of the negative pole [17]. Although this has not been shown in adult mammals, there is indirect evidence of its effects in humans. If children suffer accidental amputation of the distal phalanx, it will completely regenerate (with nail, fingerprint, etc.), provided the tissue is kept moist. The latter allows a current of injury which is negative distally and about 1 mA in amplitude [84].

In paraplegic guinea pigs, DC fields and currents have also been implicated in bone healing, plant growth, embryology, and spinal cord regeneration [128]. Preliminary studies on normal human volunteers in our laboratory indicate that needling the skin produces a decrease in local skin resistance which lasts 1–2 days [166]. A simple calculation using Ohm's law suggests to us that a small hole created by an acupuncture needle can create a current of injury (10 mA) sufficient for possible benefit to tissue growth and regeneration [17, 141]. It should be noted that these tiny currents would not be sufficient to initiate nerve impulses, and hence the mechanisms shown in Figs. 1 and 2 would not be relevant here.

Attempts to use Kirlian photography to study acupuncture cannot be trusted, as this method is so fraught with artifacts. Perhaps the most intriguing phenomenon related to the meridians are propagated sensations along the meridians (PSM). In about 10 % of the population, needling causes a sensation to radiate along the meridian away from the needle in a direction inappropriate for the direction of the nerves (i.e., paresthesias should always propagate from proximal to distal, but PSM often goes from distal to proximal). The speed of transmission of PSM is approximately 10 cm per sec, which is 10 times slower than the slowest conducting C-fibers [10, 11]. Moreover PSM does not follow somatosensory distribution of the nerves or restrict itself to one or two dermatomes. Professor Bossy has proposed a plausible mechanism which does not involve Qi transfer along the meridians but rather a neurological one [24]. He proposes that the neural message travels from the acupoint into the spinal cord and then up and down several spinal segments (i.e., dermatomes) via interneuronal networks in laminae 2 and 3 of Rexed of the dorsal horn. The brain then perceives this as a sensation traveling into these dermatomes, i.e., as an illusion.

1.6.4
Which Nerves Are Activated by Acupuncture?

Electrophysiological evidence given below indicates that stimulation of muscle afferent fibers (types II and III) produces De Qi sensations [203], which in turn send messages to the brain to release neurochemicals (endorphins, monoamines, cortisol). Perhaps acupoints are the loci of type II and III fibers.

In a review, Omura emphasized the importance of eliciting strong muscle contractions to optimize AA; this, he says, requires low frequency EA to avoid tetanic contractions [130]. Strong muscle contractions are elicited because the stimulus intensities required to activate the type III afferent fibers must be 5 to 10 times the threshold for the muscle efferents.

One of the earliest and most clear-cut papers on the subject was published by Chiang in 1973 [44]. In it he showed that the essential correlate of analgesia was a De Qi sensation: the feeling of numbness, fullness, and sometimes soreness [44]. By injecting procaine (2%) into the acupoints LI.4 and LI.10 in humans, he determined that subcutaneous injections did not block De Qi sensations, while intramuscular procaine abolished them. Moreover, whenever De Qi was blocked, so was AA. Experiments have been done in animals [27, 55, 149] showing that procaine injections also abolish AA. To rule out the role of circulating compounds released by acupuncture, he also repeated these experiments with an arm tourniquet: when the De Qi persisted, so did the AA.

Another important finding in Chiang's paper was the lack of target specificity: acupuncture of points in the arm produced equal AA in all parts of the body, as measured by skin analgesia tests [44]. (He did not test the arm itself, or he would have seen a stronger segmental effect there). Two other studies showed the same lack of target specificity in humans in acute laboratory-induced pain [103, 106]. This lack of target specificity is consistent with the mechanisms shown in Fig. 2. It must be strongly emphasized here that the authors of the last two papers mentioned may have drawn wrong conclusions from their otherwise excellent studies: they concluded that all the relief experienced was purely a placebo effect, since there was no targeting of the treatment effects to specific pain locations. Yet it is not possible that 60% of patients could have benefited from placebo: as stated previously, Beecher reports that in acute laboratory-induced pain, placebo only works in 3% of volunteers [9] and hence the 60% effect in the acute pain studies [106] could not have been mediated by placebo. Since they stimulated true acupoints, they observed widespread AA effects. We interpret all these findings as follows: the acupoint maps are essential for localizing the sites where the best De Qi can be achieved (i.e., location of type II and III muscle afferents). In that sense, the points are specific. However, the further claim of traditional Chinese medicine that the points are also target-specific may not be true.

The conclusion that point specificity is not total nonsense comes from the many studies on acute pain both in humans and animals in which sham acupuncture produces no analgesia. Here "sham" is used to mean placement of needles in nonacupoints. Remember that Lynn and Perl [106] placed needles in true acupoints but inappropriate ones for the pain targets. Their points were not truly sham in that they did not use nonacupoints.

There have been numerous studies using proper sham acupuncture. One human study acupuncturing the first dorsal interosseous muscle (LI.4) produced a rise in tooth pain threshold using signal detection theory, while sham acupuncture of the fourth dorsal interosseous muscle produced no analgesia [29]. Another study of the pain threshold in the neck produced similar results [172]. Numerous animal studies have shown the same specificity: in mice [147], cats [27, 56], horses [43], rats [186], and rabbits [55, 102]: the sham points showed no AA while real points did.

The most extensive series of experiments on sham acupuncture was performed on rats by Takeshige et al. in Japan. Not only did this group find that nonacupuncture (sham) points failed to produce AA, in contrast to true points in the same animals, but they proceeded to find a plausible explanation [54, 81, 82, 92, 122, 138, 161, 175, 176, 178, 181, 194]. In a series of elegant experiments far too complex to give in detail here, they mapped out an AA inhibitory system in the brain which is activated by stimulation of nonacupoints: this system is activated from nonacupoints via nerves to the posterior hypothalamus, then to the lateral contramedian nucleus of the thalamus, and finally to lateral PAG, where it inhibits the midbrain AA system. (For a review of this extensive research project, see [176].) Lesioning of this inhibitory system releases the suppressed AA, so that nonacupoints become effective in producing AA. Finally, Toda and Ichioka did an elegant experiment in the rat to show that lesioning of the ulnar nerve had no effect in blocking AA from LI.4 stimulation, but that radial and median nerve lesions abolished AA [186]. Conversely, electrical stimulation of radial and median nerves produced AA, but ulnar stimulation did not [186]. It thus appears that the ulnar nerve does not reach the analgesia sites of the brain. Experiments on nausea and vomiting showed that procaine into Pe.6 blocked the acupuncture effect [49].

This brings us to the most direct experiments of all: the recording of impulses from the nerves involved in producing AA. Pomeranz and Paley [149], recording from afferents from LI.4 in mice, found that type II afferents were sufficient to produce AA. But they deliberately avoided activation of pain fibers (types III and IV) in awake mice to avoid stress analgesia. Similar results were reported by Toda and Ichioka, showing that type II afferents were sufficient for AA in the rat [186], since recruiting types III and IV did not augment the AA.

Experiments in monkeys, in which A-α and A-β fibers (i.e., types I and II) of the tibial nerve were electrically stimulated, resulted in only slight inhibition of pain responses of the spinothalamic pain tract [47]. However, when the stimulus strength was increased to a level which excited A-δ (type III) fibers, a powerful inhibition was observed [47]. Moreover, it should be emphasized that increasing the stimulus strength to excite C fibers (type IV) is not necessary, as it causes unbearable pain in conscious patients.

Lu [104] showed that types II and III afferents were important in rabbits and cats for AA: dilute procaine (0.1%) blocked type IV fibers and had no effect on AA, while ischemic or anodal blockade of types II and III fibers abolished AA. Thus, types II and III mediate AA in these two species (all blockades were verified with direct electrical recordings from the blockade nerves).

Perhaps the best experiment of all was done on humans with direct microelectrode recordings from single fibers in the median nerve while acupuncture was performed distally [203]. When De Qi was achieved, the following was observed: type II muscle afferents produced numbness, type III gave sensations of heaviness, distension, and aching, and type IV (unmyelinated fibers) produced soreness. As soreness is an uncommon aspect of De Qi, we must conclude that the main components of De Qi are carried by types II and III afferents (small myelinated afferents from muscle).

A study of De Qi on 65 human volunteers supports the existence of these sensations with needling. However, they also reported a confusing finding in the same paper: it seems that sham needling at nonacupoints produces as much De Qi as is elicited from true classical acupoints [198]. More research is needed to confirm this paradox. If it is true, then acupoints may not be site-specific for AA after all, if AA is indeed always elicited by De Qi. Perhaps this could explain the moderate success rate for AA as compared to sham AA that was achieved in some studies. Unfortunately, as mentioned above, very few studies discuss the De Qi aspect of the treatment parameters used.

Finally, mention should be made of the sensation sometimes felt by the acupuncturist: the "grab" of the needle by the muscle when proper De Qi is achieved. Recordings of electromyograms around acupoints during De Qi have shown pronounced muscle activation accompanied by the therapist's noting the grab of the needle [4].

The practical importance of all this could be summarized as follows: for AA, it is important to use strong stimulation to achieve De Qi sensations; the acupuncture maps are specific in the sense of helping us find types II and III fibers needed to obtain De Qi. However, acupoints may not be target-specific, as claimed by meridian theory; the only target specificity occurs from segmental effects of Ah Shi point stimulation, in which there is an additional benefit from spinal segmental endorphins (Fig. 2, cell 7) added to the total body effect of midbrain and pituitary endorphins (Fig. 2, cells 11 and 14). Thus, of the three acupuncture effects – local, meridian, and total body – we have evidence for local (Fig. 2, cell 7) and total body effects (Fig. 2, cells 11 and 14) but so far none for meridian effects.

References

1. Abrams SE, Reynolds AC, Cusick JF (1981) Failure of naloxone to reverse analgesia from TENS in patients with chronic pain. Anesth Analg 60:81–84
2. Andersson SA (1979) Pain control by sensory stimulation. In: Bonica JJ (ed) Advances in pain research and therapy. Vol 3. Raven, New York, pp 561–585
3. Andersson S, Lundeberg T (1995) Acupuncture – from empiricism to science: Functional background to acupuncture effects in pain and disease. Med Hypotheses 45:271–281
4. Anonymous (Shanghai Institute of Physiology) (1973) Electromyographic activity produced locally by acupuncture manipulation [Chinese]. Chin Med J 53:532–535
5. Asamoto S, Takeshige C (1992) Activation of the satiety center by auricular acupuncture point stimulation. Brain Res Bull 29:157–164
6. Barber J, Mayer DJ (1977) Evaluation of the efficacy and neural mechanism of a hypnotic analgesia procedure in experimental and clinical dental pain. Pain 4:41–48
7. Basbaum AI, Fields HL (1984) Endogenous pain control systems: Brainstem spinal pathways and endorphin circuitry. Annu Rev Neurosci 7:309–338
8. Becker RO, Reichmanis M et al (1976) Electrophysiological correlates of acupuncture points and meridians. Psychoenergetic Systems 1:195–212
9. Beecher HK (1955) Placebo analgesia in human volunteers. J Am Med Assoc 159:1602–1606
10. Bensoussan A (1994) Acupuncture meridians – myth or reality? Part 1. Comp Ther Med 2:21–26
11. Bensoussan A (1994) Acupuncture meridians – myth or reality? Part 2. Comp Ther Med 2:80–85
12. Berger D, Nolte D (1975) Acupuncture – has it a demonstrable bronchospasmolytic effect in bronchial asthma? Med Klin 70:1827–1830
13. Bergland RM, Page RB (1979) Pituitary-brain vascular relations. Science 204:18–24
14. Bing Z, Villaneuva L, Le Bars D (1990) Acupuncture and diffuse noxious inhibitory controls: Naloxone-reversible depression of activities of trigeminal convergent neurons. Neuroscience 37:809–818
15. Bing Z, Le Bars D et al (1991) Acupuncture-like stimulation induces a heterosegmental release of met-enkephalin-like material in the rat spinal cord. Pain 47:71–77
16. Bloom F, Guillemin R et al (1978) Neurons containing b-endorphin in rat brain exist separately from those containing enkephalin: Immunocytochemical studies. Proc Natl Acad Sci USA 75:1591–1595
17. Borgens RB, Vanable JW, Jaffe LF (1979) Small artificial current enhances *Xenopus* limb regeneration. J Exp Zool 207:217–226

18. Bossut DF, Leshin LB, Stomberg MW (1983) Plasma cortisol and β-endorphin in horses subjected to electroacupuncture for cutaneous analgesia. Peptides 4:501–507
19. Bossut DF, et al (1986) Electroacupuncture-induced analgesia in sheep: Measurement of cutaneous pain thresholds and plasma concentrations of prolactin and beta-endorphin immunoreactivity. Am J Vet Res 47:669–676
20. Bossut DF, Mayer DJ (1991) Electroacupuncture analgesia in naive rats: Effects of brain stem and spinal cord lesions and role of pituitary-andrenal axis. Brain Res 549:52–58
21. Bossut DF, Mayer DJ (1991) Electroacupuncture analgesia in rats: Naltrexone antagonism is dependent on previous exposure. Brain Res 549:47–51
22. Bossut DF, Mayer DJ et al (1991) Electroacupuncture in rats: Evidence for naloxone and naltrexone potentiation of analgesia. Brain Res 549:36–46
23. Brockhaus A, Elger CE (1990) Hypalgesic efficacy of acupuncture on experimental pain in men. Comparison of laser acupuncture and needle acupuncture. Pain 43:181–185
24. Bossy J (1984) Morphological data concerning the acupuncture points and channel network. Acup Electrother Res 9:79–106
25. Boureau F, Willer JC, Yamaguchi Y (1979) Abolition par la naloxone de l'effect inhibiteur d'une stimulation électrique péripherique sur la composante tardive du reflex clignement. EEG Clin Neurophysiol 47:322–328
26. Chan SHH (1984) What is being stimulated in acupuncture: Evaluation of existence of a specific substrate. Neurosci Biobehav Rev 8:25–33
27. Chan SHH, Fung SJ (1975) Suppression of polysynaptic reflex by electroacupuncture and a possible underlying presynaptic mechanism in the spinal cord of the cat. Exp Neurol 48:336–342
28. Chapman CR, Benedetti C (1977) Analgesia following TENS and its partial reversal by a narcotic antagonist. Life Sci 21:1645–1648
29. Chapman CR, Chen AC, Bonica JJ (1977) Effects of intrasegmental electrical acupuncture on dental pain: Evaluation by threshold estimation and sensory decision theory. Pain 3:213–227
30. Chapman CR, Colpitts YM et al (1980) Evoked potential assessment of acupuncture analgesia: Attempted reversal with naloxone. Pain 9:183–197
31. Chapman R, Benedetti C et al (1983) Naloxone fails to reverse pain thresholds elevated by acupuncture: Acupuncture analgesia reconsidered. Pain 16:13–31
32. Charlton G (1982) Naloxone reverses electroacupuncture analgesia in experimental dental pain. South Afr J Sci 78:80–81
33. Chen XH, Han JS (1992) All three types of opioid receptors in the spinal cord are important for 2/15 Hg electroacupuncture analgesia. Eur J Pharmacol 211:203–210
34. Chen XH, Han JS (1992) Analgesia induced by electroacupuncture of different frequencies is mediated by different types of opioid receptors: Another cross-tolerance study. Behav Brain Res 47:143–149
35. Chen XH, Geller EB et al (1996) Electrical stimulation at traditional acupuncture sites in periphery produces brain opioid receptor-mediated antinociceptin in rats. J Pharm Exper Ther 277:654–660
36. Cheng R, Pomeranz B (1979) Correlation of genetic differences in endorphin systems with analgesic effects of jd-amino acids in mice. Brain Res 177:583–5870
37. Cheng R, Pomeranz B (1979) Electroacupuncture analgesia is mediated by stereospecific opiate receptors and is reversed by antagonists of type 1 receptors. Life Sci 26:631–639
38. Cheng R, Pomeranz B (1980) Electroacupuncture analgesia could be mediated by at least two pain-relieving mechanisms: Endorphin and nonendorphin systems. Life Sci 25:1957–1962
39. Cheng R, Pomeranz B (1980) A combined treatment with jd-amino acids and electroacupuncture produces a greater anesthesia than either treatment alone: Naloxone reverses these effects. Pain 8:231–236
40. Cheng R, Pomeranz B (1981) Monoaminergic mechanisms of electroacupuncture analgesia. Brain Res 215:77–92
41. Cheng R, Pomeranz B (1987) Electrotherapy of chronic musculoskeletal pain: Comparison of electroacupuncture and acupuncture-like TENS. Clin J Pain 2:143–149
42. Cheng RS, Pomeranz B, Yu G (1979) Dexamethasone partially reduces and 2 % saline treatment abolishes electroacupuncture analgesia: These findings implicate pituitary endorphins. Life Sci 24:1481–1486
43. Cheng R, Pomeranz B et al (1980) Electroacupuncture elevates blood cortisol levels in naive horses: Sham treatment has no effect. Int J Neurosci 10:95–97
44. Chiang CY, Chang CT et al (1973) Peripheral afferent pathway for acupuncture analgesia. Sci Sin 16:210–217
45. Chou J, Tang J, Yang HY, Costa E (1984) Action of peptidase inhibitors on methionine 5-enkephalin-arginine 6-phenylalanine 7 (YGGFMRF) and methionine 5-enkephalin (YGGFM) metabolism and on electroacupuncture antinociception. J Pharmacol Exp Ther 230:349–352

46. Chung JM, Willis WD et al (1983) Prolonged naloxone-reversible inhibition of the flexion reflex in the cat. Pain 15:35–53
47. Chung JM, Willis WD et al (1984) Factors influencing peripheral nerve stimulation produced inhibition of primate spinothalamic tract cells. Pain 19:277–293
48. Du HJ, Zimmerman M et al (1984) Inhibition of nociceptive neuronal responses in the cat's spinal dorsal horn by electrical stimulation and morphine microinjection in nucleus raphe magnus. Pain 19:249–257
49. Dundee JM, Ghaly RG (1991) Local anesthesia blocks the antiemetic action of P6 acupuncture. Clin Pharmacol Ther 50:78–80
50. Dung HC (1984) Anatomical features contributing to the formation of acupuncture points. Am J Acupunct 12:139–143
51. Ehrenpreis S (1985) Analgesic properties of enkephalinase inhibitors: Animal and human studies. Prog Clin Biol Res 192:363–370
52. Facchinetti F, Nappi G et al (1981) Primary headaches: Reduced circulating beta-lipotropin and beta-endorphin levels with impaired reactivity to acupuncture. Cephalalgia 1:195–201
53. Fu TC, Halenda SP, Dewey WL (1980) The effect of hypophysectomy on acupuncture analgesia in the mouse. Brain Res 202:33–39
54. Fujishita M, Hisamtsu M, Takeshige (1986) Difference between nonacupuncture point stimulation and AA after D-phenylalanine treatment [Japanese with English abstract.] In: Takeshige C (ed) Studies on the mechanism of acupuncture analgesia-based animal experiments. Showa University Press, Tokyo, p 638
55. Fung DTH, Chan SHH et al (1975) Electroacupuncture suppression of jaw depression reflex elicited by dentalgia in rabbits. Exp Neurol 47:367–369
56. Fung SJ, Chan SHH (1976) Primary afferent depolarization evoked by electroacupuncture in the lumbar cord of the cat. Exp Neurol 52:168–176
57. Goldstein A (1979) Endorphins and pain: A critical review. In: Beers RF (ed) Mechanisms of pain and analgesic compounds. Raven, New York, pp 249–262
58. Goldstein A, Hilgard EF (1975) Failure of the opiate antagonist naloxone to modify hypnotic analgesia. Proc Natl Acad Sci USA 72:2041–2043
59. Guo HF, Cui X et al (1996) C-Fos proteins are not involved in the activation of preproenkephalin gene expression in rat brain by peripheral electric stimulation (electroacupuncture). Neurosci Lett 207:163–166
60. Guo HF, Tian J et al (1996) Brain substrates activated by electroacupuncture (EA) of different frequencies (II): Role of Fos/Jun proteins in EA-induced transcription of preproenkephalin and preprodynorphin genes. Brain Res. Molecular Brain Res 43:167–173
61. Gunn CC, Milbrandt WE et al (1980) Dry needling of muscle motor points for chronic low-back pain. Spine 5:279–291
62. Ha H, Tan EC, Fukunaga H, Aochi O (1981) Naloxone reversal of acupuncture analgesia in the monkey. Exp Neurol 73:298–303
63. Hachisu M, Takeshige C et al (1986) Abolishment of individual variation in effectiveness of acupuncture analgesia [Japanese with English abstract]. In: Takeshige C (ed) Studies on the mechanism of acupuncture analgesia based on animal experiments. Showa University Press, Tokyo, p 549
64. Hammond DL (1985) Pharmacology of central pain modulating networks (biogenic amines and nonopioid analgesics). In: Fields H et al (eds) Advances in pain research and therapy. Raven, New York, pp 499–511
65. Han CS, Chou PH, Lu CC, Lu LH et al (1979) The role of central 5-HT in acupuncture analgesia. Sci Sin 22:91–104
66. Han JS, Terenius L (1982) Neurochemical basis of acupuncture analgesia. Annu Rev Pharmacol Toxicol 22:193–220
67. Han JS, Xie GX (1984) Dynorphin: Important mediator for electroacupuncture analgesia in the spinal cord of the rabbit. Pain 18:367–377
68. Han JS (1986) Physiology and neurochemical basis of acupuncture analgesia. In:Cheng TO (ed) The international textbook of cardiology. Pergamon, New York, pp 1124–1132
69. Han JS (1990) Differential release of enkephalin and dynorphin by low and high frequency electroacupuncture in the central nervous system. Acupuncture Sci Int J 1:19–27
70. Han JS, Terenius L et al (1991) Effect of low and high frequency TENS on met-enkephalin-arg-phe and dynorphin A immunoreactivity in human lumbar CSF. Pain 47:295–298
71. Han JS, Li SJ, Tang J (1981) Tolerance to acupuncture and its cross-tolerance to morphine. Neuropharmacology 20:593–596
72. Han JS, Ding XZ, Fan SG (1985) Is cholecystokinin octapeptide (CCK-8) a candidate for endogenous antiopioid substrates? Neuropeptides 5:399–402

73. Han JS, Xie GX, Terenius L et al (1982) Enkephalin and beta endorphin as mediators of electroacupuncture analgesia in rabbits: An antiserum microinjection study. In: Costa E (ed) Regulatory peptides: From molecular biology to function. Raven, New York, pp 369–377

74. Hardebo JE, Ekman R, Eriksson M (1989) Low CSF met-enkephalin levels in cluster headache are elevated by acupuncture. Headache 29:494–497

75. Hayes R, Price DD, Dubner R (1977) Naloxone antagonism as evidence for narcotic mechanisms. Science 196:600

76. He L (1987) Involvement of endogenous opioid peptides in acupuncture analgesia. Pain 31:99–121

77. He L, Lu R, Zhuang S et al (1985) Possible involvement of opioid peptides of caudate nucleus in acupuncture analgesia. Pain 23:83–93

78. He LF, Doug WQ, Wang MZ (1991) Effects of iontophoretic etorphine, naloxone, and electroacupuncture on nociceptive responses from thalamic neurones in rabbits. Pain 44:89–95

79. Heine H (1988) Akupunkturtherapie – Perforationen der oberflächlichen Körperfaszie durch kutane Gefäß-Nervenbündel. Therapeutikon 4:238–244

80. Herget HF, L'Allemand H et al (1976) Combined acupuncture analgesia and controlled respiration. A new modified method of anesthesia in open heart surgery. Anaesthesist 25:223–230

81. Hishida F, Takeshige C et al (1986) Differentiation of acupuncture point and nonacupuncture point explored by evoked potential of the central nervous system and its correlation with analgesia inhibitory system [Japanese with English abstract]. In: Takeshige C (ed) Studies on the mechanism of acupuncture analgesia based on animal experiments. Showa University Press, Tokyo, p 43

82. Hishida F, Takeshige C et al (1986) Effects of D-phenylalanine on individual variation of analgesia and on analgesia inhibitory system in their separated experimental procedures [Japanese with English abstract]. In: Takeshige C (ed) Studies on the mechanism of acupuncture analgesia based on animal experiments. Showa University Press, Tokyo, p 51

83. Ho UK, Hen HL (1989) Opioid-like activity in the cerebrospinal fluid of pain patients treated by electroacupuncture. Neuropharmacology 28:961–966

84. Illingsworth CM, Barker CT (1980) Measurement of electrical currents emerging during the regeneration of amputated fingertips in children. Clin Phys Physiol Meas 1:87–91

85. Jaffe L, Barker AT et al (1982) The glabrous epidermis of cavies contains a powerful battery. Am J Physiol 242:R358–R366

86. Janssens LA, Rogers PA, Schoen AM (1988) Acupuncture analgesia: A review. Vet Rec 122:355–358

87. Kaada B, Jorum E, Sagvolden T (1979) Analgesia induced by trigeminal nerve stimulation (electroacupuncture) abolished by nuclei raphe lesions in rats. Acupunct Electrother Res 4:221–234

88. Kenyon JM (1985) Modern techniques of acupuncture. Vol 3. Thorsons, Wellingsborough

89. Kho HG, Eijk RJ et al (1991) Acupuncture and transcutaneous stimulation analgesia in comparison with moderate-dose fentanyl anesthesia in major surgery. Clinical efficacy and influence on recovery and morbidity. Anesthesia 46:129–135

90. Kiser RS, Khatam MJ et al (1983) Acupuncture relief of chronic pain syndrome correlates with increased plasma met-enkephalin concentrations. Lancet II:1394–1396

91. Kishioka S, Miyamoto Y et al (1994) Effects of a mixture of peptidase inhibitors on met-enkephalin, β-endorphin, dynorphin (1–13), and electroacupuncture-induced antinociception in rats. Jap J Pharm 66:337–345

92. Kobori M, Mera H, Takeshige C (1986) Nature of acupuncture point and nonpoint stimulation produced analgesia after lesion of analgesia inhibitory system [Japanese with English abstract]. In: Takeshige C (ed) Studies on the mechanism of acupuncture analgesia based on animal experiments. Showa University Press, Tokyo, p 598

93. Lagerweij E, Van Ree J et al (1984) The twitch in horses: A variant of acupuncture. Science 225:1172–1173

94. Lazorthes Y, Esquerre JP et al (1990) Acupuncture meridians and radiotracers. Pain 40:109–112

95. Le Bars D, Besson JM et al (1979) Diffuse noxious inhibitory controls (DNIC). II. Lack of effect on nonconvergent neurones, supraspinal involvement, and theoretical implications. Pain 6:305–327

96. Lee JH, Beitz AJ (1993) The distribution of brainstem and spinal nuclei associated with different frequencies of electroacupuncture analgesia. Pain 52:11–28

97. Lee JH, Beitz AJ (1992) Electroacupuncture modifies the expression of c-fos in the spinal cord induced by noxious stimulation. Brain Res 577:80–91

98. Lee Peng CH, Yang MMP et al (1978) Endorphin release: A possible mechanism of AA. Comp Med East West 6:57–60

99. Lee SC, Yin SJ, Lee ML, Tsai WJ (1982) Effects of acupuncture on serum cortisol level and dopamine beta-hydroxylase activity in normal Chinese. Am J Chin Med 10:62–69
100. Leong RJ, Chernow B (1988) The effects of acupuncture on operative pain and the hormonal responses to stress. Int Anesthesiol Clin 26:213–217
101. Liao SJ (1978) Recent advances in the understanding of acupuncture. Yale J Biol Med 51:55–65
102. Liao YY, Seto K, Saito H et al (1979) Effect of acupuncture on adrenocortical hormone production: Variation in the ability for adrenocortical hormone production in relation to the duration of acupuncture stimulation. Am J Chin Med 7:362–371
103. Lim TW, Loh T, Kranz H, Scott D (1977) Acupuncture effect on normal subjects. Med J Aust 26:440–442
104. Lu GW (1983) Characteristics of afferent fiber innervation on acupuncture point zusanli. Am J Physiol 245:R606–R612
105. Lung CH, Sun AC, Tsao CJ et al (1978) An observation of the humoral factor in acupuncture analgesia in rats. Am J Chin Med 2:203–205
106. Lynn B, Perl ER (1977) Failure of acupuncture to produce localized analgesia. Pain 3:339–351
107. Madden J, Akil H, Barchas JD et al (1977) Stress-induced parallel changes in central opioid levels and pain responsiveness in rat. Nature 265:358–360
108. Malizia F, Paolucci D et al (1979) Electroacupuncture and peripheral beta-endorphin and ACTH levels. Lancet II:535–536
109. Martelete M, Fiori AM (1985) Comparative study of the analgesic effect of transcutaneous nerve stimulation (TNS), electroacupuncture (EA), and meperidine in the treatment of postoperative pain. Acupunct Electrother Res 10:183–193
110. Marx JL (1977) Analgesia: How the body inhibits pain perception. Science 196:471
111. Masala A, Satta G, Alagna S et al (1983) Suppression of electroacupuncture (EA)-induced beta-endorphin and ACTH release by hydrocortisone in man. Absence of effects on EA-induced anaesthesia. Acta Endocrinol (Copenh) 103:469–472
112. Mayer DJ, Watkins LR (1984) Multiple endogenous opiate and nonopiate analgesia systems. In: Kruger L (ed) Advances in pain research and therapy. Vol 6. Raven, New York, pp 253–276
113. Mayer DJ, Price DD, Raffii A (1977) Antagonism of acupuncture analgesia in man by the narcotic antagonist naloxone. Brain Res 121:368–372
114. McCarroll GD, Rowley BA (1979) An investigation of the existence of electrically located acupuncture points. IEEE Trans Biomed Eng 26:177–181
115. McDevitt L, Fortner P, Pomeranz B (1987) Application of weak electric field to the hindpaw enhances sciatic motor nerve regeneration in the adult rat. Brain Res 416:308 –314
116. McLennan H, Gilfillan K, Heap Y (1977) Some pharmacological observations on the analgesia induced by acupuncture. Pain 3:229–238
117. Melzack R (1984) Acupuncture and related forms of folk medicine. In: Wall PD, Melzack R (eds) Textbook of pain. Churchill Livingstone, Edinburgh, pp 691–701
118. Melzack R, Katz J (1984) Auriculotherapy fails to relieve chronic pain. JAMA 251:1041–1043
119. Melzack R, Wall PD (1965) Pain mechanism: A new theory. Science 150:971–979
120. Melzack R, Stillwell DM, Fox EJ (1977) Trigger points and acupuncture points for pain: Correlations and implications. Pain 3:3–23
121. Mezey E, de Weid D et al (1978) Evidence for pituitary-brain transport of a behaviourally potent ACTH analogue. Life Sci 22:831–838
122. Mizuno T (1986) The nature of acupuncture point investigation by evoked potential from the dorsal periaqueductal central grey in acupuncture afferent pathway [Japanese with English summary]. In: Takeshige C (ed) Studies on the mechanism of acupuncture analgesia based on animal experiments. Showa University Press, Tokyo, p 425
123. Murai M, Takeshige C et al (1986) Correlation between individual variations in effectiveness of acupuncture analgesia and those in contents of brain endogenous morphine-like factors [Japanese with English summary]. In: Takeshige C (ed) Studies on the mechanism of acupuncture analgesia based on animal experiments. Showa University Press, Tokyo, p 542
124. Nakatani Y, Yamashita K (1977) Ryodoraku acupuncture. Ryodoraku Research Institute, Osaka
125. Nappi G, Faccinetti F et al (1982) Different releasing effects of traditional manual acupuncture and electroacupuncture on propiocortin-related peptides. Acupunct Electrother Res Int J 7:93–103
126. Nogier PFM (1972) Treatise of auriculotherapy. Moulin-les-Metz, Maisonneuve, France
127. Noodergraaf, Silage D (1973) Electroacupuncture. IEEE Trans Biochem Eng 20:364–366
128. Nuccitelli R (ed) (1986) Ionic currents in development (39 papers by various authors). Liss, New York
129. Oleson TD, Kroenig RJ, Bresler DE (1980) An experimental evaluation of auricular diagnosis: The somatotopic mapping of musculoskeletal pain at acupuncture points. Pain 8:217–229

130. Omura Y (1989) Basic electrical parameters for safe and effective electrotherapeutics (electroacupuncture, TES, TENMS, TEMS, TENS, and electromagnetic field stimulation) for pain, neuromuscular skeletal problems, and circulatory disturbances. Acup Electrother Res 12:201–225

131. Patel N, Poo MM (1982) Orientation of neurite growth by extracellular electric fields. J Neurosci 2:483–496

132. Pan B, Castro-Lopes JM et al (1994) C-fos expression in the hypothalamic pituitary system induced by electroacupuncture or noxious stimulation. Neuroreport 5:1649–1652

133. Peets J, Pomeranz B (1985) Acupuncture-like transcutaneous electrical nerve stimulation analgesia is influenced by spinal cord endorphins but not serotonin: An intrathecal pharmacological study. In: Fields H et al (eds) Advances in pain research and therapy. Raven, New York, pp 519–525

134. Peets J, Pomeranz B (1987) Studies of suppression of nocifensor reflexes using tail flick electromyograms and intrathecal drugs in barbiturate-anaesthetized rats. Brain Res 416:301–307

135. Peets J, Pomeranz B (1978) CXBX mice deficient in opiate receptors show poor electroacupuncture analgesia. Nature 273:675–676

136. Pert A, Dionne R, Ng L, Pert C et al (1981) Alterations in rat central nervous system endorphins following transauricular electroacupuncture. Brain Res 224:83–93

137. Pertovaara A, Kemppainen P et al (1982) Dental analgesia produced by nonpainful, low frequency stimulation is not influenced by stress or reversed by naloxone. Pain 13:379–384

138. Pin Luo C, Takeshige C et al (1986) Inhibited region by analgesia inhibitory system in acupuncture nonpoint stimulation produced analgesia [Japanese with English summary]. In: Takeshige C (ed) Studies on the mechanism of acupuncture analgesia based on animal experiments. Showa University Press, Tokyo, p 613

139. Pomeranz B (1981) Neural mechanisms of acupuncture analgesia. In: Lipton S (ed) Persistent pain. Vol 3. Academic, New York, pp 241–257

144. Pomeranz B (1985) Relation of stress-induced analgesia to acupuncture analgesia. In: Kelly J (ed) Stress-induced analgesia. Ann NY Acad Sci:444–447

141. Pomeranz B (1986) Effects of applied DC fields on sensory nerve sprouting and motor nerve regeneration in adult rats. In: Nuccitelli R (ed) Ionic currents in development. Liss, New York, pp 251–258

142. Pomeranz B (1994) Acupuncture in America. APS Journal 3:96–100

143. Pomeranz B (1996) Scientific research into acupuncture for the relief of pain. J Alt Compl Med 2:53–60

144. Pomeranz B, Bibic L (1988) Naltrexone, an opiate antagonist, prevents but does not reverse the analgesia produced by electroacupuncture. Brain Res 452:227–231

145. Pomeranz B, Campbell JJ (1993) Weak electric field accelerates motoneuron regeneration in the sciatic nerve of 10-month-old rats. Brain Res 603:271–278

146. Pomeranz B, Cheng R (1979) Suppression of noxious responses in single neurons of cat spinal cord by electroacupuncture and its reversal by the opiate antagonist naloxone. Exp Neurol 64:327–341

147. Pomeranz B, Chiu D (1976) Naloxone blocks acupuncture analgesia and causes hyperalgesia: Endorphin is implicated. Life Sci 19:1757–1762

148. Pomeranz B, Nyguyen P (1986) Intrathecal diazepam suppresses nociceptive reflexes and potentiates electroacupuncture effects in pentobarbital rats. Neurosci Lett 77:316–320

149. Pomeranz B, Paley D (1979) Electroacupuncture hypoalgesia is mediated by afferent nerve impulses: An electrophysiological study in mice. Exp Neurol 66:398–402

150. Pomeranz B, Stux G (1989) Scientific bases of acupuncture. Springer, Berlin Heidelberg New York

151. Pomeranz B, Warma N (1988) Potentiation of analgesia by two repeated electroacupuncture treatments: The first opioid analgesia potentiates a second, nonopioid analgesia response. Brain Res 452:232–236

152. Pomeranz B, Cheng R, Law P (1977) Acupuncture reduces electrophysiological and behavioural responses to noxious stimuli: Pituitary is implicated. Exp Neurol 54:172–178

153. Pomeranz B, Mullen M, Markus H (1984) Effect of applied electrical fields on sprouting of intact saphenous nerve in adult rat. Brain Res 303:331–336

154. Price DD, Rafii A et al (1984) A psychophysical analysis of acupuncture analgesia. Pain 19:27–42

155. Reichmanis M, Marino AA, Becker RO (1975) Electrical correlates of acupuncture points. IEEE Trans Biomed Eng 22:533–535

156. Reichmanis M, Marino AA, Becker RO (1979) Laplace plane analysis of impedence on the H meridian. Am J Chin Med 7:188–193

157. Research Group of Peking Medical College (1974) The role of some neurotransmitters of brain in finger acupuncture analgesia. Sci Sin 17:112–130

158. Rossier J, Guillemin R, Bloom FE (1977) Foot shock-induced stress increases b-endorphin levels in blood but not brain. Nature 270:618–620

160. Roy BP, Cheng R, Pomeranz B et al (1980) Pain threshold and brain endorphin levels in genetically obese ob/ob and opiate receptor-deficient CXBK mice. In: Way EL (ed) Exogenous and endogenous opiate agonists and antagonists. Pergamon, Elmsford, p 297

160. Sato T, Takeshige C (1986) Morphine analgesia caused by activation of spinal acupuncture afferent pathway in the anterolateral tract [Japanese with English summary]. In: Takeshige C (ed) Studies on the mechanism of acupuncture analgesia based on animal experiments. Showa University Press, Tokyo p 673

161. Sato T, Usami S, Takeshige C (1986) Role of the arcuate nucleus of the hypothalamus as the descending pain-inhibitory system in acupuncture point and nonpoint produced analgesia [Japanese with English summary]. In: Takeshige C (ed) Studies on the mechanism of acupuncture analgesia based on animal experiments. Showa University Press, Tokyo, p 627

162. Sawynok J, Pinsky C, Labella FS (1979) Minireview on the specificity of naloxone as an opiate antagonist. Life Sci 25:1621–1632

163. Shen E, Ma WH, Lan C (1978) Involvement of descending inhibition in the effect of acupuncture on the splanchnically evoked potentials in the orbital cortex of cat. Sci Sin 21:677–685

164. Shimizu S, Takeshige C et al (1986) Relationship between endogenous morphine-like factor and serotonergic system in analgesia of acupuncture anesthesia [Japanese with English summary]. In: Takeshige C (ed) Studies on the mechanism of acupuncture analgesia based on animal experiments. Showa University Press, Tokyo, p 700

165. Shimizu T, Koja T et al (1981) Effects of methysergide and naloxone on analgesia produced by peripheral electrical stimulation in mice. Brain Res 208:463–467

166. Shu R, Pomeranz B et al (1997) Electrical impedance measurements of human skin at acupuncture points and changes produced by needling. (In press.)

167. Simon J, Giraud G et al (1988) Acupuncture meridians demystified. Contributions of radiotracer methodology. Presse Med 17:1341–1344

168. Sims J (1997) The mechanism of acupuncture analgesia: A review. Compl Therap Med 5:102–111

169. Sjolund B, Terenius L, Eriksson M (1977) Increased cerebrospinal fluid levels of endorphins after electroacupuncture. Acta Physiol Scand 100:382–384

170. Sjolund BH, Erikson BE (1979) The influence of naloxone on analgesia produced by peripheral conditioning stimulation. Brain Res 173:295–301

171. Sodipo JO, Gilly H, Pauser G (1981) Endorphins: Mechanism of acupuncture analgesia. Am J Chin Med 9:249–258

172. Stacher G, Wancura I et al (1975) Effect of acupuncture on pain threshold and pain tolerance determined by electrical stimulation of the skin: A controlled study. Am J Chin Med 3:143–146

173. Stux G, Pomeranz B (1987) Acupuncture: Textbook and Atlas. Springer, Berlin Heidelberg New York

174. Takagi J, Sawada T et al (1996) A possible involvement of monoaminergic and opioidergic systems in the analgesia induced by electroacupuncture in rabbits. Jap J Pharm 70:73–80

175. Takahashi G, Mera H, Kobori M (1986) Inhibitory action on analgesic inhibitory system and augmenting action on naloxone reversal analgesia of jd-phenylalanine [Japanese with English summary]. In: Takeshige C (ed) Studies on the mechanism of acupuncture analgesia based on animal experiments. Showa University Press, Tokyo, p 608

176. Takeshige C (1985) Differentiation between acupuncture and nonacupuncture points by association with an analgesia inhibitory system. Acupunct Electrother Res 10:195–203

177. Takeshige C, Tsuchiya M et al (1991) Dopaminergic transmission in the arcuate nucleus to produce acupuncture analgesia in correlation with the pituitary gland. Brain Res Bull 26:113–122

178. Takeshige C, Zhao WH, Guo SY (1991) Convergence from the preoptic area and arcuate nucleus to the median eminence in acupuncture and nonacupuncture stimulation analgesia. Brain Res Bull 26:771–778

179. Takeshige C, Oka K et al (1993) The acupuncture point and its connecting central pathway for producing acupuncture analgesia. Brain Res Bull 30:53–67

180. Takeshige C, Nakamura A et al (1992) Positive feedback action of pituitary beta-endorphin on acupuncture analgesia afferent pathway. Brain Res Bull 29:37–44

181. Takeshige C, Kobori M et al (1992) Analgesia inhibitory system involvement in nonacupuncture point stimulation produced analgesia. Brain Res Bull 28:379–391

182. Takishima T, Mue S, Tamura G et al (1982) The bronchodilating effect of acupuncture in patients with acute asthma. Ann Allergy 48:44–49

183. Tanaka M (1986) Studies on analgesic enhancement by D-phenylalanine [Japanese with English summary]. In: Takeshige C (ed) Studies on the mechanism of acupuncture analgesia based on animal experiments. Showa University Press, Tokyo, p 440

184. Tashkin D, Kroenig R et al (1977) Comparison of real and simulated acupuncture and isoproterenol in comparison to methacholine-induced asthma. Ann Allergy 39:379–387
185. Tay AA, Tseng CK, Pace NL et al (1982) Failure of narcotic antagonist to alter electroacupuncture modification of halothane anaesthesia in the dog. Can Anaesth Soc J 29:231–235
186. Toda K, Ichioka M (1978) Electroacupuncture: Relations between forelimb afferent impulses and suppression of jaw opening reflex in the rat. Exp Neurol 61:465–470
187. Thoren P, Floras JS et al (1989) Endorphins and exercise: Physiological mechanisms and clinical implications. Med Sci Sports Exerc 22:417–428
188. Travell J, Rinzler SH (1952) Myofascial genesis of pain. Postgrad Med J 11:425–434
189. Travell J, Simmons D (1983) Myofascial pain and dysfunction. The trigger point manual. William and Wilkins, Baltimore
190. Tsai HY, Lin JG, Inoki R (1989) Further evidence for possible analgesic mechanism of electroacupuncture: Effects of neuropeptides and serotonergic neurons in rat spinal cord. Jpn J Pharmacol 49:181–185
191. Tseng HL, Chang LT et al (1958) Electrical conductance and temperature of the cutaneous acupuncture points: A study of normal readings and bodily distributions [Chinese]. J Trad Chin Med 12:559–563
192. Tseng LF, Loh HH, Li CH (1976) Effects of systemic administration of endorphins. Nature 263:239–240
193. Tsunoda Y, Ikezono E et al (1980) Antagonism of acupuncture analgesia by naloxone in unconscious man. Bull Tokyo Med Dent 27:89–94
194. Usami S, Takeshige C (1986) The difference in analgesia producing central pathway of stress-induced analgesia and that of acupuncture point- and nonpoint-produced analgesia [Japanese with English abstract]. In: Takeshige C (ed) Studies on the mechanism of acupuncture analgesia based on animal experiments. Showa University Press, Tokyo, p 638
195. Vacca-Galloway LL et al (1985) Alterations of immunoreactive substance P and enkephalins in rat spinal cord after electroacupuncture. Peptides 6 [Suppl 1]:177–188
196. Vernejoul P de, Darras JC et al (1985) Etude des meridiens d'acupuncture par les traceurs radioactifs. Bull Acad Natl Med (Paris) 169:1071–1075
197. Vincent CA, Richardson PH (1986) The evaluation of therapeutic acupuncture: Concepts and methods. Pain 24:1–13
198. Vincent CA, Richardson PH et al (1989) The significance of needle placement site in acupuncture. J Psychosom Res 33:489–496
199. Vincent C, Lewith G (1995) Placebo controls for acupuncture studies. J R Soc Med 88:199–202
200. Walker JB, Katz RL (1981) Nonopioid pathways suppress pain in humans. Pain 11:347–354
201. Wall PD (1972) An eye on the needle. New Sci July 20, pp 129–131
202. Wall PD (1974) Acupuncture revisited. New Sci Oct 3, pp 31–34
203. Wang K, Yao S, Xian Y, Hou Z (1985) A study on the receptive field of acupoints and the relationship between characteristics of needle sensation and groups of afferent fibres. Sci Sin 28:963–971
204. Wang Q, Mao L, Han J (1990) The arcuate nucleus of hypothalamus mediates low but not high frequency electroacupuncture in rats. Brain Res 513:60–66
205. Wang Q, Mao L, Han J (1990) The role of periaqueductal grey in mediation of analgesia produced by different frequencies electroacupuncture stimulation in rats. Int J Neurosci 53:167–172
206. Watkins LR, Mayer DJ (1982) Organization of endogenous opiate and nonopiate pain control systems. Science 216:1185–1192
207. Watson SJ, Barchas JD (1979) Anatomy of the endogenous opioid peptides and related substances. In: Beers RF (ed) Mechanisms of pain and analgesic compounds. Raven, New York, pp 227–237
208. Willer JC, Boureau F et al (1982) Comparative effects of EA and TENS on the human blink reflex. Pain 14:267–278
209. Woolf CJ (1984) Transcutaneous and implanted nerve stimulation. In: Wall PD, Melzack R (eds) Textbook of pain. Churchill Livingstone, Edinburgh, pp 679–690
210. Woolf CJ, Barrett G et al (1977) Naloxone reversible peripheral electroanalgesia in intact and spinal rats. Eur J Pharmacol 451:311–314
211. Woolf CJ, Mitchell D et al (1978) Failure of naloxone to reverse peripheral TENS analgesia in patients suffering from trauma. S Afr Med J 53:179–180
212. Woolf CJ, Mitchell J, Barrett GD (1980) Antinociceptive effect of peripheral segmental electric stimulation in the rat. Pain 8:237–252
213. Wu CC, Jong SB (1989) Radionuclide venography of lower limbs by subcutaneous injection: Comparison with venography by intravenous injection. Ann Nucl Med 3:125–131

214. Wu C (1984) An experience on electroacupuncture therapy of facial palsy. (Abstract.) Proceedings of the Second National Symposium on Acupuncture and Moxibustion. All China Society of Acupuncture, Beijing, p 42
215. Wu DZ (1990) Acupuncture and neurophysiology. Clin Neurol Neurosurg 92:13–25
216. Xie GX, Han JS, Hollt V (1983) Electroacupuncture analgesia blocked by microinjection of anti-beta-endorphin antiserum into periaqueductal grey of the rabbit. Int J Neurosci 18:287–291
217. Xue JI, Yu YX et al (1995) Changes in the content of immunoreactive dynorphin in dorsal and ventral spinal cord of the rat in three different conditions. Int J Neurosci 82:95–104
218. Yang ZL, Cai TW, Wu JL (1989) Acupuncture and emotion; the influence of acupuncture anesthesia on the sensory and emotional components of pain. J Gen Psychol 116:247–258
219. Yi CC, Lu TH, Wu SH, Tsou K (1977) A study on the release of tritiated 5-HT from brain during acupuncture and morphine analgesia. Sci Sinica 20:113–124
220. Zheng M, Yang SG, Zou B (1988) Electroacupuncture markedly increases proenkephalin mRNA in rat striatun and pituitary. Sci Sin B 31:81–86
221. Zao FY, Han JS et al (1987) Acupuncture analgesia in impacted last molar extraction. Effect of clomipramine and pargyline. In: Han JS (ed) The neurochemical basis of pain relief by acupuncture. A collection of papers 1973–1989. Beijing Medical Science, Beijing, pp 96–97
222. Zhang WH, Shen YC (1981) Change in levels of monoamine neurotransmitters and their main metabolites in rat brain after electroacupuncture treatment. Int J Neurosci 15:147–149
223. Zhang AZ (1980) Endorphin and analgesia research in the People's Republic of China (1975–1979). Acupunct Electrother Res Int J 5:131–146
224. Zhou ZF, Du MY, Han JS et al (1981) Effect of intracerebral microinjection of naloxone on acupuncture- and morphine-analgesia in the rabbit. Sci Sin 24:1166–1178
225. Zou K, Yi QC, Wu SX, Lu YX et al (1980) Enkephalin involvement in acupuncture analgesia. Sci Sin 23:1197–1207
226. Zou K (1987) Neurochemical mechanisms of acupuncture analgesia. Pain Headache 9:266–282

Mechanisms of Acupuncture Analgesia Produced by Low Frequency Electrical Stimulation of Acupuncture Points

C. Takeshige

2.1
Introduction

Three noteworthy phenomena have been recognized in surgical acupuncture analgesia (AA) produced by low frequency electrical stimulation of acupuncture points: (1) consciousness is maintained, allowing the patient to talk during surgery, (2) stimulation of specific acupuncture points is essential to maintain analgesia, and (3) analgesia persists long after stimulation has been terminated, allowing the patient to move without pain after surgery. The mechanisms by which AA is produced might be clarified by investigating these phenomena. This review will explore possible mechanisms based on results from animal experiments.

Consciousness depends on activation of the brainstem ascending reticular activating system (RAS) that produces widespread stimulation of the cerebral cortex and maintains consciousness nonspecifically through the reticular nucleus in the thalamus. The RAS is activated by collateral pathways that diverge from each specific sensory afferent pathway projecting to each sensory cortex. Neurophysiological research has shown that anesthetic drugs used during surgical operations inhibit activity of the RAS. Since consciousness is diminished under this condition, sensory information reaching the sensory cortex is not translated into perception. On the other hand, it is also commonly observed that normally painful stimuli are suppressed on the battlefield and during aggressive sports such as rugby. Such analgesia is thought to be brought about by activation of the descending pain inhibitory system (DPIS) originating from the limbic system and which blocks pain information as it enters the central nervous system. Consciousness can thus be maintained in such a condition. If stimulation of a specific acupuncture point activates the DPIS through a particular pathway connected to the brain system which suppresses pain, it can be assumed that AA is produced by activation of the DPIS. This assumption has been examined in our laboratories using several animal experiments.

2.2
Classification of Acupuncture Afferent and Efferent Pathways for Producing Acupuncture Analgesia [11–13, 16, 22, 23]

The neuronal structures comprising the AA-producing brain pathway can be identified when microelectrode stimulation induces analgesia in a manner that mimics AA and by tissue ablation that results in subsequent blockage of AA. However, the nature of the analgesia produced depends upon the brain areas stimulated and can be classi-fied into two categories. The first category includes analgesia that is naloxone-reversible, disappears after hypophysectomy, persists long after stimulation of the acupoint is terminated, and exhibits individual variation in effectiveness. These fea-tures are similar to those of AA. In this category, brain potentials are evoked by stim-ulation of acupoints in the same areas that produce analgesia. Stimulation of brain areas associated with the second category produces analgesia that is not naloxone-reversible, not affected by hypophysectomy, is produced only during stimulation, and exhibits no individual variation in effectiveness. Evoked potentials are not obtained from brain regions producing analgesia of this second category, but nonsynchronized neuronal activities are obtained by stimulation of acupoints [16].

Brain regions producing analgesia of the first category appear to comprise an afferent pathway for acupuncture, since the pituitary gland is involved in this analge-sia and electrical potentials are evoked in these brain regions by stimulation of acu-points. Similarly, areas producing analgesia related to the second category appear to comprise an efferent pathway for acupuncture, since the pituitary gland is not involved and synchronized electrical potentials are not evoked in these regions by stimulation of acupoints [12, 16, 19]. All brain regions producing analgesia associated with the second category seem to be connected to the DPIS; AA is produced by acti-vation of the DPIS, which is excited by stimulation of specific acupoints through a particular pathway connected to the DPIS. This DPIS-producing analgesia related to the second category is defined as the acupuncture *efferent* pathway, whereas the par-ticular pathway from specific acupoints to the DPIS is defined as the acupuncture *afferent* pathway.

2.2.1
Acupuncture Efferent Pathway [13, 16, 24]

Acupuncture analgesia can be abolished by concurrent lesions of the Raphe nucleus and the reticular paragigantocellular nucleus that are known as the origins of the serotonergic and the noradrenergic descending pain-inhibitory systems. Stimulation of these nuclei respectively produces serotonergic and noradrenergic analgesia of the second category. The final production of AA is induced by activation of these descending pain inhibitory systems. The descending pain inhibitory pathway serves as the acupuncture efferent pathway from the hypothalamic ventromedian nucleus (HVM); it is divided into two parts that connect to the descending serotonergic and noradrenergic systems. The posterior part of the hypothalamic arcuate nucleus (P-HARN) is anatomically connected to the HVM. Analgesia produced by stimulation of both the HVM and the P-HARN is associated with the second category. Synaptic transmission from the P-HARN to the HVM is apparently dopaminergic, since anal-gesia produced by stimulation of the P-HARN is blocked by lesions of the HVM or by dopamine antagonists (Fig. 1).

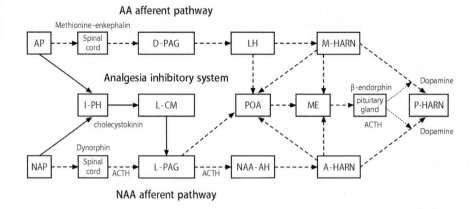

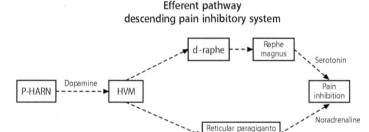

Fig. 1. Transmitters in the afferent pathway in both AA and non-AA, in the analgesia inhibitory system (*upper figure*), and in the acupuncture efferent pathway as the descending pain inhibitory systems (*bottom figure*). *AP* acupuncture point, *D-PAG* dorsal periaqueductal central gray, *L-PAG* lateral periaqueductal central gray, *LH* lateral hypothalamus, *ME* median eminence, *M-HARN, A-HARN, P-HARN* medial, anterior, and posterior hypothalamic arcuate nucleus, *NAP* nonacupuncture point, *NAA-AH* anterior hypothalamus in the NAA afferent pathway, *POA* preoptic area, *I-PH* inferior posterior hypothalamus, *L-CM* lateral centromedian nucleus of thalamus

2.2.2
Acupuncture Afferent Pathway [11, 12, 23]

The acupuncture afferent pathway (Fig. 1) starts from an acupoint, ascends through the contralateral anterolateral tract to the dorsal periaqueductal central gray, and reaches the medial part of the hypothalamic arcuate nucleus (M-HARN). Brain regions belonging to the AA afferent pathway can be identified by exhibition of analgesia of the first group related to anatomically known connections. The rostral and caudal relations between these regions have been identified by the loss of stimulation-produced analgesia of the caudal region that follows lesions of the rostral region. These relations are shown in Figs. 1 and 2 [23].

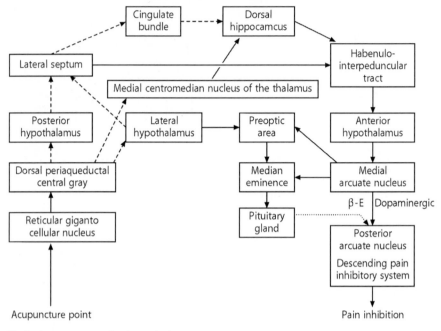

Fig. 2. Acupuncture analgesia-producing system

Fig. 3a, b. Location of lesioned and stimulated sites in the arcuate nucleus. The arcuate nucleus is bounded by the *broken line*. The *enlarged figure* shows the sites at which lesions abolished AA. Analgesia produced by stimulation (SPA) at the *open circles* was abolished by hypophysectomy. Afferent SPA at the *filled circles* was not affected by hypophysectomy. Efferent SPA at the *half-filled circles* was partially abolished by hypophysectomy. The hypothalamic arcuate nucleus (HARN) indicated by *oblique lines* was divided into three equal parts: anterior (A-HARN), medial (M-HARN), and posterior (P-HARN)

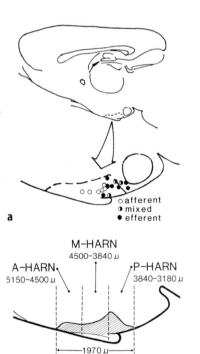

2.2.3
Synaptic Connections Between Acupuncture Afferent and Efferent Pathways
[25, 28]

The final region of the acupuncture afferent pathway is found in the M-HARN, which is anatomically close to the P-HARN, the initial region of the acupuncture efferent pathway (Fig. 3). Microinjection of the dopamine antagonist haloperidol antagonizes AA dose-dependently, while microinjection of dopamine into the P-HARN induces dose-dependent analgesia. Dopamine thus seems to serve as the neurotransmitter between the M-HARN and the P-HARN, i.e., as the neurotransmitter at the interface between the acupuncture afferent and efferent pathways. This possibility is further supported by neuronal activity in the P-HARN. Neurons in the P-HARN that respond to acupoint stimulation also respond to iontophoretically administered dopamine, whereas neurons in the P-HARN that do not respond to acupoint stimulation also do not respond to iontophoretically administered dopamine [25] (Fig. 4).

A branch of the acupuncture afferent pathway ascending to the M-HARN diverges at the lateral hypothalamus (LH) to reach the pituitary gland. Lesions of brain nuclei near this pathway to the pituitary, e.g., the preoptic area (POA) or the median eminence (ME), abolish AA. Electrical potentials are evoked in these brain areas by stimulation of acupoints, but stimulation of these particular brain structures does not produce analgesia [25, 28] (Figs. 1, 2, 5). Since acupuncture analgesia and pain relief produced by stimulation of the acupuncture afferent pathway to the M-HARN are both abolished by hypophysectomy, β-endorphin released from the pituitary gland may play an essential role in dopaminergic transmission in the P-HARN [25] (Fig. 5). Microinjection of naloxone to the P-HARN antagonizes AA dose-dependently and microinjection of β-endorphin or morphine produces analgesia dose-dependently. Analgesia produced by microinjection of β-endorphin disappears after denervation of the M-HARN, but analgesia produced by microinjection of dopamine to the P-HARN remains [25] (Fig. 6). These findings suggest that β-endorphin might act

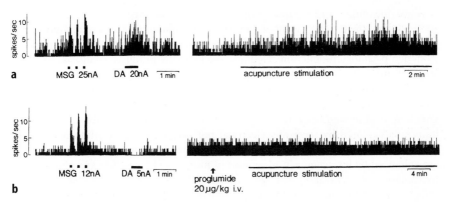

Fig. 4a, b. Rate histograms of two different typical P-HARN neurons in acupuncture-responder rats. One was excited by iontophoretically applied 25 n monosodium glutamate (MSG) and 20 nA dopamine (DA), and also by acupuncture stimulation. The other was excited by iontophoretically applied 12 nA MSG but inhibited by 5 nA DA and did not respond to acupuncture stimulation, even after IV 20 mg/kg proglumide

Fig. 5. Synaptic transmission between M-HARN and P-HARN in AA and that between A-HARN and P-HARN in non-AA. Two pathways diverge from the lateral hypothalamus (*LH*) in AA and from the L-PAG in non-AA. Both AA and non-AA are carried by dopaminergic transmission to the P-HARN. Other paths associated with release from the pituitary gland of β-endorphin (in AA) and ACTH (in non-AA) modulate the dopaminergic systems in the synapse to the P-HARN that is the initial region of the descending pain inhibitory system (*DPIS*). Convergence is necessary to activate the preoptic area (*POA*) and median eminence (*ME*). Hypophysectomy abolished analgesia produced by stimulation of M-HARN and A-HARN. Stimulation of the POA or the ME did not produce analgesia

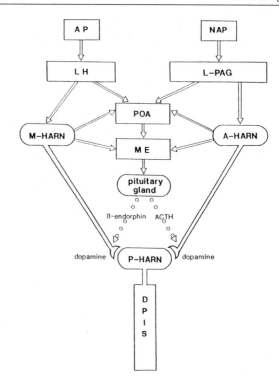

presynaptically at dopaminergic synapses in the P-HARN. This notion is further supported by the activity of P-HARN neurons. Neuronal activity in the P-HARN that occurs in response to acupuncture stimulation is not affected by iontophoretic administration of morphine or ultramicroinjection of β-endorphin via picospritzer [22] (Fig. 7).

Since morphine and β-endorphin act similarly in the P-HARN, β-endorphin released from the pituitary gland might be the neurohumoral factor acting presynaptically on axon terminals of the M-HARN neurons that innervate P-HARN neurons. Although β-endorphin microinjected into the P-HARN produces analgesia, electrical stimulation of the POA or ME in the pathway to the pituitary gland does not. Therefore, the amount of β-endorphin released by such stimulation is not sufficient to activate the P-HARN neurons without afferent impulse from the M-HARN. Morphine and β-endorphin might also act in other areas of the AA afferent pathway. This possibility was explored by recording electrical potentials evoked by stimulation of the acupoint in the final station of the AA afferent pathway, the M-HARN. Such potentials are enhanced by intravenously administered morphine (0.5 mg/kg) and abolished by hypophysectomy. The abolished evoked potentials are temporarily restored by morphine [12] (Fig. 8). Therefore, sites responsive to β-endorphin released from the pituitary gland might be widespread in the AA afferent pathway. Opioid receptors have also been reported in many regions of the acupuncture afferent pathway [1, 5, 10].

Fig. 6. Dose-dependence of analgesia caused by micro-injection of dopamine and β-endorphin into the P-HARN, and effects of denervation of the M-HARN on this dose-dependence. *Upper* control, *lower* after denervation of the M-HARN

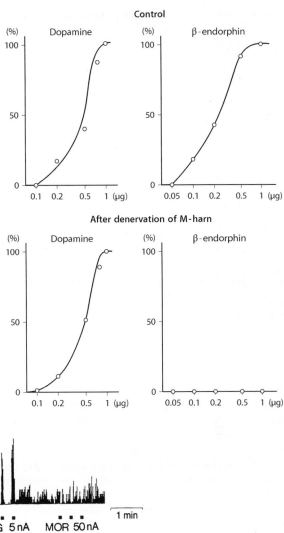

Control

After denervation of M-harn

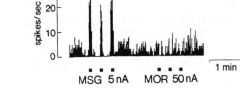

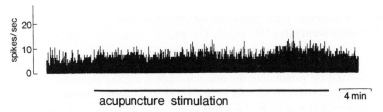

Fig. 7. Rate histograms showing typical P-HARN neuron responses in an acupuncture responder rat. The P-HARN neuron excited by iontophoretic 5 nA monosodium glutamate (MSG) did not respond to iontophoretically applied 50 nA morphine (Mor) but was excited by acupuncture stimulation (*bottom record*)

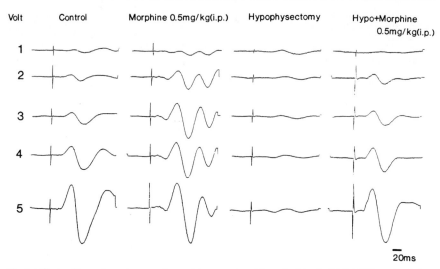

Fig. 8. Effects of hypophysectomy and morphine on potentials evoked in the M-HARN by stimulation of an acupuncture point (*AP*). *Column 1* Control. Evoked potential increased with increasing stimulus. *Column 2* Effect of intraperitoneal 0.5 mg/kg morphine on potentials 20 min after application and with 5 min intervals between successive stimuli. *Column 3* Effect of hypophysectomy on potentials. *Column 4* Effect of IP 0.5 mg/kg morphine on potentials after hypophysectomy. Note close similarity to column 1. Voltage (at 0.05 ms duration) indicated by number at left applies to all columns

2.3
Stimulation of Specific Acupoints for the Production of AA [23]

Low frequency (1 Hz) electrical stimulation of the first dorsal finger muscle and the anterior tibial muscle in rats [11, 23], which correspond to the muscles underlying the human LI.4 (Hegu) and St.36 (Zusanli) acupoints, produces behavioral analgesia, evaluated in rats by tail flick latency. The intensity of electrical stimulation must be sufficient to cause muscle contraction in order to obtain AA. In contrast, stimulation of other muscles does not produce behavioral analgesia. Hence, the Hegu and Zusanli acupoints seem uniquely able to activate the DPIS through the particular pathway connected to the DPIS [3].

2.4
Differentiation of Acupoints and Nonacupoints by Responses
of Central Neuronal Structures [11, 14, 15, 17, 18]

Potentials can be evoked specifically in the bilateral dorsal areas of the periaqueductal central gray (D-PAG) by stimulating the muscles underlying the Hegu and Zusanli acupoints but not by stimulation of other muscles (Fig. 9). Lesions of the D-PAG abolish AA. Microelectrode stimulation of this region produces analgesia of the first category that can be reversed by either naloxone or hypophysectomy. Stimulation of the auricular levator muscle beneath the X18 (Chihmo) acupoint in rabbits elicits evokes potentials in the D-PAG [11, 23]. Stimulus conditions as stated above which lead to

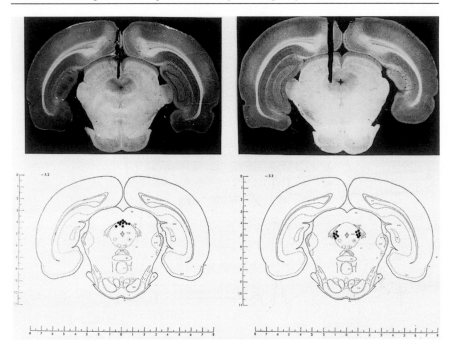

Fig. 9. Examples of scars produced by electrodes inserted into the D-PAG (*upper left*) and L-PAG (*upper right*). Sites of recordings in the D-PAG (*lower left*) and L-PAG (*lower right*)

AA were confirmed by potentials in the D-PAG. Therefore, only three acupoints for producing AA have been identified: Hegu, Zusanli, and Chihmo.

Stimulation of muscles including those beneath Hegu and Zusanli also produces *nonspecific* potentials bilaterally in the *lateral* parts of the periaqueductal central gray (L-PAG) [17] (Fig. 9). Potentials in the L-PAG are gradually decreased by repetitive 1 Hz stimulation of these muscles and disappear completely 10 minutes after the onset of stimulation [15, 17] (Fig. 10). Hence, potentials in the L-PAG are inhibited by such stimulation in a self-inhibiting fashion. Lesions of the L-PAG do not affect AA, but analgesia is produced by stimulation of the rostral L-PAG. This analgesia is largely reversible with dexamethasone, and the dexamethasone-insensitive portion is readily blocked by naloxone or hypophysectomy. Hence, acupoints are connected via the D-PAG to the particular pathway that is not self-inhibited during the production of AA. On the other hand, both acupoints and nonacupoints are connected nonspecifically to the other, self-inhibiting pathway via the L-PAG. The latter brain region belongs to a pathway distinct from the AA afferent pathway, whose analgesia production is self-inhibiting (Fig. 11). These results imply that acupoints and nonacupoints can be differentiated by their connections with different analgesia-producing central pathways [14, 17] (Figs. 1, 11).

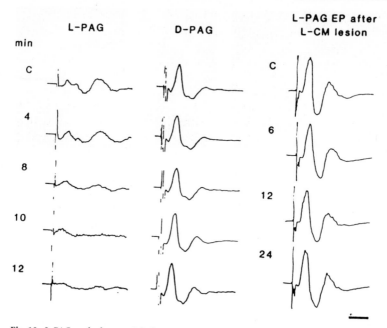

Fig. 10. L-PAG evoked potentials from a typical rat were gradually depressed and finally abolished by repetitive 1 Hz stimulation of the acupuncture points (*left*). Those in the D-PAG were not influenced (*middle*). After lesioning the L-CM, inhibition of evoked potentials in the L-PAG disappeared (*right*). Numbers by each record indicate time in minutes after start of stimulation

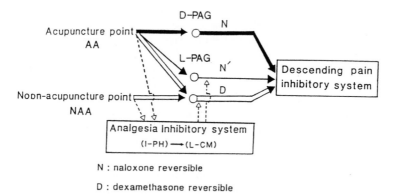

N : naloxone reversible

D : dexamethasone reversible

Fig. 11. Differentiation of acupuncture and nonacupuncture points by the analgesia inhibitory system.

2.5
Similarities Between Acupuncture Analgesia and Morphine Analgesia

Analgesia produced by intraperitoneal 0.5 mg/kg morphine is of a similar degree to that produced by low frequency electroacupuncture. In addition, both types of analgesia are abolished by hypophysectomy, lesions of the AA afferent and efferent pathways, naloxone, and antagonists of transmitters involved in the AA efferent pathway. In addition, individual variations in effectiveness between AA and morphine analgesia are highly correlated. Animals can be classified as responders or nonresponders by the presence or absence of a significant increase ($p < 0.05$) in tail flick latency.

Effects of opioid peptides antiserum on d–PAG evoked potential

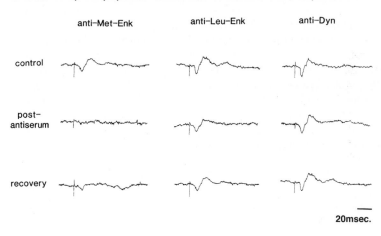

Effects of opioid peptides antiserum on l–PAG evoked potential

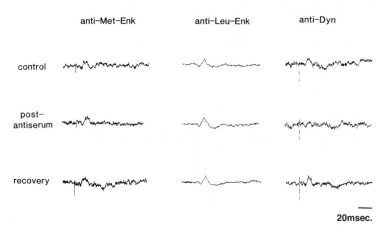

Fig. 12. Effect of intrathecal application of antisera to met-enkephalin (*left*), leu-enkephalin (*middle*), and dyn (*right*) on potentials in the D-PAG evoked by acupoint stimulation. *Top* Control, *middle* 10 min post application of the antisera of opioids, and *bottom* recovery 20 min afterward

2.6

Activation of the Spinal Acupuncture Analgesia Afferent Pathway by Morphine [8, 11, 12, 14, 18]

Potentials evoked in the D-PAG by stimulation of acupoints are blocked by contralateral lesions of the anterolateral tract or by intrathecal administration of the antiserum to methionine (met)-enkephalin. These potentials are also blocked by naloxone but not by the administration of antisera to leucine-enkephalin or dynorphin [18] (Fig. 12), supporting the involvement of a met-enkephalin pathway activated by morphine. In AA responder animals, dose-response curves of analgesia were obtained for both low and high doses of morphine administered either intraperitoneally or intrathecally. However, in nonresponding animals, only a single dose-response curve for higher doses of morphine was obtained. In AA responders, bilateral lesions of the anterolateral tract or lesions of the D-PAG that is part of the AA afferent pathway abolished dose-dependent responses to low doses of morphine without affecting the dose response to high doses of morphine. Therefore, morphine analgesia produced by lower doses is probably induced by activation of the AA afferent pathway through met-enkephalin receptors in the spinal cord [18]. Such receptors in the spinal AA afferent pathway are likely to be those activated by intraperitoneal morphine at 0.5 mg/kg or intrathecal morphine at 0.05 μg/rat that produce morphine analgesia to a degree similar to that of AA [8, 11] (Fig. 13). This mechanism may explain the reason for the similarity between AA and morphine analgesia.

Fig. 13. Morphine analgesia mediated by acupuncture analgesia-producing system

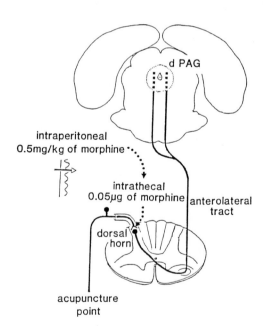

2.7
Individual Variations in Effectiveness of AA and Morphine Analgesia [21, 27]

After treatment with D-phenylalanine (DPA), an inhibitor of enzymes such as amino-peptidase and carboxypeptidase that degrade met-enkephalin, the strong correlation of individual variations in effectiveness between AA and morphine analgesia disappeared. In other words, AA and morphine analgesia were obtained at similar magnitudes in both responders and nonresponders after treatment with DPA.

Individual variation in amplitude of evoked potentials in the D-PAG also disappeared after treatment with DPA [27]. Hence, individual variations in effectiveness of both AA and morphine analgesia might be attributed to the activity of enzymes degrading met-enkephalin in the spinal cord. Higher enzyme activity might reduce met-enkephalin levels and block responses to AA, whereas lower activity might increase met-enkephalin levels, activate AA afferent pathways, and facilitate responses to AA.

2.8
Analgesia Produced by Stimulation of Nonacupoints After Lesioning of the Analgesia Inhibitory System [11, 15, 17, 26, 28]

As stated previously, potentials in the L-PAG evoked by stimulation of either acupoints or nonacupoints are self-inhibiting. However, after lesions are made in the lateral centromedian nucleus of the thalamus (L-CM) or parts of the posterior hypothalamus (I-PH), evoked potentials in the L-PAG are not self-inhibited and such stimulation results in pronounced analgesia. Analgesia produced by stimulation of nonacupoints after lesioning of these areas is referred to as nonacupuncture stimulation-produced analgesia (Fig. 11).

Since analgesia from stimulation of nonacupoints is induced by stimulation of acupoints only after lesions occur in the I-PH or the L-CM, these regions are considered part of an analgesia inhibitory system (AIS) for this type of analgesia (Figs. 1, 11). Thus, the AIS may have an important role in distinguishing between acupoints and nonacupoints, since it inhibits afferent impulses arising from stimulation of nonacupoints but not those arising from stimulation of acupoints.

2.9
Afferent and Efferent Pathways That Produce Nonacupuncture Stimulation-Produced Analgesia [26]

Nonacupuncture stimulation-produced analgesia (non-AA) can be blocked by hypophysectomy and lesions of the non-AA afferent pathway. This system is inhibited dose-dependently by dexamethasone but not by naloxone; unlike AA, non-AA does not exhibit individual variations in effectiveness [26]. Potentials in the L-PAG evoked by stimulation of nonacupoints are not abolished by intrathecal administration of antisera to met-enkephalin or leu-enkephalin but are abolished by antiserum to dynorphin (Figs. 1, 12). Hence, dynorphin is believed to be the transmitter of the spinal non-AA afferent pathway [18]. Since dynorphin is not degraded by aminopeptidase or carboxypeptidase, individual variations in effectiveness are not observed in non-AA. Descending pain inhibitory systems such as those found in the acupuncture efferent pathway are common in non-AA and AA. The afferent pathway for this system originates at nonacupoints and ends in the anterior part of the hypothalamic arcuate nucleus (A-HARN) connected to the initial region of the efferent pathway. Lesioning of the AIS augments AA produced by stimulation of acupoints; hence, the acupoint also sends fibers to the non-AA afferent pathway. The augmented component of analgesia is largely antagonized by dexamethasone, and the remainder is antagonized by naloxone [17].

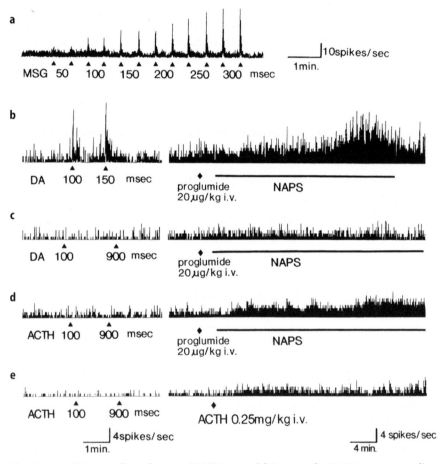

Fig. 14. a 0.1 mM monosodium glutamate (MSG) increased firing rate of P-HARN neuron as application time increased from 50 ms to 300 ms. b Firing rate of MSG-responsive neuron was increased by dopamine applied for 100 and 150 ms. This neuron also responded to nonacupoint stimulation (NAPS) after application of proglumide. c Another MSG-responsive neuron did not respond to 100 ms or 900 ms applications of dopamine. This neuron also did not respond to NAPS after application of intravenous 20 mg/kg proglumide. d Microapplication of same dose of ACTH by picospritzer for 100 and 900 ms produced no change (*left*) in NAPS-responsive neurons in the P-HARN after intravenous 20 mg/kg proglumide (*right*). e Microapplication of ACTH into the P-HARN for 100 or 900 ms produced no change in P-HARN neuron activity (*left*), but intravenous 0.25 mg/kg ACTH increased firing rate of this P-HARN neuron (*right*)

Lesions of the non-AA afferent pathway block non-AA, and stimulation of the non-AA afferent pathway produces analgesia that is largely reversible with dexamethasone. These lesions are almost completely reversible with dexamethasone plus naloxone (Fig. 11). Transmission between the A-HARN and P-HARN has been found to be dopaminergic, as is that between the M-HARN and P-HARN. Evidence supporting this conclusion is that (1) microinjection of dopamine into the P-HARN produces analgesia dose-dependently and administration of haloperidol antagonizes non-AA dose-dependently, and (2) some neurons in the P-HARN that respond to nonacupoint stimulation when the AIS is inhibited with proglumide also respond to iontophoretically administered dopamine [26] (Fig. 14).

In contrast, other neurons do not respond after either procedure. The afferent pathway of non-AA from nonacupoints divides into two pathways at the L-PAG: one pathway ascends to the A-HARN and the other ascends to the pituitary gland via the median eminence. Lesions of the latter pathway abolish non-AA, but stimulation of this pathway does not in itself produce analgesia [28] (Figs. 1, 5).

2.10
Pituitary Hormones and Nonacupuncture Stimulation-Produced Analgesia

Adrenocorticotrophic hormone (ACTH) released from the pituitary gland seems to be essential for dopaminergic transmission between the A-HARN and P-HARN. This follows, since dexamethasone microinjected into the P-HARN antagonizes non-AA dose-dependently, while ACTH administration mimics non-AA dose-dependently [26]. Therefore, two neurotransmitters are necessary for transmission between the non-AA afferent and efferent pathways in the arcuate nucleus. Dopamine has been found to act postsynaptically, while ACTH acts presynaptically at this synapse. Evidence in support of these conclusions is that after denervation of the A-HARN, analgesia produced by ACTH microinjected into the P-HARN disappears but that produced by dopamine microinjected into the P-HARN is unaffected [26] (Fig. 15).

Furthermore, neuronal activities that occur in response to stimulation of nonacupoints during administration of proglumide do not respond to iontophoretically administered ACTH [26] (Fig. 14). Beta-endorphin and ACTH released concomitantly from the pituitary gland might be the presynaptically acting neurohumoral factors in AA and non-AA, producing dopaminergic transmission in the P-HARN (Fig. 5). The possibility that ACTH acts as a neurohumoral factor in other regions of the non-AA afferent pathway has been examined by recording potentials evoked by nonacupoint stimulation after lesioning in the A-HARN, the final station of the non-AA afferent pathway. Such evoked-potentials in the A-HARN are enhanced by intraperitoneal administration of ACTH and are markedly decreased by hypophysectomy. However, these decreased potentials are restored by intraperitoneal administration of ACTH. Consequently, ACTH might act on the afferent pathway of non-AA before entering the A-HARN [22] (Fig. 16).

Microinjection of ACTH onto sites of the non-AA afferent pathway such as the L-PAG and the anterior hypothalamus produces dose-dependent analgesia. Conversely, microinjection of dexamethasone antagonizes analgesia dose-dependently [23] (Fig. 17). Furthermore, intraperitoneal ACTH produces dose-dependent analgesia, intraperitoneal dexamethasone blocks non-AA dose-dependently, and intravenous

Fig. 15. Control. Dose-response relationships for dopamine and ACTH microinjected into the P-HARN and analgesia produced. Analgesia due to ACTH disappeared after denervation of the A-HARN while that of dopamine remained unchanged

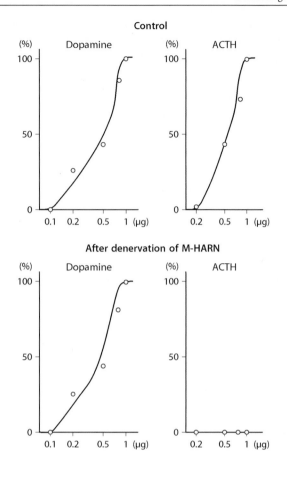

ACTH stimulates neuronal activity in some P-HARN neurons [26]. These findings suggest that ACTH acts as a synaptic neurotransmitter and dexamethasone acts as an antagonist at these sites.

2.11
Sites of Inhibition from the AIS in the Non-AA Afferent Pathway [15, 17]

Inhibition of evoked potentials and neuronal activity in the L-PAG induced by nonacupoint stimulation is observed in rostral but not caudal regions of the L-PAG. Similarly, stimulation of the I-PH or the L-CM completely inhibits nonacupoint-evoked potentials in rostral but not caudal L-PAG [17]. Therefore, the AIS exerts its inhibitory effects in the region between the rostral and caudal L-PAG in the non-AA afferent pathway. Inhibition of potentials in the rostral L-PAG evoked by nonacupoint stimulation during stimulation of the I-PH is abolished by lesions of the L-CM; hence, nonacupoint stimulation activates the I-PH first and then the L-CM [17].

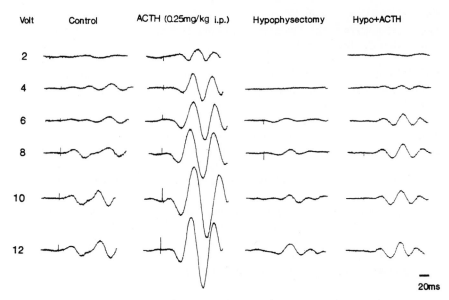

Fig. 16. Effect of 0.25 mg/kg ACTH before and after hypophysectomy on potentials in the A-HARN evoked by NAP stimulation in L-CM-lesioned rats. *Column 1* Control potentials were increased with increasing stimulus strength in volts (*V*, 0.05 ms duration) indicated by *numbers at left. Column 2* Potentials 30 min after application of ACTH. *Column 3* Effect of hypophysectomy on potentials. *Column 4* Effect of 0.25 mg/kg ACTH (*IP*) on potentials after hypophysectomy

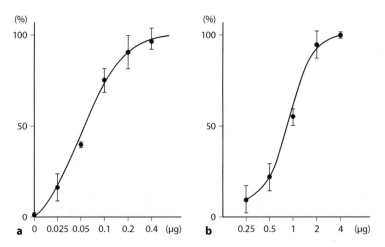

Fig. 17. a Dose response of antagonism by dexamethasone microinjected into the L-PAG. **b** Dose response of analgesia produced by ACTH microinjected into the L-PAG. Ordinate numbers: antagonism (*A*) and analgesia (*B*) in percent. *Abscissas* doses of dexamethasone (*A*) and ACTH (*B*)

2.12
Neurotransmitters in the Analgesia Inhibitory System and Nonacupuncture Stimulation-Produced Analgesia

Non-AA of the AIS is produced by stimulation of nonacupoints after intraperitoneal treatment with DPA or proglumide, an antagonist of cholecystokinin (CCK), rather than after lesions of the L-CM or I-PH [20]. Activation of the AIS by stimulation of nonacupoints is obvious during spontaneous neuronal activity of the L-CM, which increases markedly 10 minutes after the onset of nonacupoint stimulation. Such enhancement of neuronal activity is blocked by treatment with proglumide, suggesting that CCK is a neurotransmitter in the AIS [2].

The timing of the onset of enhancement of neuronal activity in the L-CM (Fig. 18) corresponds fairly well with the timing of the onset of self-inhibition of evoked potentials in the L-PAG after the onset of nonacupoint stimulation [14] (Fig. 10). This finding is supported by the increase in CCK-like immunoreactivity in perfusate collected from the L-CM with the push-pull method. Stimulation both of acupoints and nonacupoints significantly increased CCK-like immunoreactivity in the L-CM but produced no increase in the cerebral cortex [31] (Fig. 19). After microinjection of proglumide or DPA into the I-PH or L-CM, analgesia is produced by stimulation of nonacupoints. Of several CCK antagonists microinjected into the L-CM, L365,250 was the most effective in producing non-AA. These results further support the suggestion that CCK-8 is a principal neurotransmitter in the L-CM [2].

2.13
Effects of Adrenalectomy on AA and Non-AA [7]

Acupuncture analgesia and non-AA are abolished 12 and 24 hours after adrenalectomy, respectively. However, both are restored 1 hour after IV or IP administration of 1–2 ml of 5 % NaCl. Sodium ions are required for the action of met-enkephalin and dynorphin in both the AA and non-AA afferent pathways in the spinal cord. Sodium

Fig. 18. Changes of L-CM neuronal activity during nonacupuncture point stimulation and antagonistic action of proglumide. Neuronal activity (*A*) during nonacupuncture point stimulation. *Ordinate numbers* integrated spikes/2 s. *Abscissa* time in minutes. Time scale 4 min. Effect of IV 20 mg/kg proglumide on neuronal activity changes. Effect of 20 mg/kg proglumide 6 min prior to onset of nonacupuncture point stimulation on the L-CM neuronal activity. *Arrow* indicates application of proglumide. *Solid lines* under records indicate nonacupuncture point stimulation (NAPS)

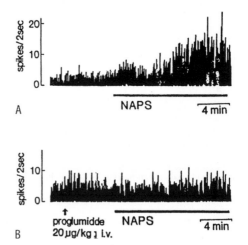

Fig. 19. Effect of 1 Hz peripheral stimulation on release of CCK-like immunoreactivity (*CCK-LI*) from medial thalamic and cerebral cortex. *Dotted Column* from thalamus by stimulation of Zusanli, *Hatched column* from thalamus by stimulation of abdominal muscle, *Open column* from cortex by stimulation of abdominal muscle. The concentration of CCK-LI in thalamic dialysate before stimulation was lower than the detection limit (5 pg/100 g)

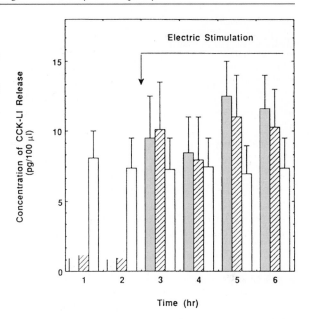

is also needed for the presynaptic actions of β-endorphin and ACTH in the P-HARN. These conclusions are supported by the abolition of acupoint- or nonacupoint-evoked potentials in either D-PAG or L-PAG, respectively. They are also supported by the analgesia produced following microinjection of β-endorphin or ACTH into the P-HARN after adrenalectomy and by their recovery after application of sodium chloride. Therefore, the adrenal gland plays a prominent role in production of both AA and non-AA by maintaining sodium levels in the blood independently of the action of the pituitary gland.

2.14
Aftereffects of AA and Non-AA [30]

Acupuncture analgesia characteristically persists long after termination of acupuncture stimulation. This aftereffect becomes dominant 60 min after stimulation and is still marked at 120 min post stimulation at 1 Hz. The same pattern is observed with non-AA [2] (Fig. 20). The presence of long-lasting effects in both AA and non-AA suggests that an analgesic mechanism is activated without afferent impulses produced by stimulation of acupoints and nonacupoints. As stated earlier, hypophysectomy abolishes both AA and non-AA, and this procedure abolishes potentials in the M-HARN and A-HARN evoked by stimulation of the acupoints and nonacupoints, respectively. However, abolished potentials in these final regions of the AA and non-AA afferent pathways are temporarily restored by intravenously administered morphine and ACTH, respectively. This finding implies that an increased amount of β-endorphin and ACTH results in a longer period of analgesia. Acupoint or nonacupoint stimulation restores the transmission in the regions of the AA and non-AA afferent pathways.

Fig. 20. a Changes of acupuncture point stimulation-produced analgesia as related to stimulation period ($n = 6$). **b** Changes of nonacupuncture point stimulation-produced analgesia as related to stimulation period ($n = 6$). *Ordinate numbers* percent increase of tail flick latency, *Abscissa* time in minutes, *Bars under figure* indicate stimulation period

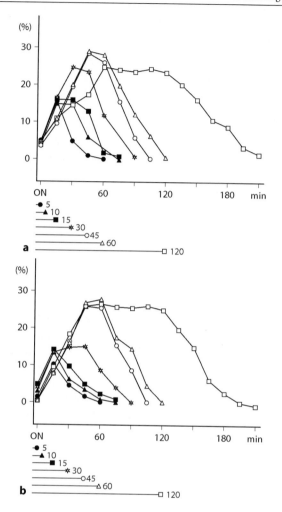

During electroacupuncture, major increases of β-endorphin and ACTH have been detected in peripheral blood [5]. Both peptides show a continual increase up to 80 minutes after termination of acupuncture stimulation. Furthermore, an analgesic effect was induced in cross-circulation recipient rats after electroacupuncture was applied to donor rats [4]. An increase of endorphins in the cerebrospinal fluid after electroacupuncture [9] suggests a correlation between cerebral and peripheral β-endorphin levels [5]. The characteristic, frequency-analyzed EEG changes in the deep structure of the brain induced by acupoint stimulation of donor rabbits also appears in cross-circulation recipient rabbits [29]. Since met-enkephalin is a putative neurotransmitter in the AA afferent pathway of the spinal cord, ACTH may be the transmitter in the L-PAG and the anterior hypothalamus in the non-AA afferent pathway. Beta-endorphin and ACTH, coreleased from the pituitary gland, are likely to reach levels high enough to activate these regions. Extended periods of stimulation might also activate the AA and non-AA afferent pathways in which excitability may increase due to post-tetanic potentiation without ongoing afferent impulses.

2.15
Conclusions

Acupuncture analgesia is produced by activation of the DPIS through a specific pathway connected to the acupoints while still allowing maintenance of consciousness. In contrast, the AIS is activated by stimulation of acupoints or nonacupoints, leading to nonspecific inhibition of different interconnected pathways. Therefore, acupoints and nonacupoints can be distinguished by their anatomically distinct brain pathways. The aftereffects of AA might be produced by the actions of an increased amount of β-endorphin released from the pituitary gland on components of the AA-producing pathway.

References

1. Atweh SF, Kuhar MJ (1997) Autoradiographic localization of opiate receptors in rat brain: The brainstem. Brain Res 129:1–12
2. Arai T, Guo SY, Takeshige C (1992) Cholecystokinin in the analgesia inhibitory system and its antagonists in this system. J Showa Med Assoc 52:58–67
3. Huang SF, Luo CP, Takeshige C (1998) Identity of a central analgesia-producing mechanism in Hoku point stimulation compared with that in Tsusanli point stimulation. J Showa Med Assoc 48:485–492
4. Lung CH, Sun AC, Tsao CJ, Chang,YL, Fan L (1974) An observation of the humoral factor in acupuncture analgesia in rats. Amer J Chin Med 2:203–205
5. Malizia E, Andreucci G, Paolucci D, Grescenzi F, Fabbri A, Fraioli F (1979) Electroacupuncture and peripheral β-endorphin and ACTH levels. Lancet 535–536
6. Pert CB, Snyder SH (1973) Opiate receptor: Demonstration in nervous tissue. Science 179:1011–1014
7. Sato T, Hishida F, Luo CP, Tsuchiya M, Takeshige C (1989) Relations of adrenal gland and sodium ions in production of acupuncture and nonacupuncture points stimulation-produced analgesia. J Showa Med Assoc 49:286–294
8. Sato T, Takeshige C, Shimizu S (1991) Morphine analgesia mediated by activation of the acupuncture analgesia-producing system. Acupunct Electrother Res 16:13–26
9. Sjolund B, Terenius L, Erikson M (1977) Increased cerebrospinal fluid levels of endorphins after electroacupuncture. Acta Physiol Scand 100:382–384
10. Snyder SH (1955) Opiate receptor in normal and drug-altered brain function. Nature 257:185–189
11. Takeshige C (1990) Mechanism of acupuncture analgesia based on animal experiments. In: Pomeranz B, Stux G (eds) Scientific bases of acupuncture. Springer-Verlag, Berlin Heidelberg New York, pp 53–78
12. Takeshige C (1990) Mechanism of acupuncture analgesia (AA) caused by low frequency stimulation of the acupuncture point based on animal experiments. Part 1: Acupuncture afferent and efferent pathways and the nature of AA. Acupunct Scient Int J 1:75–88
13. Takeshige C, Sato T, Komugi H (1980) Role of periaqueductal central gray in acupuncture analgesia. Acupunct Electrother Res 5:323–337
14. Takeshige C (1985) Differentiation between acupuncture and nonacupuncture points by association with analgesia inhibitory system. Acupunct Electrother Res 10:195–203
15. Takeshige C (1987) Inhibition associated with acupuncture analgesia. In: Charlazonits N, Gola M (eds) Inactivation of hypersensitive neurons. Alan R. Liss, New York, pp 255–262
16. Takeshige C, Kamada Y, Hisamatu T (1981) Commonly responsive neurons in the periaqueductal gray matter and midbrain reticular formation of rabbits to acupuncture stimulation, inversion, pressure on body parts, and morphine. Acupunct Electrother Res 6:57–74
17. Takeshige C, Kobori M, Hishida F, Luo CP, Usamai S (1992) Analgesia inhibitory system involvement in nonacupuncture point stimulation-produced analgesia. Brain Res Bull 28:379–391
18. Takeshige C, Luo CP, Hishida F, Igarashi O (1990) Differentiation of acupuncture and nonacupuncture points by difference of associated opioids in the spinal cord in production of analgesia

by acupuncture and nonacupuncture point stimulation, and relations between sodium and those opioids. Acupunct Electrother Res 15:193–209

19. Takeshige C, Luo CP, Kamada Y, Oka K, Murai M, Hisamatu T (1979) Relation between midbrain neurons (periqueductal central gray and midbrain reticular formation) and acupuncture analgesia, animal hypnosis. Advances Pain Res Ther 3:615–621

20. Takeshige C, Mera H, Hisamatu T, Tanaka M, Hishida F (1991) Inhibition of the analgesia inhibitory system by D-phenylalanine and proglumide. Brain Res Bull 26:385–391

21. Takeshige C, Murai M, Tanaka M, Hachisu M (1983) Parallel individual variations in effectiveness of acupuncture, morphine analgesia, and dorsal PAG-SPA, and their abolition by D-phenylalanine. Adv Pain Res Ther 5:563–569

22. Takeshige C, Nakanura A, Asamoto S, Arai T (1992) Positive feedback action of pituitary β-endorphin on acupuncture analgesia afferent pathway. Brain Res Bull 29:37–44

23. Takeshige C, Oka K, Mizuno T, Hisamatu T, Luo CP, Kobori M, Mera H, Fang TQ (1993) The acupuncture point and its connecting central pathway for producing acupuncture analgesia. Brain Res Bull 30:53–67

24. Takeshige C, Sato T, Mera T, Hisamitsu T, Fang TO (1992) Descending pain inhibitory system involved in acupuncture analgesia. Brain Res Bull 29:617–634

25. Takeshige C, Tsutiya M, Guo SY, Sato T (1991) Dopaminergic transmission in the hypothalamic arcuate nucleus to produce acupuncture analgesia in correlation with the pituitary gland. Brain Res Bull 26:113–122

26. Takeshige C, Tsutiya M, Zhao W, Guo S (1991) Analgesia produced by pituitary ACTH and dopaminergic transmission in the arcuate. Brain Res Bull 26:779–788

27. Takeshige C, Tanaka M, Sato T, Hishida F (1990) Mechanism of individual variation in effectiveness of acupuncture analgesia based on animal experiments. Eur J Pain 11:109–113

28. Takeshige C, Zhao WH, Guo SY (1991) Convergence from the preoptic area and arcuate nucleus to the median eminence in acupuncture and nonacupuncture point stimulation analgesia. Brain Res Bull 26:771–778

29. Takeshige C, Luo CP, Kamada Y (1976) Modulation of EGG and unit discharges of deep structure of brain during acupunctureal stimulation and by hypnosis of rabbits. Adv Pain Res Ther 1:781–785

30. Toyoda I, Takeshige C (1992) Changes in characteristics of analgesia produced by difference in duration of stimulation of acupuncture points. J Showa Med Assoc 52:1–7

31. Xu M, Aiuchi T, Nakaya K, Arakawa H, Maeda M, Tsuji A, Kato T, Takeshige C, Nakamura Y (1990) Effect of low frequency electric stimulation on in vivo release of cholecystokinin-like immunoreactivity in medial thalamus of conscious rat. Neurosci Let 118:205–207

CHAPTER 3

Opioid and Antiopioid Peptides:
A Model of Yin-Yang Balance in Acupuncture
Mechanisms of Pain Modulation

J.-S. Han

3.1
Introduction

At first glance, sharp differences exist between medicinal practices originating in the east and in the west. While Western medicine is more technological, relies on quantitative measurements, and is increasingly evidence-based, Eastern medicine is minimally invasive, relies on qualitative assessments, and remains largely experience-based. However, one concept shared by both medical systems is that most if not all physiological functions are regulated by activities possessing opposite effects. To consider only a few examples, blood sugar is decreased by insulin and increased by glucagon, calcitonin and parathyroid hormone act in opposing directions to regulate calcium levels in blood and tissues, and, generally speaking, the sympathetic and parasympathetic systems have contrasting functions in regulating many aspects of our internal environment. These phenomena can be regarded as reflections of the yin-yang balance described in traditional Chinese medicine. Thus, the "homeostasis" of Western medicine has long been recognized as "dynamic balance" in the classical texts of Chinese medicine.

The discovery of enkephalins, the first family of endogenous opioids, by Hughes et al. in 1975 [1] triggered the search for endogenous substrates with antiopioid activities. Ungar et al. [2] were among the first to present evidence for antiopioid substances [AOS]. At present, an array of AOS has been reported, the most widely studied and probably the most potent of which is cholecystokinin octapeptide (CCK-8) [3].

Studies of the interactions between opioid peptides and antiopioid peptides are of considerable pharmacological and physiological interest, especially when the ever-increasing functions of endogenously released peptides are considered. As with all peptides, the endogenous opioids and antiopioids have been best studied in animal models. Using such models, acupuncture (manipulation of metal needles inserted in specific body sites known as acupoints) and electroacupuncture, or EA (electrical stimulation administered via the needles placed at acupoints), have been shown to be reliable approaches for inducing release of endogenous opioid peptides in the CNS [4]. More recently, animal studies have also demonstrated the acupuncture-induced release of antiopioid substances and examined the functional interactions between these opposing classes of peptides in producing acupuncture analgesia (AA). The aims of the present chapter are to review (a) the current understanding of the involvement of endogenous opioid peptides in AA, (b) the role of CCK in determining the effectiveness of AA and its possible mechanisms, and (c) the role of other putative antiopioid peptides in the CNS, including the newly characterized opiate-like peptide orphanin FQ (OFQ) [5] and angiotensin II.

3.2
Opioid Mechanisms for Acupuncture Analgesia

The role of endogenous opioids in AA has been examined at three different levels; the opiate receptors, the opioid peptides, and the neural pathways mediating opioid effects.

3.2.1
Opiate Receptors

3.2.1.1
Receptor Blockade

The first evidence suggesting the involvement of opioid receptors in AA, provided by Pomeranz et al. in 1976 [6] and Mayer et al. in 1977 [7], was that effects of AA in mice and humans could be abolished or at least markedly attenuated by treatment with the powerful opiate receptor antagonist, naloxone. Further studies revealed that naloxone reversibility of electroacupuncture analgesia (EAA) is dependent on the frequency of EA. Thus, the dose of naloxone needed for 50% inhibition (ID_{50}) of the analgesic effect of EA in the rat is 0.53 mg/kg for 2 Hz EA, 1.02 mg/kg for 15 Hz EA, and 24.0 mg/kg for 100 Hz EA [8]. Since the sensitivity of different types of opiate receptors to naloxone blockade is known to be $\mu > \delta > \varkappa$, the relative resistance of 100 Hz EAA to naloxone reversibility suggests the involvement of $\varkappa$ opioid receptors in mediating high frequency EA effect. In contrast, since 2 Hz as well as 15 Hz EAA are very sensitive to naloxone, μ and δ receptors are implicated.

3.2.1.2
Cross-Tolerance Study

Cross-tolerance provides another useful clue for identifying the type or subtype of opioid receptors involved in EAA. When rats were given consecutive sessions of 100 Hz EA for 6 h (30 min on, 30 min off) and the tail flick latency (TFL) measured at the end of each session to assess the potential change of EAA with time, analgesia decreased with the prolongation of stimulation, suggesting the development of tolerance. This is not attributable to either tissue damage surrounding the needle tip or depletion of relevant neurotransmitters in the CNS, since the effect of EAA resumed when the EA frequency was lowered to 2 Hz. Similarly, rats made tolerant to 2 Hz EA were still responsive to 100 Hz EA. The lack of cross-tolerance between 2 Hz EA and 100 Hz EA suggests involvement of different types of receptor mechanisms. Further studies revealed that rats made tolerant to 2 Hz EA were still reactive to intrathecal injection of dynorphin A (1–13), a selective $\varkappa$ opioid agonist, but not to OMF and DPDPE and selective μ and δ receptor agonists, respectively [9]. These results are

Fig. 1. Summary of electro-acupuncture frequency-specific release of endogenous opioid peptides. *EM* endomorphin, *β-EP* β-endorphin, *ENK* enkephalin, *DYN* dynorphin, *EA* electroacupuncture, *EOP* endogenous opioid peptide, *OR* opioid receptor

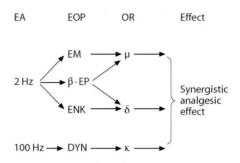

consistent with the suggestion that 2 Hz EAA is mediated by μ and δ receptors. In contrast, rats made tolerant to 100 Hz EA showed full response to OMF and DPDPE but not to dynorphin A (1–13), implying that 100 Hz EAA is mediated by ϰ opioid receptors (Fig. 1).

To summarize, 2 Hz EA uses μ and δ receptors to induce the analgesic effect, whereas 100 Hz EA is mediated by ϰ opioid receptors. When 2 Hz and 100 Hz or 15 Hz EA are administered alternately for 3 seconds each (the so-called dense-and-disperse mode), all three types of opioid receptors are involved [10]. This is an important example of how basic research has led to improved clinical treatment, since most electrostimulation devices used for EA now include a setting that automatically toggles between high and low frequency output.

3.2.2
Opioid Peptides

The framework of a three-member opioid peptide family, the enkephalins [1], endorphins [11], and dynorphins [12], remained for more than 2 decades, when Zadina et al. isolated and characterized the novel endogenous μ-selective agonists, the endomorphins [13]. Evidence will be presented to characterize the respective roles of the four opioid peptides involved in EAA.

3.2.2.1
Antibody Microinjection Study

While receptor blockade and cross-tolerance studies are powerful techniques for identifying the receptor entities that mediate AA, they provide no information as to the chemical nature of the mediators. To solve this problem, we developed the antibody microinjection technique. Antibodies against specific opioid peptides were developed and injected into the brain or spinal cord (Fig. 1). Each of these antibodies would recognize and bind to its target peptide, resulting in selective blockage of the function of the specific peptide by preventing peptide-receptor interaction. Such studies revealed that low frequency (2 Hz) EA analgesia is attenuated by enkephalin antibodies but not by dynorphin antibodies microinjected into the spinal subarachnoid space. In contrast, 100 Hz EAA is markedly attenuated by intrathecal injection of antibodies against dynorphin but not by antibodies against enkephalin [8]. The results provide strong support for the hypothesis that endogenously released enkephalin and dynorphin are responsible for mediating low and high frequency EA effects, respectively. Furthermore, microinjection of β-endorphin antiserum into the periaqueductal gray (PAG) of rat selectively blocked the analgesic effect induced by 2 Hz EA but not by 100 Hz, suggesting that β-endorphin plays a significant role in mediating low frequency EAA in the PAG of the midbrain [14, 21].

In summary, 2 Hz EA uses β-endorphin in the midbrain and enkephalin in the spinal cord to produce analgesic effects, whereas 100 Hz EA uses dynorphin in the spinal cord (Fig. 1). But what of the newly characterized opioid peptide, endomorphin? In a recent study, we used endomorphin-1 (EM1) antiserum in different dilutions for intrathecal injection in a fixed volume of 10 μl and found that EM1 antiserum could suppress 2 Hz EAA at 1:10 and 1:100 dilutions but not at 1:1000 dilution [15]. In contrast, 100 Hz EAA was not affected by EM1 antiserum even when undiluted. The data clearly suggest that endomorphin-1 is involved in 2 Hz EAA but not 100 Hz EAA, at least in rat spinal cord.

3.2.2.2
Radioimmunoassay of Spinal Perfusate

Neuropeptides released from the spinal cord may diffuse into the CSF, where they can be detected by radioimmunoassay (RIA). The CSF level of a peptide is assumed to be related to its rate of release. In experiments with rats, a dramatic increase of immunoreactive (IR) enkephalin was detected during 2 Hz EA but not 100 Hz [16]. In contrast, 100 Hz EA was accompanied by an increase of IR dynorphin but not IR enkephalin. Similar results were obtained in humans [17]. Low frequency (2 Hz) electrical stimulation applied on the skin at the hand acupoint Hegu (LI.4) produced a 367 % ($p<0.05$) increase of a peptide encoded in the enkephalin gene, with no concomitant increase in dynorphin A. In contrast, 100 Hz EA induced a moderate but highly significant 49 % ($p<0.01$) increase in dynorphin A with no change in IR enkephalin. These animal and human findings of RIA-detectable changes of opioid peptides in spinal perfusates are consistent with the results described above from antibody microinjection studies.

3.2.3
Neural Pathways

Neurons containing β-endorphin aggregate in the arcuate nucleus of the hypothalamus (ARH). This is in sharp contrast to the widespread distribution of enkephalins and dynorphins in both brain and spinal cord. Focal lesion and stimulation (mechanical, chemical, and electrical) have been used to characterize the neural pathways involved in electroacupuncture analgesia (EAA) that use opioid peptides as mediators.

3.2.3.1
ARH Mediates Low Frequency EA Analgesia

To identify the neural substrate within the diencephalon, lesions were placed in several nuclei in the thalamus and hypothalamus [18]. Restricted electrolytic lesioning of the ARH or microinjection of kainic acid, which selectively attacks neuronal cell bodies rather than passing fibers, produced a dramatic reduction of EAA induced by 2 Hz, with no effect at 100 Hz EAA. Additional evidence supporting the importance of ARH in mediating low frequency EAA derives from the observation that cross-tolerance exists between 2 Hz EAA and ARH stimulation-produced analgesia [19]. In fact, the latter could be fully prevented by intrathecal (ITH) administration of naloxone or the δ-selective antagonist ICI 174,864, implying that analgesia induced by ARH stimulation is mediated by the release of endogenous δ opioid agonists, most probably enkephalins. Together with results presented above – that intra-PAG injection of antiserum against β-endorphin prevents 2 Hz EAA – these findings indicate that signals induced by 2 Hz EA reach ARH, which sends axons to PAG to release β-endorphin, from which site fibers descend to the spinal cord to release enkephalins, resulting in the production of analgesia.

3.2.3.2.
Parabrachial Nucleus Mediates High Frequency EA Analgesia

Gross anatomical studies have revealed that (a) removal of the whole forebrain (telencephalon and diencephalon) abolishes 2 Hz EAA but not 100 Hz EAA [20] and (b) EAA is totally abolished in spinal rats. It is logical to speculate that the key element for mediating high frequency EAA is located at a supraspinal, intradiencephalic level, i.e., in the lower brainstem.

On the basis of this reasoning, discrete electric lesions were placed in several candidate areas of the lower brainstem. Electrolytic or kainate lesions placed within the parabrachial nucleus (PBN) were found to produce a selective reduction of the analgesic effect induced by 100 Hz EA without affecting that of 2 Hz EA. On the other hand, intra-PBN injection of glutamate produced profound analgesia [22].

In contrast to PBN lesions that selectively block high frequency EAA, electrolytic and kainate lesion of the ventral portion of the PAG (vPAG) produce an almost total abolishment of EAA (at 2 Hz or 100 Hz), although the baseline pain threshold (TFL) remained essentially intact. Thus, the vPAG seems to be a common pathway for low and high frequency EAA [22].

A key question is: why should the ARH be activated by 2 Hz EA and PBN by 100 Hz EA? A likely explanation is that while afferent neural impulses reach widespread areas in the CNS, only those neurons that can follow the frequency of the afferent impulses can be effectively activated.

3.3
CCK-8 and Acupuncture Analgesia

3.3.1
Initial Findings

In order to study the mechanisms of AA, we established an animal model in the rat [24]. One animal response that attracted our attention was the gradual decline of analgesic effect when EA stimulation was prolonged for more than 3 h. The similarity of this phenomenon to morphine tolerance led us to refer to it tentatively as "acupuncture tolerance." Since the content of opiate-like substances remained high in the brain of rats subjected to this prolonged EA, their tolerance was unlikely due to a depletion of endogenous opiate-like substances. We speculated initially on whether the antiopioid substance (AOS) might act directly as an opioid receptor antagonist or might act via their own receptor to trigger a negative feedback response to dampen the release of opiate-like substance(s).

A potentially fruitful approach was to test brain extracts from EA-tolerant rats for antiopiate activity. In an in vitro system, mouse vas deferens exhibited a morphine-induced contraction that was antagonized by either naloxone or a brain extract prepared from morphine- or EA-tolerant rats. Brain extract from untreated control rats had no effect. In an in vivo study in the rat, intracerebroventricular (ICV) injections of the same "tolerant" brain extracts produced a powerful suppression of morphine analgesia [25]. Further purification yielded a peptide (sensitive to the broad-spectrum proteolytic action of pronase) with a molecular weight of around 1000, but the chemical structure was not characterized.

In a seminar presented at St. Louis University School of Medicine in 1982, I was pleased to receive comments from the audience that CCK-8 might well be the AOS mentioned in my talk, since this peptide was already known to antagonize β-endorphin's stimulation of feeding behavior. Dr. M. C. Benfield kindly provided me with CCK antiserum and Dr. R. Y. Wang enthusiastically encouraged me to test CCK-8 in our studies. This was the starting point of a series of experiments performed in my laboratory aimed at examining the possible role of CCK-8 as an endogenously released AOS in the modulation of opioid analgesia [26–28].

3.3.2
CCK-8 as a Potent Endogenous Antiopioid Peptide

3.3.2.1
Behavioral Studies

Using the tail flick assay as an index of nociception, a stable level of analgesia induced by morphine or EA can be established. Experiments in rats have shown that ICV or ITH injection of 1–4 ng (1–4 pmol) of CCK-8 antagonizes EA analgesia or morphine analgesia dose-dependently (Fig. 2) [3]. The doses of CCK-8 needed for 50 % reversal (ID_{50}) of EA analgesia are 1.0 ng ICV and 1.5 ng ITH, respectively, suggesting that CCK-8 exerts a somewhat more potent antiopioid action in brain than in spinal cord. Corresponding values for antagonizing morphine analgesia were 1.7 ng and 3.1 ng, respectively. The potency of CCK-8 as an opioid antagonist can be compared with that of naloxone. On a molar basis, the dose of naloxone needed for complete antagonism of morphine analgesia (6–30 nmol) is 6000–8000 times greater than the corresponding dose of CCK-8 (1–4 pmol).

3.3.2.2
Electrophysiological Study

The results obtained from behavioral studies appear straightforward and relatively easy to interpret. However, since the end point of nociception depends on the occurrence of a motor response (tail flick, for example), the results may be subject to mis-

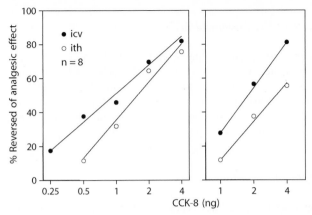

Fig. 2. Dose-dependent reversal of electroacupuncture (EA)-induced analgesia (*left*) and morphine analgesia (*right*) by ICV or ITH injection of cholecystokinin-8 (CCK-8). In the EA study, eight rats were given EA stimulation of 15 Hz, 3V, 10 min, on hind limb acupoints ST 36 and SP 6. Immediately prior to EA stimulation, four rats received injection of CCK-8; the other four received unsulfated CCK-8 as control. In the morphine study, morphine sulfate, 5 mg/kg was injected SC. CCK-8 or unsulfated CCK-8 were injected 25 min after morphine injection [3]

interpretation (analgesia versus motor paralysis). To test this possibility, the phenomenon was examined in pain-related neurons in the CNS using single cell recording techniques. Among the brain nuclei involved in nociception, the nucleus parafascicularis (PF) has received special attention. Most of the PF neurons reveal an increase of spikes in response to noxious stimuli. These spikes are inhibited by subcutaneous injection of morphine and this effect of morphine is reversed by ITH injection of CCK-8. Likewise, the noxious stimulation-induced spikes of PF neurons is suppressed by EA, and this effect of EA is reversed by ICV injection of CCK-8 [29]. Since the results of these electrophysiological studies reproduced almost every aspect observed in behavioral studies, it can be concluded that the antinociceptive effects of morphine or EA can be antagonized by CCK-8 at nanogram doses.

3.3.2.3
Sites of Action in the CNS

To locate the sites of action of CCK-8 in CNS, microinjection techniques were employed to administer the octapeptide into discrete brain areas at doses equal to 1 %–10 % of parenteral doses. For example, microinjection of 0.25 ng of CCK-8 into rat PAG produced a 50 % decrease of morphine analgesia [30]. This effect of CCK-8 was readily reversed by the CCK receptor antagonist, proglumide, indicating that CCK-8 is indeed acting via CCK receptors. Similar results were obtained when CCK-8 was injected into the amygdala or nucleus accumbens. These nuclei have been shown to be the central sites that mediate morphine analgesia [31, 32].

3.3.2.4
Types of CCK Receptors Involved in Antiopioid Activity

Two types of CCK receptors designated as types A and B have been characterized. When rat brain or spinal cord slices were incubated with ^{125}I-labeled CCK-8, that can bind to both types of CCK receptors, subsequent incubation with selective CCK-A or CCK-B antagonists demonstrated that the CCK receptors in the PAG, nucleus accumbens, amygdala, and spinal cord of the rat belong to the CCK-B type [33]. In contrast, CCK-A receptors appear to predominate in the CNS of the monkey.

3.3.2.5
Types of Opiate Receptor Interacting with CCK Receptor

Opiate receptors have been classified into three types: μ, δ, and $\varkappa$, with all three types mediating analgesic effects. However, CCK-8 suppresses analgesia mediated by the μ and $\varkappa$ receptors, not that mediated by δ receptor [34], findings that have been confirmed by Dickenson et al. [35]. In summary, the results obtained from behavioral, electrophysiological, and morphological studies have amply demonstrated that nanogram levels of CCK-8 can interact with CCK-B receptors in specific sites in the CNS to interfere with the function of μ and $\varkappa$ opiate receptors, resulting in antiopioid effects.

3.3.3
Biochemical Mechanisms of Opiate/CCK Interaction

3.3.3.1
Interaction (Cross Talk) at the Receptor Level

Firstly we used ^{3}H-etorphine, which binds to all three types of opiate receptors, and found that CCK suppresses total opiate receptor binding in a dose-dependent manner [36]. In subsequent studies, we used selective ligands for μ, δ, and $\varkappa$ opiate receptors and found that CCK-8 decreased the total receptor number (Bmax) of the μ receptor without changing its binding affinity (Kd). In contrast, CCK-8 decreased the affinity of the $\varkappa$ receptor without changing its Bmax [37]. CCK-8 had no effect on binding characteristics of the δ receptor, which is consistent with results obtained in the behavioral studies described above [34].

3.3.3.2
Coexistence of Opiate and CCK Receptors on the Same Neuron

Electrophysiological experiments were performed on small dorsal root ganglion (DRG) neurons using the whole cell patch clamp technique to record voltage-gated calcium currents. The μ and $\varkappa$ opioid receptor agonists produced a marked decrease in the calcium current that was readily reversed by CCK-8. The effect of CCK-8, in turn, was reversed by the CCK-B antagonist L-365260, suggesting that CCK-8 acts via the CCK receptor rather than directly as an opioid receptor antagonist [38, 39]. These results favor the interpretation that opioid receptors and CCK receptors coexist on one and the same neuron.

3.3.3.3
Uncoupling of Opiate Receptor from G Protein

It has been established that GTPγ S, the long acting GTP analog, can induce an uncoupling of the opiate receptor from the G protein, resulting in a lowering of the receptor affinity to opiates. Similar activity was found for CCK-8 [41]. Since combination of GTPγ S with CCK-8 produced no additive effect, it is reasoned that they may act at the same postsynaptic site, i.e., uncoupling the receptor from the G protein and thus lowering the efficacy of signal transduction.

3.3.3.4
Involvement of the Phosphoinositol System

As mentioned previously, antiopiate effects of CCK-8 are induced only by small doses (ng level), in contrast to large doses, which may induce an analgesic effect. It is of interest that an increase in IP$_3$ production is induced by small, but not large, doses of CCK-8 [40, 41]. In addition, evidence that the antiopiate effect of CCK can be reversed by lithium seems to favor the involvement of the phosphoinositol system [42].

3.3.3.5
Interaction at the Intracellular Free Calcium Level

Three types of experiments were performed to examine the role of intracellular free calcium in mediating CCK-8 actions:
1. Experiments using rat brain synaptosomal preparations revealed that the suppressive effect of morphine on synaptosomal ^{45}Ca uptake is reversible by low concentrations (10–100 nmol) of CCK-8.
2. Studies with dissociated neonatal rat brain cells demonstrated that ^{45}Ca uptake could be suppressed by agonists of all three types of opioid receptors, whereas CCK-8 antagonized the effect produced by μ- and $\varkappa$- but not δ opioid agonists [43], findings that are consistent with in vivo results.
3. CCK-8 increases intracellular free calcium concentration ($[Ca^{2+}]_i$) [41], in contrast to the effect of opiates that decrease $[Ca^{2+}]_i$. This effect of CCK-8 can be observed even in calcium-free medium, suggesting that it is due to mobilization of intracellular calcium stores rather than increased calcium influx. In fact, the increase of intracellular IP$_3$ induced by CCK-8 would accelerate the release of free calcium from calcium storage.

3.3.4
CCK in Morphine and Electroacupuncture Tolerance

3.3.4.1
CCK-8 and Morphine Tolerance

Subcutaneous injection of morphine (5 mg/kg) produced an 89 % increase of CCK-8 content in spinal perfusates, suggesting an increase in CCK release [44]. Further studies revealed that CCK-8 release can be activated by μ and $\varkappa$ but not δ opioid ago-

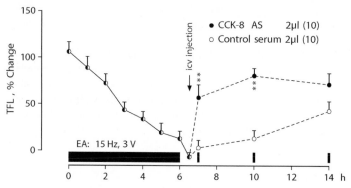

Fig. 3. Reversal of electroacupuncture (EA) tolerance by ICV injection of CCK-8 antiserum. Twenty rats were given continuous EA stimulation of 15 Hz, 3V, 6 h. Thirty minutes after cessation of EA, 10 rats received ICV injection of CCK-8 antiserum, while 10 rats received normal rabbit serum as control. All rats were given EA, 15 Hz, 3V, 10 min, at 0.5, 3.5, and 7.5 h after the ICV injection. *TFL* tail flick latency. **$P<0.01$ relative to control [3]

nists [45]. Continuous injection of morphine for 6 days resulted in an increase in brain content of CCK-8 [28] together with an increase in CCK gene expression [46, 47]. That an increase in CCK biosynthesis and release plays a role in the development of morphine tolerance is inferred from findings that ICV injection of CCK-8 antiserum can reverse, at least partly, the morphine tolerance [48].

3.3.4.2
CCK-8 and Electroacupuncture Tolerance

Experiments in rats have demonstrated that (a) EA for 1 h produces a marked increase of CCK-8 content in the CSF, suggesting an accelerated CCK release in the CNS, (b) EA for 2 h produces a moderate increase in CCK-8 content in midbrain PAG, suggesting an accelerated enzymatic processing of CCK precursor to form the functionally active octapeptide, and (c) continuous EA for 8 h elicits a significant increase in the abundance of CCK mRNA in the brain, indicating an acceleration of gene expression [49]. That increased biosynthesis and release of CCK-8 plays an important role in the development of EA tolerance is suggested by findings that tolerance induced by continuous EA for 6 h is reversed by ICV injection of antiserum against CCK-8 (Fig. 3) [3, 50].

3.3.5
CCK as a Negative Feedback Mechanism for Opioid Analgesia

3.3.5.1
Efficacy of EA Analgesia Determined by Opioid/CCK Balance in the CNS

As mentioned in Section 3.2.2.2, the efficacy of EA analgesia correlated positively with the availability of opioid peptides in the CNS [16]. Here we emphasize the *negative* correlation between EA analgesia and the availability of CCK-8 in the CNS. Using cluster analysis, Liu et al. [51] separated 168 rats into two groups according to their response to EA (100 Hz, 3 mA, 30 min). A demarcation in response to EA was calculated at 50 % increase of tail flick latency (TFL). Rats showing a TFL increase of less than 40 % were designated as low responders (LR), while high responders (HR) were those showing an increase of more than 60 %. Spinal perfusion was performed and the perfusate used for measurement of CCK-8 immunoreactivity (IR). No difference was found in the baseline concentration of CCK-8 in spinal perfusate between LR and HR. A marked difference, however, was found in CCK-8 levels during the period of EA stimulation. While HR showed no significant increase in CSF CCK-8 levels, the LR showed a dramatic increase, suggesting an immediate and robust release of CCK-8 from the spinal cord. It is thus clear that LR release a large amount of CCK-8 during EA stimulation (to antagonize opioid analgesia). In contrast, those rats producing no increase in CCK-8 release are the HR. CCK-8 in the CNS thus functions as a brake, or negative feedback mechanism, limiting the magnitude of EA analgesia. The sensitivity and extent of the feedback mechanism form the key determinants for the efficacy of EA analgesia.

Taken together, the findings give rise to the following description: EA stimulation accelerates the release of a whole array of neurotransmitters, including the endogenous opioid peptides. The latter in turn stimulate relevant neurons to release CCK-8 as a negative feedback mechanism. This model is supported by findings that morphine-induced spinal CCK-8 release can be totally abolished by the intrathecal injection of the opiate receptor blocker, naloxone [52]. On the other hand, a direct activation of CCK neurons by EA stimulation cannot be completely ruled out.

Zhang et al. [54] made a detailed study to clarify whether the rat phenotypes HR and LR are genetically determined. They found a strain (P77PMC) derived from Wistar rats that exhibits genetically determined audiogenic seizures. These rats also happen to exhibit an extraordinarily high analgesic response to 100 Hz EA. Radioimmunoassay (RIA) revealed that brain CCK-8 content is approximately 50 % lower in this rat strain as compared to Wistar rats [54], a finding that may serve as the common denominator for the high response to EA and the high vulnerability to acoustically evoked seizures in these animals.

3.3.5.2
Effect of CCK Gene Manipulation on the Efficacy of EA Analgesia

P77PMC rats that exhibit both audiogenic epileptic seizures and an extraordinarily high analgesic response to EA were used for gene manipulation studies in which brain content of CCK-8 was altered. Since the brain level of CCK-8 is very low in these rats, we tried to correct this genetic defect by ICV injection of the pSV2 expression vector containing an insert of CCK cDNA (pSV2-CCK). An increase of brain CCK content, appearing 2–4 days after the ICV injection of pSV2-CCK, was accompanied by a decrease in seizure attacks [53] as well as a lowered response to EA analgesia [28]. These effects reverted to preinjection levels in 9 days. In another experiment, LR rats – identified from a large population – were given ICV injections of antisense CCK expression vector (pSV2-CCK^{AS}). A decrease in brain CCK-8 content observed 4–6 days after the ICV injection was accompanied by a marked augmentation of EA analgesia, an effect that subsided in 9 days [55]. The results indicate that effects of EA analgesia can be modulated by manipulation of genes that encode opioid or antiopioid peptides, a phenomenon that fits the concept of yin-yang balance in traditional Chinese medicine.

3.4
Other Antiopioid Peptides

3.4.1
Orphanin FQ and Nocistatin

Since the discovery of three families of opioid peptides in the 1970s, scientists have not ceased looking for other endogenous opioid peptides and their receptors. The successful cloning of the δ opioid receptor in 1993 led to the discovery of an opioid receptor-like (ORL1) receptor in 1994 [56]. While the ORL1 receptor shows approximately 50 % identity with the μ, δ, and κ opioid receptors, it has a very low affinity with typical opioid ligands; hence it was also referred to as the "orphan receptor." An endogenous ligand for ORL1 receptor, characterized in 1995 on the basis of its hyperalgesic effect in mice after ICV injection, was named orphanin FQ (OFQ) or nociceptin [5, 56]. Subsequently, it was observed that the apparent hyperalgesic effect of OFQ/nociceptin in mice was in fact a reversal of opioid-mediated stress analgesia. This finding led to the notion that OFQ might belong in the category of antiopioid peptides, at least in brain. We undertook a detailed survey to ascertain the effects of exogenously injected OFQ on morphine analgesia and EA analgesia and the relevant role played by endogenously released OFQ in the CNS.

3.4.1.1
OFQ in Morphine Analgesia and Morphine Tolerance

When injected into the cerebral ventricle of the rat, OFQ shows no significant direct effect on baseline TFL at any dose between 4 fmol and 10 nmol, but it antagonizes morphine-induced analgesia in a dose-dependent manner over a range 0.4–50 nmol. Injected intrathecally, OFQ displays an analgesic effect and *potentiates* morphine analgesia [57], suggesting opposite roles for OFQ in spinal cord and brain.

In order to study the possible role of endogenous OFQ in the development of morphine tolerance, rats made tolerant to morphine were given an ICV injection of antiserum against OFQ to sequester putative OFQ from the synaptic cleft. Intracerebroventricular injection of OFQ antiserum but not of normal rabbit serum restored the sensitivity to morphine, suggesting that endogenously released OFQ in the brain plays an important role in the mechanisms underlying morphine tolerance [58]. In a recent study, Yuan et al. [59] administered increasing doses of morphine to rats for 5 days and found a gradual increase of OFQ content in the PAG and amygdala, up to 50 % more than controls, and more than 50 % increased levels of OFQ in the cerebroventricular perfusate, suggesting increased biosynthesis and release of OFQ in the brain.

These results imply that OFQ in brain is antagonistic to morphine-induced analgesia. It may also play an important role in the development of morphine tolerance, forming a link – in addition to CCK – in the negative feedback control for morphine analgesia.

3.4.1.2
OFQ in EA Analgesia and EA Tolerance

That brain OFQ may also play an antagonistic role in EA analgesia is supported by three lines of evidence: (a) analgesia induced by 100 Hz EA, as measured by radiant heat tail flick latency, is antagonized by ICV injection of OFQ in a dose-dependent manner [60], (b) EA analgesia is potentiated by ICV injection of antisense oligonucleotides complementary to the OFQ receptor, possibly by interfering with the expression of OFQ receptors in brain [60], but is not affected by injection of mis-sense oligonucleotide [60], and (c) LR rats were converted to HR by the ICV injection of antiserum against OFQ at 1:1 and 1:10 dilutions but not at 1:100; in addition, HR rats changed to LR following intrathecal injection of OFQ antiserum at 1:1 and 1:10 dilutions but not at 1:100 [58]. Taken together, these results support the notion that endogenous OFQ plays contradictory roles in brain versus spinal cord in affecting EA analgesia. In other words, while brain OFQ is partially responsible for the LR phenotype in rats, spinal OFQ may be a determining factor for the HR phenotype.

Tian et al. studied the role of brain OFQ in the development of EA tolerance [58]. Tolerance to EA analgesia can be induced by continuous administration of EA for 6 h (acute EA tolerance) or by one session of EA (30 min) per day for 6 consecutive days (chronic EA tolerance). Both acute and chronic EA tolerance can be reversed by ICV injection of IgG antiserum against OFQ. These results suggest that brain OFQ is recruited to function as an antiopioid peptide within a period of 6 h, and the effect of OFQ may last as long as 24 h and accumulate gradually during a period of 6 days, thus contributing to the formation of chronic EA tolerance.

3.4.1.3
Nocistatin: Endogenous Antagonist for OFQ/Nociceptin?

It was of interest that the nociceptin precursor designated as nocistatin [61] comprises another bioactive peptide that blocks OFQ-induced allodynia and hyperalgesia in mice. We were interested in determining whether ICV nocistatin would reverse the antimorphine effect of OFQ in rats, using TFL as nociceptive index. Nocistatin ICV produced no significant changes in basal TFL nor did it affect morphine analgesia. However, it significantly reversed the antagonistic effect of OFQ on morphine analgesia. The dose-response curve was bell-shaped and the most effective dose was 0.5 ng [62]. According to Okuda-Ashitaka et al. [61], nocistatin does not bind to the OFQ receptor, although it does bind to membranes of mouse brain and spinal cord with a high affinity in a saturable manner, suggesting the existence of its own receptor. The occurrence of two peptides with opposite functions in the same precursor protein would certainly engender considerable interest from the viewpoint of yin-yang balance.

3.4.2
Angiotensin II

Kaneko et al. purified an antiopioid substance from bovine brain that was characterized as a peptide chemically identical with angiotensin II (A II) [63]. In rats, we injected A II ICV into CSF of brain and ITH into spinal cord and found that A II antagonized morphine analgesia dose-dependently in brain but not spinal cord [64]. Further studies revealed that A II antagonizes morphine analgesia in the PAG of the midbrain but not in the nucleus accumbens [65], suggesting that PAG is an important site for A II to exert an antiopioid effect.

3.4.2.1
Involvement of Brain A II in EA Tolerance

To assess the role of endogenous A II in the development of EA tolerance, rats were given ICV injections of A II antiserum or the A II antagonist, saralasin. The antiserum as well as the antagonist led to postponement or reversal of EA tolerance, while radioimmunoassay revealed 1.7-fold (at 1 h continuous EA), 3.3-fold (2 h), and 1.3-fold (6 h) increases in CSF content of immunoreactive A II [66]. The results suggest that synthesis and release of brain A II contribute to the decreased efficacy of EA in producing analgesia when EA stimulation is prolonged.

3.4.2.2
Involvement of Brain A II in Morphine Tolerance

Acute morphine tolerance was induced in the rat by six successive injections of morphine at 2-hour intervals. Similar to the findings with EA-induced tolerance described above, acute morphine tolerance was postponed by ICV injection of either A II IgG or saralasin [67]. Chronic tolerance to morphine was achieved by injecting increasing doses of morphine 3 times a day for 5 days. This tolerance was partially (50 %) reversed by ICV injection of A II IgG [67]. Radioimmunoassay revealed a 1.2-fold increase in CSF content of A II in rats receiving three or six successive injections of morphine. Likewise, repeated administration of morphine for 3 or 5 days produced 1.1-fold and 2.8-fold increases of CSF A II relative to the control level [67].

Observation of the dynamic changes in A II biosynthesis induced by long-term EA stimulation revealed that: (a) CSF content of A II increased within 1 h, suggesting an accelerated release, (b) brain content of A II started to increase at 2 h, (c) the A II peak in the gel filtration profile of brain extract shifted markedly to the right after 3 h of continuous EA stimulation, suggesting a shift from the larger, precursor molecule angiotensinogen to the smaller A II molecule [68], and (d) a significant increase of angiotensinogen mRNA was observed after continuous EA for 6 h or after repeated injections of morphine for 4 consecutive days [69].

3.4.2.3
Spinal A II: Antagonist of 100 Hz EA

We reported in our first study that A II antagonizes morphine analgesia after ICV injection but not after ITH injection [64]. Of related interest, we subsequently found that ITH administration of the A II antagonist, saralasin, produces a significant augmentation of the analgesic effect induced by 100 Hz EA analgesia but not that resulting from 2 Hz or 15 Hz EA [70]. In addition, only 100 Hz EA produces a significant increase in the release of A II in spinal cord. Since 100 Hz EA is known to trigger the release of dynorphin in spinal cord, it can be inferred that spinal A II plays a negative feedback role in dynorphin-induced analgesia but not in enkephalin- or morphine-induced analgesia.

3.4.2.4
Mechanisms Underlying the Antiopioid Effect of A II

Several lines of evidence suggest that A II exerts its antiopioid effect at a postreceptor site rather than at the opiate receptor level: (a) A II does not bind to opiate receptors to a significant extent, as determined by radio receptor assay [70], (b) ICV A II increased brain content of cyclic AMP, whereas the level of this cofactor was decreased by SC morphine [71], and (c) A II increased synaptosomal ^{45}Ca uptake and completely reversed the morphine-induced *decrease* in Ca uptake [72].

3.5
Concluding Remarks

While only about a dozen classic neurotransmitters have been identified, neuropeptides with synaptic modulatory effects may well exist in 10-fold greater numbers. Interactions among the neuropeptides within the narrow synaptic cleft is well-documented, with additive, synergistic, and antagonistic effects being described. Studies of two families of peptides, the opioids and the antiopioids, as manifested in pain control are proving to create an excellent model for understanding neuropeptide interactions.

It is theoretically interesting to explore the varied underlying mechanisms by which neuropeptides have evolved into groups with opposite functions. We know, for example, that the opioid peptide dynorphin and the putative antiopioid peptide OFQ have 50 % homology in their amino acid structures [5], suggesting a common origin at the genomic level. We also know that adrenocorticotropic hormone (ACTH) and β-endorphin are derived from the common precursor, POMC, and antiopioid activity is one the many functions of ACTH [73]. Equally interesting is that when the carboxy-terminal 4 amino acids of β-endorphin (1–27) are truncated, this peptide's function changes from opioid to antiopioid [74]. Similarly, as discussed in Section 3.4.1.3, nociceptin (also known as OFQ) has an action opposite from that of its precursor peptide, nocistatin.

It is also of interest that, although no structural similarity has been found between CCK-8, A II, and OFQ, a functional synergism was revealed to exist between CCK-8 and A II [75] and between CCK-8 and OFQ (Yuan L et al., unpublished observation). In contrast to the heterogeneity in chemical structure among antiopioid peptides, most opioid peptides bear a common N-terminal structure of Tyr-Gly-Gly-Phe, thus an interaction of either synergism or antagonism between them becomes plausible.

Unlike exogenously administered chemical agents, the dose of which can be readily varied by several orders of magnitude, the endogenous release of neurotransmitters and neuropeptides is limited to a narrower physiological range. However, thanks to the evolutionary development of synergistic mechanisms, amplification of function can be reached by the simultaneous release of several related transmitters or peptides. The biological economy of these mechanisms is clear. One can safely predict that the biochemical mechanisms underlying neuropeptide interactions will be a major target of research in this millennium and that such research is likely to result in important medical applications.

Acknowledgement. This work was supported by the National Natural Science Foundation of China and a grant from the U. S. National Institute of Drug Abuse (DA 03983).

References

1. Hughes J, Smith TW, Kosteritz HW et al (1975) Identification of two related pentapeptides from the brain with potent opiate agonist activity. Nature 258:577–579
2. Ungar G, Ungar A, Malin DH et al (1977) Brain peptides with opiate antagonistic action: TheIR possible role in tolerance and dependence. Psychoneuroendocrinol 2:1–10
3. Han JS, Ding XZ, Fan SG (1985) Is CCK-8 a candidate for endogenous antiopioid peptide substrate? Neuropeptides 5:399–402
4. Han JS, Terenius L (1982) Neurochemical basis of acupuncture analgesia. Annu Rev Pharmacol Toxicol 22:193–220
5. Meunier JC, Mollereau C, Toll L et al (1995) Isolation and structure of the endogenous agonist of opioid receptor-like ORL1 receptor. Nature 377:532–535
6. Pomeranz B, Chiu D (1976) Naloxone blocks acupuncture analgesia and causes hyperalgesia: Endorphin is implicated. Life Sci 19:1757–1762
7. Mayer DJ, Price DD, Rafii A (1977) Antagonism of acupuncture analgesia in man by the narcotic antagonist naloxone. Brain Res 121:368–372
8. Han JS, Wang Q (1992) Mobilization of specific neuropeptides by peripheral stimulation of identified frequencies. News Physiol Sci USA 7:176–180
9. Chen XH, Han JS (1992) Analgesia induced by electroacupuncture of different frequencies is mediated by different types of opioid receptors: Another cross-tolerance study. Beh Brain Res 47:143–149
10. Chen XH, Han JS (1992) All three types of opioid receptors in the spinal cord are important for 2–15 Hz electroacupuncture analgesia. Eur J Pharmacol 211:203–210
11. Cox BA, Goldstein A, Li CH (1976) Opiate activity of a peptide, β-lipotropin (61–91) derived from β-lipotropin. Proc Natl Acad Sci USA 73:1821–1823
12. Goldstein A, Tachibana S, Lowrey LI et al (1979) Dynorphin (1–13), an extraordinary potent opioid peptide. Proc Natl Acad Sci USA 76:6666–6670
13. Zadina JE, Lackler L, Ge LJ, Kastin AJ (1997) A potent and selective endogenous agonist for μ-opiate receptor. Nature 386:499–502
14. He CM, Han JS (1990) Attenuation of low rather than highfrequency electroacupuncture analgesia by microinjection of β-endorphin antiserum into the periaqueductal gray in rats. Acupuncture. Sci Intl J 1:94–99
15. Han Z, Jiang YH, Wan Y, Wang Y, Chang JK, Han JS (1999) Endomorphin 1 mediates 2 Hz but not 100 Hz electroacupuncture analgesia in the rat. Neurosci Lett 274:75–78
16. Fei H, Xie GX, Han JS (1987) Low and high frequency electroacupuncture stimulation releases met-enkephalin and dynorphin A in rat spinal cord. Chin Sci Bull 1987 34:703–705
17. Han JS, Chen XH, Sun SL et al (1991) Effect of low and highfrequency TENS on met-enkephalin-Arg-Phe and dynorphin A immunoreactivity in human lumbar CSF. Pain 47:295–298
18. Wang Q, Mao LM, Han JS (1990) The arcuate nucleus of hypothalamus mediates low but not high frequency electroacupuncture analgesia in rats. Brain Res 513:60–66
19. Wang Q, Mao LM, Han JS (1990) Analgesic electrical stimulation of the hypothalamic arcuate nucleus: Tolerance and its cross-tolerance to 2 Hz or 100 Hz electroacupuncture. Brain Res 518:40–46
20. Wang Q, Mao LM, Han JS (1990) Diencephalon as a cardinal neural structure for mediating 2 Hz but not 100 Hz electroacupuncture-induced tail flick latency suppression. Behav Brain Res 37:149–156
21. Wang Q, Mao LM, Han JS (1990) The role of PAG in mediation of analgesia produced different frequencies electroacupuncture stimulation in rats. Intl J Neurosci 53:167–172
22. Wang Q, Mao LM, Han JS (1991) The role of parabrachial nucleus in high frequency electroacupuncture analgesia in rats. Chin J Physiol Sci 7:363–367
23. Han JS, Tang J, Huang BS (1979) Acupuncture tolerance in rats: Antiopiate substrates implicated. Chin Med J 92:625–627
24. Ren MF, Han JS (1979) Rat tail flick acupuncture analgesia model. Chin Med J 92:576–582

25. Han JS, Tang J, Huang BS et al (1979) Acupuncture tolerance in rats: Antiopiate substrates implicated. Chin Med J 92:625–627
26. Han JS (1992) The role of CCK in electroacupuncture analgesia and electroacupuncture tolerance. In: CT Dourish, SJ Cooper, SD Iversen, LL Iversen (eds) Multiple cholecystokinin receptors in the CNS. Oxford University Press, Oxford, pp 480–502
27. Han JS (1995) Molecular events underlying the antiopioid effect of CCK-8 in the central nervous system. In: AC Cuello, B Collier (eds) Pharmacological sciences: Perspectives for research and therapy in the late 1990s. Birkhauser Verlag, Basel, pp 199–207
28. Han JS (1995) Cholecystokinin octapeptide (CCK-8): A negative feedback control mechanism for opioid analgesia. Prog Brain Res 105:263–271
29. Bian JT, Sun MZ, Xu MY, Han JS (1993) Antagonism by CCK-8 of the antinociceptive effect of electroacupuncture on pain-related neurons in nucleus parafascicularis of the rat. Asia Pacific J Pharmacol 8:90–97
30. Li Y, Han JS (1989) Cholecystokinin octapeptide antagonizes morphine analgesia in periaqueductal gray of the rat. Brain Res 480:105–110
31. Zhou ZF, Du MY, Jian Y et al (1981) Effect of intracerebral microinjection of naloxone on acupuncture- and morphine-analgesia in the rabbit. Sci Sinica 24:1166–1178
32. Zhou ZF, Xuan YT, Han JS (1984) Analgesic effect of morphine injected into habenula, nucleus accumbens, or amygdala of rabbits. Acta Pharmacol Sin 5:150–153
33. Pu SF, Zhuang HX, Han JS (1994) CCK-8 antagonizes morphine analgesia in nucleus accumbens of the rat via the CCK-B receptor. Brain Res 657:159–164
34. Wang XJ, Wang XM, Han JS (1990) CCK-8 antagonize opioid analgesia mediated by μ- and κ- but not δ-receptors in the spinal cord of the rat. Brain Res 523:5–10
35. Dickenson AH, Sullivan AF, Magnuson DS (1992) CCK and opioid interaction in the spinal cord. In: CT Dourish, SJ Cooper, SD Iversen et al (eds) Multiple CCK receptors in the CNS. Oxford University Press, Oxford, pp 503–510
36. Wang XJ, Fan SG, Ren MF, Han JS (1989) Cholecystokinin-8 suppressed 3H-etorphine binding to rat brain opiate receptors. Life Sci 45:117–123
37. Wang XJ, Han JS (1990) Modification by CCK-8 of the binding of μ-, δ-, and κ opioid receptors. J Neurochem 55 1379–1382
38. Liu NJ, Xu T, Xu C, Li CQ et al (1995) Cholecystokinin octapeptide reverses μ opioid receptor-mediated inhibition of calcium current in rat dorsal root ganglion neurons. J Pharmacol Exp Ther 1995 275:1293–1299
39. Xu T, Liu NJ, Li CQ et al (1996) Cholecystokinin octapeptide reverses the κ opioid receptor-mediated depression of calcium current in rat dorsal root ganglion neurons. Brain Res 730:207–211
40. Zhang LJ, Lu XY, Han JS (1992) Influence of CCK-8 on phosphoinositide turnover in neonatal rat brain cells. Biochem J 285:847–850
41. Zhang LJ, Wang XJ, Han JS (1993) Modification of opioid receptors and uncoupling of receptors from G protein as possible mechanisms underlying suppression of opioid binding by CCK-8. Chin Med Sci J 8:1–4
42. Zhang LJ, Han JS (1994) Regulation by lithium of the antagonistic effect of CCK-8 on ohmefentanyl-induced antinociception. Neuropharmacol 33:123–126
43. Wang JF, Ren MF, Han JS (1992) Mobilization of calcium from intracellular store as a possible mechanism underlying the antiopioid effect of CCK-8. Peptides 13:947–951
44. Zhou Y, Sun YH, Zhang ZW et al (1993) Increased release of immunoreactive CCK-8 and enhancement of electroacupuncture analgesia by CCK-8 antagonist in rat spinal cord. Neuropeptides 24:139–144
45. Sheng S, Tian JB, Han JS (1995) Electroacupuncture induces spinal CCK release via μ- and κ opioid receptors. Chin Sci Bull 40:555–557
46. Pu SF, Xhuang HX, Han JS (1994) CCK-8 gene expression in rat amygdaloid neurons: Normal distribution and effect of morphine tolerance. Mol Brain Res 21:183–189
47. Zhou Y, Sun YH, Zhang ZW, Han JS (1992) Accelerated expression of CCK gene in the brain of rats rendered tolerant to morphine. NeuroReport 3:1121–1123
48. Ding XZ, Fan SG, Zhou JP, Han JS (1986) Reversal of tolerance to morphine analgesia but no potentiation of morphine-induced analgesia by antiserum against CCK-8. Neuropharmacol 25:1155–1160
49. Sun YH, Zhou Y, Han JS (1995) Accelerated release and production of CCK-8 in CNS of rats during prolonged electroacupuncture stimulation. Chin J Neurosci 2:83–88
50. Bian JT, Sun MZ, Han JS (1993) Reversal of electroacupuncture tolerance by CCK-8 antiserum: An electrophysiological study on pain-related neurons in nucleus parafascicularis of the rat. Intl J Neurosci 72:15–29

51. Liu SX, Luo F, Shen S et al (1999) Relationship between the analgesic effect of electroacupuncture and CCK-8 content in spinal perfusate in rats. Chin Sci Bull 44:240–243
52. Zhou Y, Sun YH, Zhang ZW, Han JS (1993) Increased release of immunoreactive CCK-8 by morphine and potentiation of opioid analgesia by CCK-B receptor antagonist L-365260 in rat spinal cord. Eur J Pharmacol 234:147–154
53. Zhang LX, Wu M, Han JS (1992) Suppression of audiogenic epileptic seizure by intracerebral injection of a CCK gene vector. NeuroReport 03:700–702
54. Zhang LX, Li XL, Wang L, Han JS (1997) Rats with decreased brain CCK levels show increased responsiveness to peripheral electrical stimulation-induced analgesia. Brain Res 745:158–164
55. Tang NM, Dong HW, Wang XM et al (1997) Cholecystokinin antisense RNA increases the analgesic effect induced by electroacupuncture or low dose morphine: Conversion of low responders into high responders. Pain 71:71–80
56. Darland T, Heinricher MM, Grandy DK (1998) Orphanin FQ nociceptin: A role in pain and analgesia, but so much more. Trends Neurosci 21:215–221
57. Tian JH, Xu W, Fang Y et al (1997) Bidirectional modulatory effect of OFQ on morphine-induced analgesia: Antagonism in brain and potentiation in spinal cord of the rat. Br J Pharmacol 20:676–680
58. Tian JH, Zhang W, Fang Y et al (1998) Endogenous orphanin FQ: Evidence for a role in the modulation of electroacupuncture analgesia and development of tolerance to analgesia produced by morphine and electroacupuncture. Br J Pharmacol 124:21–26
59. Yuan L, Han Z, Chang JK, Han JS (1999) Accelerated release and production of orphanin FQ in brain of chronic morphine tolerant rats. Brain Res 826:330–334
60. Tian JH, Xu W, Zhang W et al (1997) Involvement of endogenous orphanin FQ in electroacupuncture-induced analgesia. NeuroReport 8:497–500
61. Okuda-Ashitaka E, Minami T, Tachibana S et al (1998) Nocistatin, a peptide that blocks nociceptin action in pain transmission. Nature 392:286–289
62. Zhao CS, Li BS, Zhao GY et al (1999) Nocistatin reversed the effect of orphanin FQ nociception in antagonizing morphine analgesia. NeuroReport 10:297–299
63. Kaneko S, Tamura S, Takagi H (1985) Purification and identification of endogenous antiopioid substance from bovine brain. Biochem Biophys Res Commun 587–593
64. Wang KW, Han JS (1987) Angiotensin II antagonizes morphine analgesia: Effective by intracerebroventricular injection but not by intrathecal injection. Chinese Sci Bull 33:123–128
65. Wang XM, Han JS (1989) Antagonism to morphine analgesia and involvement in morphine tolerance of angiotensin II in periaqueductal gray of the rabbit. Chinese Sci Bull 33:149–152
66. Wang KW, Han JS (1989) Evidence for involvement of brain angiotensin II in tolerance to electroacupuncture analgesia in rats. Chin J Appl Physiol 5:32–36
67. Wang KW, Han JS (1989) Evidence for brain angiotensin II being involved in morphine tolerance in the rat. Chin J Pharmacol Toxicol 3:7–11
68. Wang KW, Han JS (1999) Accelerated synthesis and release of angiotensin II in the rats brain during electroacupuncture tolerance. Sci Sinica (B) 33:686–693
69. Gao RW, Wang KW, Han JS (1989) Accelerated angiotensinogen gene expression in the brain of the rat made tolerance to morphine and electroacupuncture analgesia. Acta Physiol Sin 41:299–303
70. Sheng S, Li J, Wang XM et al (1989) Angiotensin II release and antielectroacupuncture analgesia in spinal cord. Acta Physiol Sin 41:179–183
71. Wang KW, Han JS (1989) Possible mechanisms of the antiopioid activity of angiotensin II. J Beijing Med Univ 21:7–9
72. Wang XM, Wang XJ, Han JS (1989) Antagonistic effects of angiotensin II and morphine on synaptosomal calcium uptake. Acta Physiol Sin 41:179–183
73. Smock T, Fields HL (1989) ACTH1–24 blocks opiate-induced analgesia in the rat. Brain Res 212:202–206
74. Hammonds RG, Li CH (1984) Beta-endorphin (1–27) is an antagonist of beta-endorphin analgesia. Proc Natl Acad Sci (USA) 81:1389–1390
75. Han NL, Bian ZB, Luo F, Han JS (1997) Antagonistic effect of CCK-8 and angiotensin II in antagonizing morphine-induced analgesia in rats. Chin J Pain Med 3:233–237

CHAPTER 4

The Past, Present, and Future of Meridian System Research

C. Shang

4.1
Acupuncture and the Meridian System

In 1996, the U.S. Food and Drug Administration reclassified acupuncture needles and substantially equivalent devices from class III (premarket approval, investigational use) to class II (special controls), which includes medical devices for general use such as scalpels and syringes [1]. Hundreds of randomized controlled trials on acupuncture have been published [2]. Positive results of acupuncture were demonstrated in a variety of conditions such as renal colic [3], migraine [4], osteoarthritis [5], Raynaud's syndrome [6], stroke [7, 8], and low sperm quality [9]. A systematic review of the high quality randomized controlled trials for acupuncture antiemesis showed consistent positive results across different investigators, different groups of patients, and different forms of acupuncture point stimulation such as electroacupuncture, laser, acupressure, and manual acupuncture [10]. The success of acupuncture has sparked many studies on the nature of the meridian system – the foundation of traditional acupuncture theory. According to the Standard Acupuncture Nomenclature proposed by the World Health Organization (WHO) [11], there are about 400 acupuncture points and 20 meridians/vessels connecting most of the points. Since the 1950s, it has been discovered and confirmed by researchers in several countries with refined techniques [12] that most acupuncture points correspond to the high electric conductance points on the body surface [13–17] and vice versa [18]. The high skin conductance of the meridian system is further supported by the finding of a high density of gap junctions at the sites of acupuncture points [19–22]. Gap junctions are hexagonal protein complexes that form channels between adjacent cells. It is well-established in cell biology that gap junctions facilitate intercellular communication and increase electric conductivity. Acupuncture and meridian points have also been found to have higher temperature [23], metabolic rates, and carbon dioxide release [24].

4.2
Neurobiology and Acupuncture

In acupuncture analgesia, the peripheral nervous system has been shown to be crucial in mediating the effect. The analgesia can be abolished if the acupuncture site is affected by postherpetic neuralgia [25] or injection of local anesthetics [26]. In other effects of acupuncture such as antihyperglycemic effects, studies have shown that local blockade of peripheral nerves or denervation did not interfere with the acupuncture effect [27]. In the 1970s, the relation between cerebral cortex and acupuncture alteration of visceral function was explored by examining the cortical evoked potentials, single unit discharges, and neurochemistry associated with acupuncture. For example, the projecting area of Pe. 6 was mapped at the cortex and found to overlap with the cortical splanchnic projection area. It was proposed that the cerebral cortex plays an important role in the mechanism of acupuncture inhibition of visceral pain [28]. These studies brought forth the meridian-cortex-viscera correlation hypothesis [29], which states that the meridian system (1) is an independent system connected via the nervous system to the cerebral cortex and (2) acts through neuro-humoral mechanisms [30]. Recently, the activation of visual cortex by stimulation of Bl. 67 was mapped by functional MRI [31]. The result showed that the activation of visual cortex by stimulation of Bl. 67 – a point at the little toe used to treat eye-related disorders – is similar to that of visual light stimulation. A generalized acupoint-brain-organ model was proposed in which acupuncture stimulates the corresponding brain cortex via the nervous system, thereby controlling the chemical or hormone release to the disordered organs for treatment.

In the mid-1970s, the discovery of endorphin induction in acupuncture analgesia and its blockade by naloxone marked a milestone in establishing the validity of acupuncture in mainstream science [32, 33]. Animals that respond poorly to acupuncture analgesia can be rendered good responders by treatment with D-phenylalanine, which inhibits the degradation of met-enkephalin [34]. A close relation between acupuncture and nervous system is also indicated by the considerable overlap between acupuncture points and trigger points – points of maximum tenderness in myofascial pain syndrome [35]. These results have led some practitioners to believe that the meridian system as described in the classic acupuncture literature does not exist and that all the effects of acupuncture are mediated through the nervous system [36, 37]. Other scholars regard the neurally mediated acupuncture phenomena as possibly "minor or secondary effects" and "not the central core of the mechanism of acupuncture" [38]. The neurohumoral theory of acupuncture has been mostly descriptive, with little predictive power.

4.3
Developmental Biology and the Meridian System

The traditional concepts of the meridian system have been studied from the perspective of morphogenesis. The relation between the meridian system and embryogenesis has been noted for decades [39]. The "gap junction embryonic epithelial signal transduction model" in the mid-1980s [19] proposed that the meridian system contains relatively underdifferentiated epithelial cells connected by gap junctions which transduce signals and play a central role in mediating acupuncture effects. The *morphogenetic singularity theory* [40] published in the late 1980s applied the singularity theory of mathematics to explain the origin, distribution, and nonspecific activation phenomena of the meridian system, as described below.

4.3.1
Acupuncture Points Are Singular Points in the Surface Bioelectric Field

Epithelia usually maintain a 30–100 mV voltage difference [41]. This voltage is the potential difference across cell layers, not membrane potential. An acupuncture point with high density of gap junctions and high electric conductance will also have local maximum electric current density – a converging point of surface current. This is a singular point of abrupt change in electric current flow. A singular point is a point of discontinuity as defined in mathematics and indicates a point of abrupt transition from one state to another. Small perturbations around singular points can have decisive effects on a system. As James Maxwell observed: *"Every existence above certain rank has its singular points... At these points, influence whose physical magnitude is too small to be taken account of by a finite being may produce results of the greatest importance"* [42]. The electromagnetic field pattern on the human scalp mapped by a superconducting quantum interference device (SQUID) [43] shows a singular point at the surface electromagnetic field where the surface magnetic flux trajectories converge and enter the body. This point coincides with the acupuncture point GV20 Baihui (Dr. Magnus Lou, personal communication). The converging pathway of magnetic flux on the scalp coincides with the governor vessel in the meridian system. This is a separatrix dividing the surface magnetic field into two symmetrical domains of different flow directions. A separatrix is a trajectory or boundary between different spatial domains [44] and often connects singular points. Morphologically, the governor vessel is also the axis of symmetry on the scalp. This pattern is consistent with the pattern of the meridian system but different from the distribution of any major nerve, lymphatic, or blood vessel on the scalp.

4.3.2
The Role of Electric Field in Growth Control and Morphogenesis

A variety of cells are sensitive to electric fields of physiological strength [45]. Somite fibroblasts migrate to the negative pole in a voltage gradient as small as 7 mV/mm [46]. Asymmetric calcium influx is crucial in the migration, which can be blocked or even reversed by certain calcium channel blockers and ionophores [47]. In most cases, there is enhanced cell growth toward the cathode and reduced cell growth toward the anode in electric fields of physiological strength [48, 49]. Fast-growing cells tend to have relatively negative polarity. This polarity is due to the increased negative membrane potential generated by the mitochondria at a high level of energy metabolism [50]. Imposed electric fields can cause polarization of mouse blastomeres [51]. The anterior-posterior polarity [52] and dorsal-ventral polarity [53] in lower animal morphogenesis can be reversed when the polarity of the imposed external electric field is opposite to that of the intrinsic bioelectric field.

4.3.3
Organizing Centers Have High Electric Conductance

In development, the fate of a larger region is frequently controlled by a small group of cells which is termed an organizing center [54]. Organizing centers are the high

Fig. 1. Illustration of singular points and separatrices (modified from Fig. 2.1 [117] (courtesy of John Wiley and Sons)) This also approximates the pattern of acupuncture points and meridians – the singular points and separatrices of electromagnetic field on the body surface

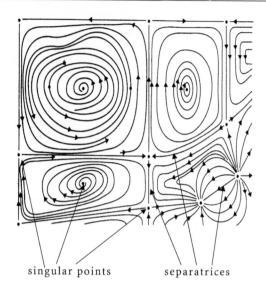

singular points   separatrices

electric conductance points on the body surface [40]. The amphibian blastopore, a classic organizing center, has high electric conductance and current density [55]. Similar phenomena have also been observed in higher vertebrates [56]. The high conductance phenomenon is further supported by the finding of high density of gap junctions at the sites of organizing centers [57–60]. At the macroscopic level, organiz-

Fig. 2. Ionic currents traversing an embryo [118] (courtesy of John Wiley and Sons) The blastopore, a classic organizing center, has high electric conductance and current density. A steady blastopore current persists after early embryogenesis. The electric fields polarize the embryo and serve as cues for morphogenesis. These results confirmed earlier predictions [116]

blastopore

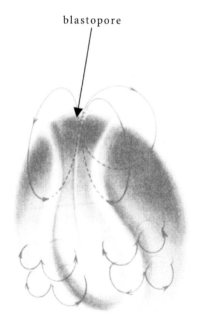

ing centers are singular points in the morphogen gradient and electromagnetic field [40]. The electric potential gradient and chemical morphogen gradient are likely to enhance each other, as morphogens are usually charged molecules or ions and can form a more stable gradient over long range guided by electric field than by reaction-diffusion alone. The effect of morphogens on ion channels and pumps can modify the electric field. Disruption of the intrinsic electric field at the organizing center can cause malformation [55]. A change of electric activity at the organizing centers correlates with signal transduction and can precede morphologic change [61, 62]. For example, an outward current can be detected at the site of a future limb bud (an organizing center) in amphibians several days before the first cell growth [63].

4.3.4
Acupuncture Points – Organizing Centers

Both acupuncture points and organizing centers have high electric conductance, current density, high density of gap junctions, and can be activated by nonspecific stimuli. A therapeutic effect of acupuncture can be achieved by a variety of stimuli [10, 64], including electricity, needling, temperature variation, laser [65], and pressure. Similarly, morphogenesis of organizing centers can be induced by various stimuli such as mechanical injury and injection of nonspecific chemicals [54, 66].

Based on the phase gradient model in developmental biology [40, 67], many organizing centers are expected to be at the extreme points of curvature on the body surface, such as the locally most convex points (e.g., the apical ectodermal ridge and other growth tips) or concave points (e.g., the zone of polarizing activity). Similarly, almost all the extreme points of the body surface curvature are acupuncture points. For example, the convex points include EX-UE11 Shixuan, EX-LE12 Qiduan, St.17 Ruzhong, St.42 Chongyang, St.45 Lidui, SP.1 Yinbai, SP.10 Xuehai, GV25 Suliao, and more. The concave points include CV17 Danzhong, KI.1 Yongquan, SI.19 Tinggong, GB.20 Fengchi, BL.40 Weizhong, HT.1 Jiquan, BL.1 Jingming, CV8 Shenque, among others. These similarities between acupuncture points and organizing centers suggest that acupuncture points originate from organizing centers.

4.3.5
Why Do Auricles Have the Highest Density of Acupuncture Points?

The distribution of acupuncture points and organizing centers is closely related to the morphology of the organism. For example, the auricle, which has the most complex surface morphology, also has the highest density of acupuncture points. According to the WHO, 43 auricular points have proven therapeutic value [11] and comprise 10 % of the acupuncture points of the whole body. Although an auricle has no important nerves or blood vessels and no significant physiological function other than sound collection, auricular morphology is one of the most sensitive indicators of malformations in other organs. Auricular malformation has been observed in Turner's syndrome, Potter's syndrome, Treacher-Collins syndrome, Patau's syndrome, Edwards' syndrome, Noonan's syndrome, maternal diabetes, atherosclerosis [68], Goldenhar's syndrome, Beckwith's syndrome, DiGeorge syndrome, cri du chat syndrome, and fragile X syndrome. It is recommended in a standard textbook of pediatrics that any auricular anomaly should initiate a search for malformations in other parts of the body [69].

4.3.6
Meridian-Separatrix Boundary

At early stages of embryogenesis, gap junction-mediated cell-to-cell communication is usually diffusely distributed, which results in the entire embryo becoming linked as a syncytium. As development progresses, gap junctions become restricted at discrete boundaries, leading to the subdivision of the embryo into communication compartment domains [70]. These high conductance boundaries or separatrices are also major pathways of bioelectric currents and likely to be the precursors of meridians. Separatrices can be folds on the surface or boundaries between different structures [40, 71]. It was proposed that interconnected cells in the meridian system remain underdifferentiated and maintain their regulatory function in a partial embryonic state [20, 40]. Consistent with this theory, it has been observed that the most apical parts of folds remain undifferentiated in morphogenesis [72], as well as organizing centers such as the zone of polarizing activity [73] and the apical ectodermal ridge [74]. The separatrix attributes are consistent with the observation in the *Inner Classic* (Nei Jing) that meridians are distributed along the boundaries between different muscles. For example, part of the lung meridian runs along the borders of the biceps and brachioradialis. Part of the pericardium meridian runs between the palmaris longus and flexor carpi radialis. Part of the gallbladder meridian runs between the sternocleidomastoid and trapezius. Trigger points also tend to be located at the free borders of muscles [75]. The governor vessel and the conception vessel are the axis of symmetry on the body surface. They form the boundaries between many different structures. They are also regarded as the convergence of all meridians in traditional acupuncture.

4.3.7
The Role of the Meridian System in Evolution and Physiology

In ontogeny, the development of organizing centers in the growth control system precedes the development of the nervous system and other physiological systems. The formation and maintenance of all the physiological systems are directly dependent on the activity of the growth control system. Based on the morphogenetic singularity theory, the meridian system originates from a network of organizing centers. As the individual embryonic development recapitulates the evolution of the species, (ontogeny recapitulates phylogeny), the evolutionary origin of the meridian system is likely to have preceded all the other physiological systems, including the nervous, circulatory, and immune systems. Its genetic blueprint might have served as a template from which the newer systems evolved. Consequently, it overlaps and interacts with other systems but is not simply part of them. The growth control signal transduction is embedded in the activity of the function-based physiological systems. Many neural, circulatory, and immune processes are regulated through growth control mechanisms such as hypertrophy, hyperplasia, atrophy, apoptosis with shared messenger molecules and common signal transduction pathways involving growth control genes such as proto-oncogenes [76–80]. Acupuncture also induces the expression of proto-oncogene c-fos [81, 82]. Many "nonexcitable" cells have shown electrochemical oscillation, coupling, long range intercellular communication [62, 83, 84], and can participate in the meridian signal transduction

4.3.8
Unified Basis of the Meridian and Chakra Systems

Based on the morphogenetic singularity theory, the distribution of the meridian system is related to both internal and external structures and not solely determined by nerves, muscles, or blood vessels. The distribution is a result of morphogenesis. Therefore, acupuncture points which are not at obvious extreme points of surface curvature or meridians which are not at obvious boundaries can be vestigial or more related to internal structures. The underdifferentiated, interconnected cellular network is not limited to the body surface. One type of least differentiated cell is the germ cell. The primary tumor distribution pattern of a certain cell type reflects the distribution of its normal counterpart. For example, the distribution of primary pheochromocytoma reflects the distribution of normal sympathetic ganglion cells. The germ cell tumors [85, 86] have a midline and para-axial distribution pattern which extends from the sacrococcygeal region, through the anterior mediastinum, tongue, and nasopharynx to the pineal gland. It appears to concentrate at seven locations: sacrococcygeal region, gonads, retroperitoneum, thymus [87], thyroid [88], suprasellar region, and pineal gland [89]. The pattern resembles the chakra system

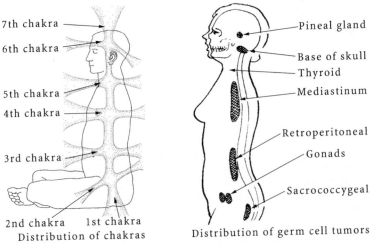

7th chakra
6th chakra
5th chakra
4th chakra
3rd chakra
2nd chakra   1st chakra
Distribution of chakras

Pineal gland
Base of skull
Thyroid
Mediastinum
Retroperitoneal
Gonads
Sacrococcygeal
Distribution of germ cell tumors

Fig. 3. Just as the distribution of pheochromocytoma correlates with the distribution of sympathetic ganglions, the distribution of germ cell tumors correlates with undifferentiated cells in human body which are likely to be involved in the regulation of growth control and physiology as part of the "inner meridian system". This distribution also correlates well with the chakra system used in yoga and acupuncture, suggesting a unified structural basis for chakra system and meridian system. Figure modified from: Govan ADT, MacFarlane PS, Callander R et al (1995) Pathology illustrated, 4th edn. Churchill Livingstone, London, p 150 and from: Stux (1997) Basics of acupuncture, 4th edn. Springer, Berlin, p 287. Courtesy of Churchill Livingstone and Dr. Gabriel Stux

used in yoga and acupuncture [90], suggesting the existence of underdifferentiated cells which may be highly interconnected in a normal state as part of the "inner meridian system" and provide important regulatory functions [91]. It is likely that there is a hierarchy in the degree of cell differentiation and function in the meridian system, with the germ cell system (major chakra system) as the least differentiated and constituting the central core of the regulatory system. The more superficial meridians and acupuncture points are more differentiated and lower in the hierarchy.

4.3.9
Mechanism of Meridian System-Based Diagnosis and Therapy

As the electric conductance of organizing centers varies with morphogenesis, the conductance of acupuncture points also varies and correlates with physiological change [13] and pathogenesis [92, 93]. The facts that the change in electric field precedes morphologic change [63] and that manipulation of the electric field can affect the change [94] may shed light on the diagnosis [93, 95] and treatment of many diseases. According to the morphogenetic singularity theory [40], the network of organizing centers retains its regulatory function through high levels of intercellular communication correlated with relatively low levels of cell differentiation during and after embryonic development. This prediction is consistent with the finding that underdifferentiation and high electric conductance persists at the organizing centers after early embryogenesis [96]. The organizing centers communicate with other parts of the body to maintain proper forms and functions. Gap junctional communication has been shown to play a crucial role in morphogenesis [97]. The gap junction genes can also behave as classical tumor suppressor genes in both culture and animal tests in restoring growth regulatory properties to metastatic cancer cells [98]. An anomaly inside the organizing center network may be detected by measuring the electric parameters of some points on its surface at the early signal transduction stage and treated by manipulation of the interconnected organizing centers.

The activation of organizing centers is likely to be involved in the restoration of proper form and function in wound healing and stress response. Acupuncture can speed up the wound healing process [99] and cause an exaggerated systemic wound healing and stress response [100, 101]. The response can include excessive release of endorphin, which stimulates epithelial cell growth [102] as well as analgesia. Other neurohumoral factors induced by acupuncture such as serotonin [103] and ACTH [104] also have effects on growth control [105].

In acupuncture, the often nonspecific perturbation at singular points (acupuncture points) may not directly antagonize a pathological process but may indirectly adjust the process and restore normal function by activating the network of organizing centers in the organism. For example, acupuncture at ST36 suppresses hyperfunction and stimulates hypofunction of gut motility [106]. The activation of organizing centers to elicit a normalizing function as explained above is less likely to cause the side effects resulting from directly antagonizing a pathological process which often overlaps with other normal and beneficial physiological processes. Therefore, proper use of these meridian system-based techniques causes few side effects [107–110], as demonstrated in randomized controlled trials [3, 4].

A principle in electroacupuncture is that positive (anode) pulse stimulation of a point inhibits its corresponding function while negative (cathode) pulse stimulation enhances that function [111]. This polarity effect is similar to the finding that cell growth is enhanced toward cathode and reduced toward anode [48, 49] and consistent with the theory that the mechanism underlying acupuncture overlaps with that of growth control.

4.4
Conclusions

The morphogenetic singularity theory outlines the common ground shared by the meridian and chakra systems and modern science. It is compatible with the findings from neurohumoral studies. It explains several phenomena and puzzles in developmental biology and acupuncture research, including the distribution of the meridian and chakra systems and germ cell tumors, the nonspecific activation of acupuncture points and organizing centers, the high electric conductance of acupuncture points, the polarity effect and side effect profile of electroacupuncture, and the ontogeny, phylogeny, and physiological function of the meridian system. Most of these have not been explained by any neurohumoral theory. In several prospective blind trials [55, 57–59, 71], researchers unaware of the theory confirmed its corollary on the role of singularity and separatrix in morphogenesis and its predictions of the high electric conductance and high density of gap junctions at organizing centers such as blastopores and zones of polarizing activity.

Techniques involving the stimulation of the meridian system such as acupuncture and qigong [112, 113] may activate the self-organizing system of an organism and improve its structure and function at a more fundamental level than symptomatic relief. Development of these techniques may enable the diagnosis and treatment of a pathologic process at the early signal transduction stage prior to the anatomical or morphological change.

4.5
Prospects

The advances reviewed above have broad implications in biomedicine beyond acupuncture. The current stage of meridian system research is analogous to that of physics in the early nineteenth century – during the transition from Newtonian mechanics to electromagnetics. More spectacular advances similar to those of relativity and quantum physics may await in the twenty-first century and will depend on the further development of meridian "electromagnetics." Many other areas related to the meridian system such as psychophysiology, chronobiology [114], and pulse analysis [115] await more rigorous studies. Many details of the current theories remain to be clarified and tested.

Besides neurohumoral studies, the following directions of research are likely to be important in further understanding acupuncture and the meridian system:
1. Mapping of the meridian system and the dynamics of its electromagnetic field with high resolution techniques such as SQUID

2. The relation between the physical parameters of the meridian system and various pathological or physiological changes, including changes during acupuncture and qigong practice
3. Development of acupuncture-related techniques of early diagnosis and treatment and establishing their cost effectiveness
4. Clarifying the role of the meridian system in morphogenesis and growth control
5. Exploring cell differentiation and signal transduction in the meridian system
6. Mapping the body surface curvature through embryonic development and study of its relation to the meridian system

Acknowledgements. I thank Drs. David Diehl, James Gordon, Richard Hammerschlag, Magnus Lou, and San Wan for their help and Drs. Mesterton-Gibbons and Gabriel Stux for permission to use figures from their books.

References

1. Food and Drug Administration (1996) Medical devices: Reclassification of acupuncture needles for the practice of acupuncture. Federal Register 61: 64616–64617
2. Kaptchuk TJ, Edwards RA, Eisenberg DM (1996) Complementary medicine: Efficacy beyond the placebo effect. In: Ernst E (1996) Complementary medicine – an objective appraisal. Butterworth-Heinemann, Oxford, pp 42–70
3. Lee YH, Lee WC, Chen MT, Huang JK, Chung C, Chang LS (1992) Acupuncture in the treatment of renal colic. J Urol 147:16–18
4. Hesse J, Mogelvang B, Simonsen H (1994) Acupuncture versus metoprolol in migraine prophylaxis: A randomized trial of trigger point inactivation. J Intern Med 235:451–456
5. Christensen BV, Iuhl IU, Vilbek H, Bulow HH, Dreijer NC, Rasmussen HF (1992) Acupuncture treatment of severe knee osteoarthrosis. A long-term study. Acta Anaesthesiol Scand. 36(6):519–525
6. Appiah R, Hiller S, Caspary L, Alexander K, Creutzig A (1997) Treatment of primary Raynaud's syndrome with traditional Chinese acupuncture. J Intern Med 241:119–124
7. Naeser MA, Alexander MP, Stiassny-Eder D, Galler V, Hobbs J, Bachman D (1992) Real versus sham acupuncture in the treatment of paralysis in acute stroke patients: A CT scan lesion site study. J Neuro Rehab 6:163–173
8. Hu HH, Chung C, Liu TJ, Chen RC, Chen CH, Chou P et al (1993) A randomized controlled trial on the treatment for acute partial ischemic stroke with acupuncture. Neuroepidemiology 12:106–113
9. Siterman S, Eltes F, Wolfson V, Zabludovsky N, Bartoov B (1997) Effect of acupuncture on sperm parameters of males suffering from subfertility related to low sperm quality. Arch Androl 39:155–161
10. Vickers AJ (1996) Can acupuncture have specific effects on health? A systematic review of acupuncture antiemesis trials. J R Soc Med 89:303–311
11. World Health Organization (1991) A proposed standard international acupuncture nomenclature: Report of a WHO scientific group. World Health Organization, Geneva
12. Pomeranz B (1997) Scientific basis of acupuncture. In: Stux G (ed) Basics of acupuncture. Springer-Verlag, New York, pp 30–32
13. Comunetti A, Laage S, Schiessl N, Kistler A (1995) Characterisation of human skin conductance at acupuncture points. Experientia 51:328–331
14. Bergsman O, Wooley-Hart A (1973) Differences in electric skin conductivity between acupuncture points and adjacent skin areas. Am J Acupunct 1:27–32
15. Wensel LO (1980) Acupuncture in medical practice. Reston Publishing, Reston, p 128
16. Nakatani Y, Yamashita K (1977) Ryodoraku acupuncture. Ryodoraku Research Institute, Osaka
17. Reichmanis M (1988) Electroacupuncture. In: Marino AA (ed) Modern Bioelectricity. Dekker, New York, pp 762–765
18. Eory A (1984) In-vivo skin respiration (CO_2) measurements in the acupuncture loci. Acupunct Electrother Res 9:217–223
19. Mashansky VF, Markov UV et al (1983) Topography of the gap junctions in the human skin and their possible role in the non-neural signal transduction. Arch Anat Histol Embryol 84:53–60

20. Cui H-M (1988) Meridian system—specialized embryonic epithelial conduction system. Shanghai J Acupunct 3: 44–45
21. Fan JY (1990) The role of gap junctions in determining skin conductance and their possible relationship to acupuncture points and meridians. Am J Acupunct 18:163–170
22. Zheng JY, Fan JY, Zhang YJ, Guo Y, Xu TP (1996) Further evidence for the role of gap junctions in acupoint information transfer. Am J Acupunct 24:291–6
23. Zhang D, Fu W, Wang S, Wei Z, Wang F (1996) Displaying of infrared thermogram of temperature character on meridians [Chinese]. Chen Tzu Yen Chiu Acupuncture Research 21:63–67
24. Eory A (1984) In vivo skin respiration (CO_2) measurements in the acupuncture loci. Acupunct Electrother Res 9:217–223
25. Bowsher D (1998) Mechanisms of acupuncture. In: Filshie J, White A, (eds) Medical Acupuncture. Churchill Livingston, Edinburgh, pp 69–80
26. Chiang CY, Chang CT (1973) Peripheral afferent pathway for acupuncture analgesia. Scientia Sinica 16:210–217
27. Liu Z (1998) Meridian pharmacology research [Chinese]. Jinluo Luntan Meridian Forum 5:1–4
28. Chen P, Chen Z, Weng J, Ren H, Zhang J, Zhang J, Feng J (1986) Relationship between cerebral cortex and acupuncture inhibition of visceral pain. In: Zhang X (ed) Research on acupuncture, moxibustion, and acupuncture anesthesia. Science Press, Beijing and Springer-Verlag, Berlin, p 227
29. Anonymous (1976) A preliminary investigation of the mechanism of antipain and counterinjury effects of acupuncture anaesthesia. Scientia Sinica. 19:529–556
30. Chang HC, Xie YK, Wen YY, Zhang SY, Qu JH, Lu WJ (1983) Further investigation on the hypothesis of meridian-cortex-viscera interrelationship. Am J Chin Med 11:5–13
31. Cho ZH, Chung SC, Jones JP, Park JB, Park HJ, Lee HJ et al (1998) New findings of the correlation between acupoints and corresponding brain cortices using functional MRI. Proc Natl Acad Sci USA 95:2670–2673
32. Pomeranz B, Chiu D (1976) Naloxone blocks acupuncture analgesia and causes hyperalgesia: Endorphin is implicated. Life Sci 19:1757–1762
33. Mayer DJ, Price DD, Raffii A (1977) Antagonism of acupuncture analgesia in man by the narcotic antagonist naloxone. Brain Res 121:368–372
34. Takeshige C, Tanaka M, Sato T, Hishida F (1990) Mechanism of individual variation in effectiveness of acupuncture analgesia based on animal experiment. Eur J Pain 11:109–113
35. Melzack R, Stillwell DM, Fox EJ (1977) Trigger points and acupuncture points for pain: Correlations and implications. Pain 3:3–23
36. Ulett GA (1992) Beyond yin and yang: How acupuncture really works. Warren H. Green, St. Louis
37. Mann F (1998) A new system of acupuncture. In: Filshie J, White A, (eds) Medical acupuncture. Churchill Livingston, Edinburgh, p 63
38. Pearson P (1987) An introduction to acupuncture. MTP Press, Norwell. p 75
39. Mann F (1971) Acupuncture. Random House, New York, p 40
40. Shang C (1989) Singular point, organizing center, and acupuncture point. Am J Chin Med 17:119–127
41. Jaffe LF (1977) Electrophoresis along cell membranes. Nature 265:600–602
42. Winfree AT (1980) The geometry of biological time. Springer-Verlag, New York, p 71
43. Cohen D, Palti Y, Cuffin BN, Schmid SJ (1980) Magnetic fields produced by steady currents in the body. Proc Natl Acad Sci USA 77:1447–1451
44. Vinogradev IM, Adyan SI, Alesandrov PS, Bakhvalov NS et al (1992) Encyclopaedia of mathematics Norwell, MA: Kluver Academic, Norwell, pp 276, 346
45. Erickson CA (1985) Morphogenesis of the neural crest. In: Browder LW (ed),Developmental biology. Plenum, New York, p 528
46. McGinnis ME, Vanable JW jr (1986) Voltage gradients in newt limb stumps. Prog Clin Biol Res 210:231–238
47. Cooper MS, Schliwa M (1986) Transmembrane Ca^{2+} fluxes in the forward and reversed galvanotaxis of fish epidermal cells. Prog Clin Biol Res 210:311–318
48. Nuccitelli R (1984) The involvement of transcellular ion currents and electric fields in pattern formation. In: Malacinski GM (ed),Pattern formation. Macmillan, New York
49. McCaig CD (1987) Spinal neurite regeneration and regrowth in vitro depend on the polarity of an applied electric field. Development 100:31–41
50. Chen LB (1989) Fluorescent labeling of mitochondria. Methods in Cell Biology 29:103–120
51. Wiley LM, Nuccitelli R (1986) Detection of transcellular currents and effect of an imposed electric field on mouse blastomeres. Prog Clin Biol Res 210: 97–204

52. Marsh G, Beams HW (1952) Electric control of morphogenesis in regenerating Dugesia tigrina. J Cell Comp Physiol 39:191
53. Kolega J. The cellular basis of epithelial morphogenesis. In: Browder LW (eds),Developmental Biology. Plenum, New York, pp 112–116
54. Meinhardt H (1982) Models of biological pattern formation. Academic, London, p 20
55. Hotary KB, Robinson KR (1994) Endogenous electric currents and voltage gradients in Xenopus embryos and the consequences of their disruption. Dev Biol 166:797
56. Jaffe LF, Stern CD (1979) Strong electric currents leave the primitive streak of chick embryos. Science 206:569–571
57. Laird DW, Yancey SB, Bugga L, Revel JP (1992) Connexin expression and gap junction communication compartments in the developing mouse limb. Dev Dyn 195:153–161
58. Yancey SB, Biswal S, Revel JP (1992) Spatial and temporal patterns of distribution of the gap junction protein connexin 43 during mouse gastrulation and organogenesis. Development 114:203–212
59. Coelho CN, Kosher RA (1991) A gradient of gap junctional communication along the anterior-posterior axis of the developing chick limb bud. Dev Biol 148:529–535
60. Meyer RA, Cohen MF, Recalde S, Zakany J, Bell SM, Scott WJ jr, Lo CW (1997) Developmental regulation and asymmetric expression of the gene encoding Cx43 gap junctions in the mouse limb bud. Dev Genet 21:290–300
61. Nelson PG, Yu C, Fields RV, Neale EA (1989) Synaptic connections in vitro modulation of number and efficacy by electric activity. Science 244:585–587
62. Shang C (1993) Bioelectrochemical oscillations in signal transduction and acupuncture—an emerging paradigm. Am J Chin Med 21:91–101
63. Nuccitelli R (1988) Ionic currents in morphogenesis. Experientia 44:657–666
64. Altman S (1992) Techniques and instrumentation. Probl Vet Med 4:66–87
65. Hornstein OP (1997) Melkersson-Rosenthal syndrome—a challenge for dermatologists to participate in the field of oral medicine. J Dermatol 24:281–296
66. Toivonen S (1978) Regionalization of the embryo. In: Nakamura O, Toivonen S (eds) Organizer—A milestone of a half-century from Spemann. Elsevier, Amsterdam, p.132
67. Winfree AT (1984) A continuity principle for regeneration. In: Malacinski GM (ed) Pattern formation. Macmillan, New York, pp.106–107
68. Petrakis NL (1995) Earlobe crease in women: Evaluation of reproductive factors, alcohol use, and quetelet index and relation to atherosclerotic disease. Am J Med 99:356–361
69. Cotton RT (1996) The ear, nose, oropharynx, and larynx. In: Rudolph AM, Hoffman JIE, Rudolph CD (eds) Rudolph's Pediatrics. Appleton and Lange, Stamford, p 945
70. Lo CW (1996) The role of gap junction membrane channels in development. J Bioenerg Biomembr 28:379–385
71. Lee D, Malpeli JG (1994) Global form and singularity: Modeling the blind spot's role in lateral geniculate morphogenesis. Science 263:1292–1294
72. Toivonen S (1978) Regionalization of the embryo. In: Nakamura O, Toivonen S (eds) Organizer—a milestone of a half-century from Spemann. Elsevier, Amsterdam, p.124
73. Ros MA, Sefton M, Nieto MA (1997) Slug, a zinc finger gene previously implicated in the early patterning of the mesoderm and the neural crest, is also involved in chick limb development. Development 124:1821–1829
74. Carlson MR. Bryant SV. Gardiner DM (1998) Expression of Msx-2 during development, regeneration, and wound healing in axolotl limbs. J Experimental Zool 282:715–723
75. Baldry P (1998) Trigger point acupuncture. In: Filshie J, White A (eds),Medical Acupuncture. Churchill Livingston, Edinburgh, p 35
76. Baldwin AS jr (1996) The NF-kappa B and I kappa B proteins: New discoveries and insights. Annu Rev Immunol 14:649–683
77. Berczi I (1994) The role of the growth and lactogenic hormone family in immune function. Neuroimmunomodulation 1:201–216
78. Bailey CH, Bartsch D, Kandel ER (1996) Toward a molecular definition of long-term memory storage. Proc Natl Acad Sci USA 93:13445–13452
79. Miano JM, Topouzis S, Majesky M, Olson EN (1996) Retinoid receptor expression and all-trans retinoic acid-mediated growth inhibition in vascular smooth muscle cells. Circulation 93:1886–1895
80. Tanaka H, Samuel CE (1994) Mechanism of interferon action: Structure of the mouse PKR gene encoding the interferon-inducible RNA-dependent protein kinase. Proc Natl Acad Sci USA 91:7995–7999
81. Pan B, Castro-Lopes JM, Coimbra A (1996) Activation of anterior lobe corticotrophs by electro-acupuncture or noxious stimulation in the anaesthetized rat, as shown by colocalization of Fos

protein with ACTH and beta-endorphin and increased hormone release. Brain Res Bull 40:175–182

82. Lee JH, Beitz AJ (1993) The distribution of brainstem and spinal cord nuclei associated with different frequencies of electroacupuncture analgesia. Pain 52:11–28
83. Rink TJ, Jacob R (1989) Calcium oscillations in nonexcitable cells. Trends Neurosci 12:43–46
84. Nedergaard M (1994) Direct signaling from astrocytes to neurons in cultures of mammalian brain cells. Science 263:1768–1771
85. Azizkhan RG, Caty MG (1996) Teratomas in childhood. Curr Opin Pediatr 8:287–292
86. Kountakis SE, Minotti AM, Maillard A, Stiernberg CM (1994) Teratomas of the head and neck. Am J Otolaryngol 15:292–296
87. Dehner LP (1990) Germ cell tumors of the mediastinum. Semin Diagn Pathol 7:266–284
88. Gonzalez-Crussi F (1982) Extragonadal teratomas. Armed Forces Institute of Pathology, Washington, p.118
89. Kretschmar CS (1997) Germ cell tumors of the brain in children: A review of current literature and new advances in therapy. Cancer Invest 15:187–198
90. Stux G (1997) Chakra acupuncture. In: Stux G (ed) Basics of acupuncture. Springer-Verlag, New York, pp 298–302
91. Nichols CR, Timmerman R, Foster RS, Roth BJ, Einhorn LH (1997) Neoplasms of the testis. In:. Holland JF, Basst RC jr, Morton DL, Frei E III, Kufe DW, Weichselbaum RR (eds),Cancer medicine. Fourth edn. Williams and Wilkins, Baltimore, p.2206
92. Saku K, Mukaino Y, Ying H, Arakawa K (1993) Characteristics of reactive electropermeable points on the auricles of coronary heart disease patients. Clin Cardiol 16:415–419
93. Oleson TD, Kroenig RJ, Bresler DE (1980) An experimental evaluation of auricular diagnosis: The somatotopic mapping of musculoskeletal pain at acupuncture points. Pain 8:217–229
94. Smith SD (1988) Limb regeneration. In:Marino AA (ed),Modern bioelectricity. Dekker, New York, p.526–555
95. Ishchenko AN, Kozlova VP, Shev'yev PP (1991) Auricular diagnostics used in the system of screening surveys. Med Prog Technol 17:29–32
96. Shi R, Borgens RB (1996) Three-dimensional gradients of voltage during development of the nervous system as invisible coordinates for the establishment of embryonic pattern. Dev Dynamics 202:101–114
97. Ewart JL, Cohen MF, Meyer RA, Huang GY, Wessels A, Gourdie RG et al (1997) Heart and neural tube defects in transgenic mice overexpressing the Cx43 gap junction gene. Development 124:1281–1292
98. Hirschi KK, Xu CE, Tsukamoto T, Sager R (1996) Gap junction genes Cx26 and Cx43 individually suppress the cancer phenotype of human mammary carcinoma cells and restore differentiation potential. Cell Growth Differ 7:861–870
99. King GE, Scheetz J, Jacob RF, Martin JW (1989) Electrotherapy and hyperbaric oxygen: Promising treatments for postradiation complications. J Prosthet Dent 62:331–334
100. Wong WH, Brayton D (1982) The physiology of acupuncture: Effects of acupuncture on peripheral circulation. Am J Acupunct 10:59–63
101. Lin MT, Liu GG, Song JJ, Chen YF, Wu KM (1980) Effects of stimulation of acupuncture Ta-Churi, Nei-Kuan, and Tsu-San-Li points on physiological function of normal adults. Acupunct Res Quarterly 4:11–19
102. Kishi H, Mishima HK, Sakamoto I, Yamashita U (1996) Stimulation of retinal pigment epithelial cell growth by neuropeptides in vitro. Curr Eye Res 15:708–713
103. Cheng RS, Pomeranz B (1979) Electroacupuncture analgesia mediation by endorphin and nonendorphin systems. Life Sci 25:1957–1962
104. Malizia E, Andreucci G, Paolucci D (1979) Electroacupuncture and peripheral endorphin and ACTH levels. Lancet 2:535–536
105. Pakala R, Benedict CR (1998) Effect of serotonin and thromboxane A2 on endothelial cell proliferation: Effect of specific receptor antagonists. J Lab Clin Med 131:527–537
106. Li Y, Tougas G, Chiverton SG, Hunt RH (1992) The effect of acupuncture on gastrointestinal function and disorders. Am J Gastroenterol 87:1372–1381
107. Holden C (1994) Acupuncture: Stuck on the fringe. Science 264:770
108. Carneiro NM, Li SM (1995) Acupuncture technique. Lancet 345:1577
109. Shiraishi T, Onoe M, Kojima T, Sameshima Y, Kageyama T (1995) Effects of auricular stimulation on feeding-related hypothalamic neuronal activity in normal and obese rats. Brain Res Bull 36:141–148
110. Marwick C (1997) Acceptance of some acupuncture applications. JAMA 278:1725–1727
111. Kenyon JN (1983) Modern techniques of acupuncture. Thorsons, Wellingborough, pp 51–58

112. McGee CT, Sancier K, Chow EPY (1996) Qigong in traditional Chinese medicine. In: Micozzi MS (ed),Fundamentals of complementary and alternative medicine. Churchill-Livingston, New York, pp.225–226
113. Lu Z (1997) Scientific qigong exploration. Amber Leaf Press, Malvern
114. Li L, Chen H, Xi Y, Wang X, Han G, Zhou Y, Yang D et al (1994) Comparative observation on effect of electric acupuncture of PC6 at 7–9 AM vs. 7–9 PM on left ventricular function in patients with coronary artery disease. J Tradit Chin Med 14:262–265
115. Wang WK, Hsu TL, Wang YY (1998) Liu-wei-dihuang: A study by pulse analysis. Am J Chin Med 26:73–82
116. Shang C (1989) Singular point, organizing center, and acupuncture point. Am J Chin Med 17:119–127
117. Mesterton-Gibbons M (1995) A concrete approach to mathematical modeling. Wiley, New York
118. Shi R, Borgens RB (1996) Three-dimensional gradients of voltage during development of the nervous system as invisible coordinates for the establishment of embryonic pattern. Dev Dynamics 202:102

Functional Magnetic Resonance Imaging of the Brain in the Investigation of Acupuncture

Z.-H. Cho · C.-S. Na · E. K. Wang · S.-H. Lee · I.-K. Hong

5.1
Introduction

Medical imaging techniques that allow noninvasive observation of the structure and function of the human brain have improved dramatically during the past few decades. The relatively poor resolution of the biohazardous two-dimensional x-ray technique has been effectively replaced by safer and far more sensitive optical scanning techniques, including x-ray computed tomography (CT), positron emission tomography (PET), and magnetic resonance imaging (MRI). These modern advances in brain imaging routinely provide critical diagnostic information in such conditions as stroke, multiple sclerosis, and Parkinson's disease as well as basic insights into how we experience, respond to, and even think about the world [2, 5–8, 12, 15, 18, 22–24, 27].

The application of this state of the art medical technology to the low tech, millennia-old practice of acupuncture seems at first to represent scientific overkill. But several preliminary explorations in this "west meets east" field of inquiry have yielded extremely promising results. For example, just as brain imaging is used on acute ischemic stroke patients to assess the need for administering so-called clot busting drugs [21], CT scans also have been effectively used to predict which stroke patients are likely to benefit from acupuncture treatment [20]. In addition, noninvasive imaging techniques have obvious potential for corroborating the brain pathways mediating acupuncture analgesia that have been identified in animals by microelectrode recordings, focal application of pharmacological agents, and ablation studies (see chapters 1.3).

The present chapter will focus in detail on the recent use of functional magnetic resonance imaging (fMRI) to test oriental medical theory [9, 10]. These studies have detected activity in the visual and auditory lobes of the brain during needling of distal acupoints on the leg and foot that Oriental medicine selects for treating eye and ear dysfunctions.

5.2
Brain Imaging for Identifying Neural Correlates of Acupuncture Analgesia

Several imaging techniques, including PET, its related procedure single photon emission computed tomography (SPECT), and fMRI are used to measure neural activity as reflected in the uptake of cerebral blood glucose or increased cerebral blood flow.

(Unlike most other cells, neurons have little stored glucose and rely on uptake of blood glucose as well as blood oxygen to sustain their high levels of activity.) The first two of these techniques are based on the use of radioisotopes that undergo predictable and detectable decay that can be resolved to specific brain regions. In a pilot study of five chronic pain patients, SPECT was employed to examine patterns of cerebral blood flow in various brain regions before and after acupuncture treatment [1]. The most striking finding was that four of the five patients had a marked left/right asymmetry in pretreatment blood flow in the thalamus, a major site in the neural integration of pain sensation. Following acupuncture treatment that resulted in all five patients reporting pain relief, the thalamic asymmetry was greatly reduced. Control subjects showed no blood flow asymmetries either before or after acupuncture.

The main advantage of MRI (for anatomical imaging) and fMRI (for physiological imaging) is their production of images without the use of radioisotopes. Since neural activity is critically dependent on oxygen derived from cerebral blood supplies, fMRI is an extremely sensitive means of measuring deoxyhemoglobin, the paramagnetic, oxygen-depleted carrier molecule. (Oxyhemoglobin is, fortuitously, nonmagnetic.) Functional MRI has been widely used for mapping changes in brain activity in response to specific sensory stimuli, motor tasks, or cognitive challenges as well as for detecting brain hemorrhages associated with pathological conditions [7, 8, 18, 23, 27].

Laboratories in Boston [16, 17] and Taiwan [33] have begun using fMRI to examine brain activity in response to needling at acupoints LI.4 and St.36 in normal subjects. Significantly greater levels of brain activity were detected during periods of acupoint stimulation than during periods of rest, shallow needling, or superficial pricking on the leg. A wide variety of brainstem, midbrain, and cerebral cortical structures showed reproducible patterns of increased or decreased activity; changes were especially related to structures associated with ascending nociceptive and descending antinociceptive pathways. Once stronger magnets become available, the activity patterns and the pathways they reflect will be identifiable with greater spatial and temporal resolution.

5.3

Functional Magnetic Resonance Imaging for Examining Correlations Between Brain Cortical Activity and Acupoint Function

Several of the studies seeking anatomical bases for acupuncture points and meridians support the possibility that meridians, the classically defined "energy transporting channels," are largely related to peripheral nerves [3, 4]. In fact, comparisons of acupoints with the peripheral nervous system given in many anatomical books [30] show that many acupoints correspond with the sites where small nerve bundles penetrate the fascia [14]. According to recently published reports, as many as 300 acupoints are situated on or very close to nerves, while an almost equal number are on or very close to major blood vessels that are surrounded by small nerve bundles [3]. This study, which also confirms that the acupoints lie along the peripheral nerves, leads us to hypothesize that acupuncture signals are projected to the brain via the spinal cord and brainstem. Such signals could terminate in subcortical areas, while many are likely to reach the higher cortical areas, including the sensory cortex.

Fig. 1. Conceptual relationships in the brain, organs, and acupoints that can be examined by fMRI. These relationships suggest functional interactions between acupoints and the cortical areas related to disease treatment by each acupoint. As examples, cortical areas are indicated that may be activated by eye- or ear-related acupoints

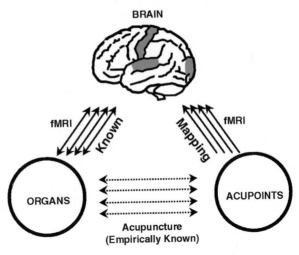

Acupoint/brain cortex relationships have been described in the Oriental acupuncture literature [11, 19, 31] and observed by experienced acupuncturists. More specifically, it has been hypothesized that the disease treatment claimed for acupuncture points may have somatotopic or sensory-related cortical correspondence (Fig. 1). We became interested in experimental testing of this hypothesis using fMRI to monitor cerebral cortical activity in areas functionally related to sensory conditions classically treated by selected acupoints. For example, visual dysfunctions that are localized and treated by Western medicine at sites along the retina/optic-nerve/occipital-lobe axis can, according to Oriental medicine, often be diagnosed by alterations in radial pulses corresponding to the urinary bladder (UB) and gallbladder (GB) channels. Such conditions can be treated, in turn, by needling along these meridians at distal acupoints localized on specific aspects of a toe, foot, and lower leg [11, 19]. More specifically, the UB meridian starts at the inner canthus of the eye, has 67 acupoints along its route, and ends on the lateral side of the little toe, while the GB channel starts at the outer canthus of the eye, has 44 acupoints, and ends at the lateral side of the fourth toe. The fMRI technique can therefore be used to explore quantitative correlations between acupoint stimulation and activation of functional areas of the brain. If aspects of Oriental medicine theory not predicted by the biomedical view of the body can be validated, e.g., correlations between sites of acupuncture stimulation and cerebral cortical activity not linked by known neural pathways, then an expanded theory of physiology may be required to combine aspects of both the Oriental and allopathic medical models.

To test our hypothesis that sensory-related acupoints have brain cortical correspondence, fMRI signals were sought in the visual cortex following needling of acupoints GB.37 (used to treat eye-related diseases such as itchiness or pain in the eyes, cataracts, night blindness, and optic atrophy) and in the auditory cortex following needling of GB.43 (known to be effective for treating ear-related diseases such as deafness and tinnitus). We examined brain activity associated with stimulation of both acupoints and compared the results to our initial findings with another eye-

Table 1. Acupoints, target organs, and functionally activated areas

Acupoint	Target area	Cortical activation area	Indications
UB.67 Zhiyin	Eye	Visual cortex	Conditions of head and sense organs: headache, neck pain, ophthalmalgia
GB.37 Guangmin	Eye	Visual cortex	Conditions of head and sense organs Primary: itching or painful eyes, cataracts, night blindness, optic atrophy Secondary: ear disease
GB.43 Xiaxi	Ear	Auditory cortex	Conditions of head and sense organs Primary: deafness, tinnitus, dizziness, dacryorrhea Secondary: eye disease

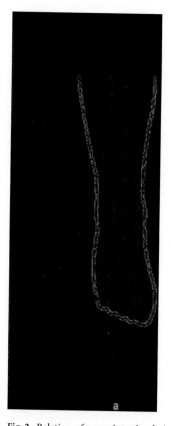 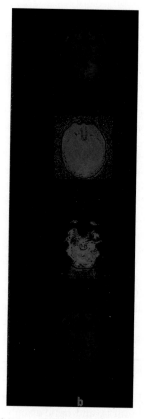

Fig. 2. Relation of acupoint stimulation and fMRI activity in visual cortex. **a** Two eye-related acupoints and a nonacupoint overlaid on the nervous system. **b** Activation maps of the brain due to (i) direct retinal stimulation by flashing light, (ii) acupuncture stimulation of UB.67, (iii) acupuncture stimulation of GB.37, and (iv) acupuncture-like stimulation of a nonacupoint

related acupoint, UB.67 [9]. For each of these three acupoints, the disease-related information and the cortical area expected to be activated are listed in Table 1. Distal acupoints on the lower leg and foot were chosen for ease of access, since subjects undergoing fMRI have their head, torso, and upper legs inside the magnet.

In our initial studies, we tested whether needling of UB.67, an acupoint traditionally used for treating eye disorders, would produce brain activity in the visual cortex that is detectable by fMRI (Fig. 2). Surprisingly, needling of this point led to reproducible increases in blood flow, i.e., increased fMRI signals, in Brodmann's areas 17, 18, and 19 of the visual cortex (Fig. 2b, ii). The effects were comparable to the changes in blood flow in the visual cortex produced by stimulation of the retina with flashing light (Fig. 2b, i). Needling of proximal acupoints UB.66 and UB.65 on the same channel also produced visual cortex activation [9]. In contrast, no visual cortex activity was detectable following needling either nonacupoints on the foot 2–5 cm from the vision-related acupoints (Fig. 2b, iv) or acupoint Sp.1 on the large toe (Fig. 2a), which is irrelevant to the treatment of eye disorders. Of considerable interest, needling of GB.37, on a separate meridian but another of the most effective acupoints for the treatment of eye disorders (Fig. 3), again produced strong fMRI activity in the

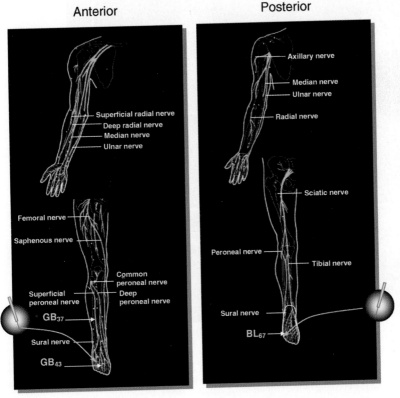

Fig. 3. Acupuncture points overlaid on the peripheral nervous system as seen from anterior and posterior views

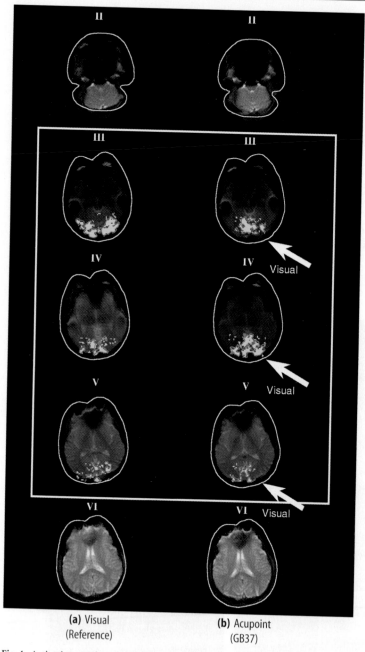

(a) Visual
(Reference)

(b) Acupoint
(GB37)

Fig. 4. Activation results of acupuncture stimulation of vision-related acupoint GB.37 observed by fMRI optical slice imaging. Cortical activation is shown due to (a) direct retinal stimulation by flashing light and (b) needling of the vision-related acupoint GB.37

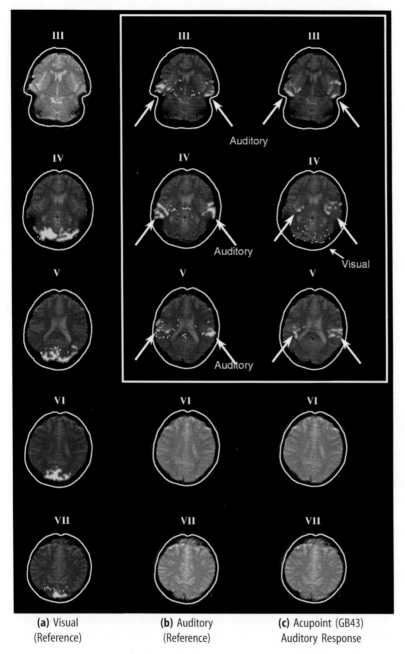

(a) Visual
(Reference)

(b) Auditory
(Reference)

(c) Acupoint (GB43)
Auditory Response

Fig. 5. Activation results of acupuncture stimulation of a hearing-related acupoint GB.43. Cortical activation due to (a) flashing light, (b) music, and (c) acupuncture at GB.43. In (c), note the primary activation of the auditory cortex similar to that detected during listening to music (b) but also the small activation in the visual cortex similar to that detected during flashing light (a). This, we believe, is a secondary effect, since GB.43 is also used for the treatment of eye-related disease (Table 1)

visual cortex (Fig. 2b, iii). Activation of the visual cortex following stimulation of GB.37 is also shown in a series of "optical slices" (Fig. 4).

As a further exploration of this phenomenon in other cortical areas, activity in the auditory cortex detectable by fMRI was examined following stimulation of GB.43, one of the best-known acupoints for the treatment of ear-related disease (Fig. 5). Interestingly, needling this acupoint resulted in strong activation of the auditory cortex in a manner similar to direct auditory stimulation with music but also led to weak activation of the visual cortex. It has been empirically observed and noted in acupuncture texts that some acupoints are relatively specific while others have more diverse functions. According to experienced acupuncturists, such primary and secondary responses may also be dependent on the health status of the patient.

5.4
Implications and Hypotheses

Our results provide the first scientific evidence that acupuncture "signals" are projected to neocortical areas of the brain for central processing. These observations of the cortical projections of "signals" following stimulation of several acupoints strongly support the notion that many effects of acupuncture are mediated through the central nervous system. This concept of CNS involvement is supported by a considerable body of experimental evidence in the area of acupuncture analgesia, where correlations have been observed between acupoint stimulation, analgesia onset, and release of a variety of neurotransmitters, endogenous opioids, and hormones in the brain, spinal cord, and peripheral circulation [11, 13, 25, 26, 32] (see chapters 1.3).

Projections to the brain's sensory cortices and the eventual effect on diseased organs by the brain's higher centers may occur in concert with other functional centers in the body. The well-known homunculus of the human cortex illustrates just such a somatotopic possibility [28, 29]. To gain additional support for the theory of a CNS-mediated mechanism relating acupoints with disease sites as proposed from our preliminary findings, it seems necessary to study effects of many more prominent acupoints related to somatosensory and visceral organ systems. However, current observations may lead to some useful new hypotheses.

For example, we may hypothesize that stimulation of a specific acupoint delivers information to the corresponding cortical area(s), enabling the higher centers of the brain to make necessary decisions to regulate activities controlled by the endocrine and autonomic nervous systems. For this to occur, we believe that the hypothalamus and the amygdala play a key role, both in mediating the sensory input to the prefrontal cortex by integrating limbic information and in retrieving it from the prefrontal cortex. Information thus received from the amygdala would then be acted upon by the hypothalamus. The hypothalamus has unusually rich connections (both afferent and efferent) to many higher cortical areas such as the prefrontal cortex (both directly and via the amygdala), the limbic areas, and the brainstem and spinal cord.

One of the hypotheses postulated to explain acupuncture phenomena in terms of these neurobiological mechanisms is known as the beta-endorphin theory, which is presented schematically in Fig. 6 [13, 25, 32]. It is interesting to note that, in this model, the hypothalamus interacts with the higher cortical areas, especially the prefrontal cortex. A further extension of this acupuncture therapy model depicts the sen-

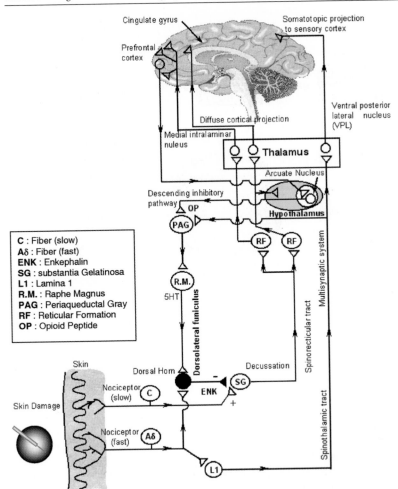

Fig. 6. A pain relief hypothesis involving higher cortical areas. In this example, the hypothalamus and other higher cortical areas are involved in secretion of beta-endorphin as well as other opioids and neurotransmitters. This hypothesis suggests involvement of higher cortical areas such as the sensory cortex as well as the frontal cortex, especially the prefrontal cortex and the limbic areas [11]

sory hierarchy coupled to the motor hierarchy via the limbic-hypothalamus or great limbic system (Fig. 7). In this schema, the final executive center is the hypothalamus where three survival-related systems involving endocrine, autonomic (ANS), and neuromodulatory functions are controlled.

The thrust of the present findings is that acupuncture stimulation is projected to higher brain areas such as the visual and auditory cortices. It is postulated that information is relayed from these sites to other key processing areas including the prefrontal cortex and limbic system. It is likely that acupuncture signals projected to these higher cortical areas will induce pain modulation as previously postulated but may also affect other survival-related functions. These latter mechanisms may shed light

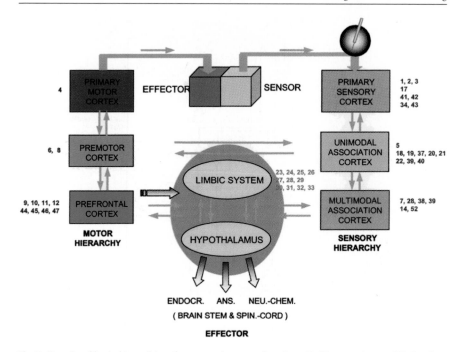

Fig. 7. Functional brain hierarchies of motor and sensory functions. To illustrate the possible involvement of the acupuncture disease treatment effect, the limbic system is inserted as a mediator between the prefrontal cortex and the multimodal sensory association cortex. Here we hypothesize that acupuncture signals are projected to the sensory cortex and that the hypothalamus controls three major survival-related systems: endocrine, ANS, and diffuse modulatory neurochemical functions

on what has been a mystery for many acupuncture investigators, namely how acupuncture treats various diseases beyond the level of pain relief. In Fig. 8, an overall acupuncture disease treatment model is shown that contains but goes beyond current endorphin-mediated theories of pain control.

We may conclude that clues to the basic mechanisms underlying the several thousand-year-old practice of acupuncture will be revealed through modern scientific imaging techniques such as PET and fMRI. The careful and systematic examination of the hundreds of currently known acupoints and the mapping of corresponding cortical activation may well reveal evidence of homeostatic regulatory mechanisms not yet understood by Western physiology and medicine. Furthermore, future research with stronger magnetic fields will allow greater temporal and spatial resolution so that more subtle acupuncture signals can be detected. Such research will also contribute significantly to creating more accurate and reliable treatment for the millions of patients who may benefit from alternative medical therapies such as acupuncture.

Acknowledgements. The present work is the product of many coworkers and their generous support. We are especially indebted to Drs. Heoung-Keun Kang and Gwang-Wu Chung in the Department of Diagnostic Radiology of Chun Nam University School of Medicine, Kyangju, Korea for their support of our use of MRI scanners.

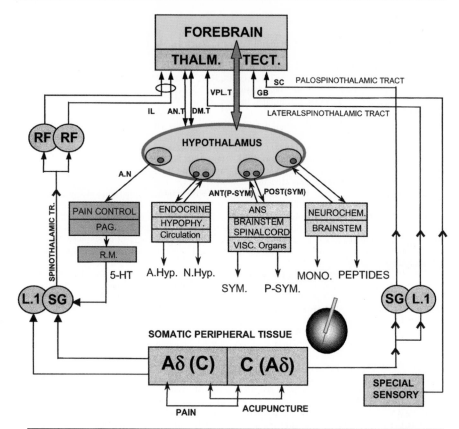

Fig. 8. Model of the therapeutic effects of acupuncture analgesia. As diagrammed in this model, the importance of cortical projection of acupuncture stimuli is the possibility it presents of integrating the endocrine, ANS, and neurochemical regulation by the hypothalamus with activities of other higher cortical centers such as the prefrontal cortex and the limbic system

References

1. Alavi A, LaRiccia P, Sadek H, Lattanand C, Lee L, Reich H, Mozley PD (1996) Objective assessment of the effects of pain and acupuncture on regional brain function with Tc99 mm HMPAO SPECT imaging. J Nucl Med 37 [Suppl 5]:278
2. Bandettini PA, Wong EC, Hinks RS, Tikofsky RS, Hyde JS (1992) Time course EPI of human brain function during task activation. Magn Reson Med 25:390–397
3. Chan SH (1984) What is being stimulated in acupuncture: Evaluation of the existence of a specific substrate. Neurosci Behav Rev 8:25–33
4. Chiang CY, Chang CT, Chu HL, Yang IL (1973) Peripheral afferent pathways for acupuncture analgesia. Sci Sin 16:210–217
5. Cho ZH, Chan JK, Ericksson L (1976) Circular ring transverse axial positron camera for 3D reconstruction of radionuclides distribution. IEEE, Trans Nucl Sci 23:613–622
6. Cho ZH, Ro YM, Lim TH (1992) NMR venography using the susceptibility effect produced by deoxyhemoglobin. Magn Reson Med 28:25–38
7. Cho ZH, Ro YM, Chung SC (1995) Susceptibility effect – enhanced functional MR imaging using tailored RF gradient echo (TRFGE) sequence. Int J Imag Syst Technol 6:164–170
8. Cho ZH, Ro YM, Park ST, Chung SC (1996) NMR functional imaging using a tailored RF gradient echo sequence: A true susceptibility measurement technique. Magn Reson Med 35:1–5
9. Cho ZH, Chung SC, Jones JP, Park JB, Park HJ, Lee HJ, Wong EK, Min BI (1998) New findings of the correlation between acupoints and corresponding brain cortices using functional MRI. Proc Natl Acad Sci, USA 95:2670–2673
10. Cho ZH, Lee SH, Hong IK, Wong EK, Na CS (1999) Further evidence for the correlation between acupuncture stimulation and cortical activation. Proceedings, New Directions in the Scientific Exploration of Acupuncture. University of California, Irvine
11. Filshie J, White A (1998) Medical Acupuncture: A Western scientific approach. Churchill Livingstone, Edinburgh, pp 225–294
12. Gilman S (1998) Imaging the brain. New Engl J Med 338:812–820, 889–896
13. Han JS (1993) Acupuncture and stimulation-produced analgesia. Handbook Exp Pharmacol 104/II:105–125
14. Heine H (1988) Anatomical structure of acupoints. J Trad Chin Med 8:207–212
15. Hennig J, Janz C, Speck 0, Ernst T (1995) Functional spectroscopy of brain activation following a single light pulse: Examinations of the mechanism of the fast initial response. Int J Imag Syst Technol 6:203–213
16. Hui KKS, Liu J, Wu M-T, Wang KKK (1996) Functional mapping of the human brain during acupuncture with magnetic resonance imaging. Proc Fourth World Conf Acupunct 4:71
17. Hui KK, Liu J, Makris N, Gollub RL, Chen AJ, Moore CI, Kennedy DN, Rosen BR, Kwong KK (2000) Acupuncture modulates the limbic system and subcortical gray structures of the human brain: evidence from fMRI studies in normal subjects. Human Brain Mapping 9:13–25
18. Kwong KK, Belliveau JW, Chester DA, Goldberg IE, Weisskoff RM et al (1992) Dynamic magnetic resonance imaging of human brain activity during primary sensory stimulation. Proc Natl Acad Sci USA 89:5675–5679
19. Liu G (1996) Acupoints and meridians. Huaxia Publishing House, Huaxia, China
20. Naeser MA, Alexander MP, Stiassny-Eder D, Galler V, Hobbs J, Bachman D (1992) Real vs. sham acupuncture in the treatment of paralysis in acute stroke patients: A CT scan lesion site study. J Neurol Rehab 6:163–173
21. National Institute of Neurological Disorders and Stroke rt-PA Study Group (1995) Tissue plasminogen activator for acute ischemic stroke. New Engl J Med 333:1581–1587
22. Ogawa S, Lee TM, Kay AR, Tank DW (1990) Brain magnetic resonance imaging with contrast dependent on blood oxygenation. Proc Natl Acad Sci USA 87:9868–9872
23. Ogawa S, Tank DW, Menon R, Ellermann JM, Kim SG et al (1992) Intrinsic signal changes accompanying sensory stimulation: Functional brain mapping with magnetic resonance imaging. Proc Natl Acad Sci USA 89:5951–5955
24. Phelps ME, Hoffman EJ, Mullani NA, Ter-Pogossian MM (1975) Application of annihilation coincidence detection to transaxial reconstruction tomography. J Nucl Med 16:210–224
25. Pomeranz B (1987) Scientific basis of acupuncture. In: Stux G, Pomeranz B (eds) Acupuncture. Textbook and atlas. Springer, Berlin, pp 1–34
26. Pomeranz B (1996) Scientific research into acupuncture for the relief of pain. J Alt Compl Med 2:53–60
27. Raichle ME (1998) Behind the scenes of functional brain imaging: A historical and physiological perspective. Proc Natl Acad Sci USA 95:765–772

28. Ramachandran VS (1994) Phantom limbs, neglected syndromes, repressed memories, and Freudian psychology. Int Rev Neurobiol 37:291–333
29. Ramachandran VS (1998) Phantoms in the brain. William Morrow, New York
30. Rohen JW, Yokochi C, Lutjen-Drecoll E (1987) Color atlas of anatomy. Fourth edn. Williams and Wilkins, Baltimore
31. Stux G, Pomeranz B (1987) Acupuncture. Textbook and atlas. Springer, Berlin
32. Takeshige C, Sato T, Mera T, Hisamitsu T, Fang J (1992) Descending pain inhibitory system involved in acupuncture analgesia. Brain Res Bull 29:617–634
33. Wu MT, Hsieh JC, Xiong J, Yang CF, Pan HB et al (1999) Central nervous pathway for acupuncture stimulation: Localization of processing with functional MR imaging of the brain – preliminary experience. Radiol 212:133–141

CHAPTER 6

Neurophysiological Basis of Auricular Acupuncture

T. Oleson

6.1
Introduction

Of all the areas of acupuncture, one of the most challenging aspects for acceptance by Western trained scientists is the use of acupuncture points on body organs that are distant from the site of pathology. One such remote system is the application of needles, electrical stimulation, or applied pressure to specific regions of the external ear or auricle. Western scientists are particularly skeptical of the concept that the organization of auricular acupoints can be seen as configured like an inverted fetus. Upper regions of the external ear are used to alleviate conditions in the legs and feet, middle regions represent chest problems and back pain, while lower regions relieve headaches and neurological disorders. The purpose of this chapter is to review the history, theories, clinical studies, and neurophysiological research which has examined this field of auricular acupuncture. There is growing scientific evidence which not only supports its use as an effective clinical modality but also suggests that acupuncture points on the external ear have specific connections to the central nervous system, which then affect reflexes in other parts of the body.

6.2
Somatotopic Organization of Auricular Acupuncture Points

Classic acupuncture theory attributes chronic pain and pathological disease to the blockage of energy flow along acupuncture meridians, invisible lines of force extending over the surface of the body. Ancient Oriental medical texts described direct energy connections between the yang acupuncture meridians on the body and acupuncture points on the external ear [22]. However, the Chinese revised their use of auricular acupuncture in 1958 after they learned of the inverted fetus map of the ear first described by Dr. Paul Nogier of Lyon, France (Fig. 1). While familiar with an energy perspective of the human body [17], Nogier's theory for the spatial arrangement found on the external ear [34] was based primarily on the proposition that there are neurophysiological connections between auricular reflex points and the central nervous system. The somatotopic pattern said to exist on the external ear is configured in a manner similar to the neurological homunculus demonstrated for the human cerebral cortex [43]. Neurophysiological research has not yet revealed a connection between Nogier's auricular map and the somatotopically organized neurons in the brain, but this remains an exciting area for future investigations.

Fig. 1. Inverted fetus map
represented on the auricle
of the external ear

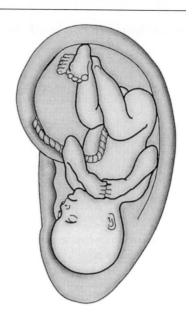

Nogier suggested that there are three different zones on the external ear which are related to different types of neural innervation and different categories of embryological tissue [35]. A picture of the external ear identifying the nomenclature for different anatomical regions of the auricle is shown in Fig. 2, whereas the specific functional zones of the ear are represented in Fig. 3. The central concha of the ear is innervated by the vagus nerve and serves as the region for autonomic regulation of pain and pathology originating from internal organs. The surrounding antihelix and antitragus ridges of the ear represent somatic nerve processing of myofascial pain, backaches, and headaches. The outer helix tail and earlobe represent the spinal cord and brain regions which affect neuropathic pain such as peripheral neuropathies and trigeminal neuralgia. The body organs represented on the external ear can be viewed as three concentric rings: the embryologically based endodermal organs are "found" at the center of the ear, the mesodermal tissue that becomes the somatic musculature is represented on the middle ridges of the auricle, and the ectodermal skin and nervous system tissue are found on the outer ridges. Each of these three auricular regions depicts body orientation in an inverted somatotopic pattern. Higher organs of the actual lungs, shoulder, or cerebral cortex are represented on lower areas of the auricle, whereas lower organs of the actual intestines, leg, or lumbar spinal cord are represented farther up on the auricle (Fig. 4).

It has been proposed by Oleson [36] that the relief of pain by auricular acupuncture can be best understood by the theory of stimulation-produced analgesia. Liebeskind et al. [30] developed this theory to account for the pain relieving effects following electrical stimulation of neurons in the brain. In addition to the classically known, ascending pain sensation pathway, there is a descending pain inhibitory pathway. The latter travels from the brainstem down the spinal cord; it then activates pain suppressive cells in the dorsal horn of the spinal cord. In their gate control theory of

Fig. 2. Nomenclature for anatomical regions of the external ear

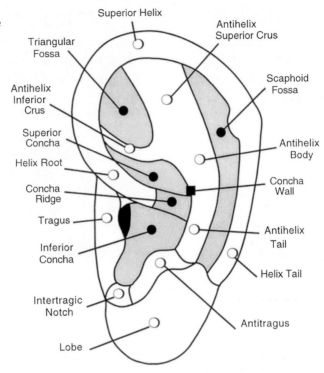

Fig. 3. Functional zones represented on the auricle. An endodermal region is shown in the central concha of the ear, representing vagus nerve control of autonomic disorders. A mesodermal region is shown in the middle ridges of the antihelix and antitragus, representing somatic nerve control of myofascial pain. An ectodermal region is shown in the outer helix and lobe of the auricle, representing central nervous system regulation of neuropathic pain

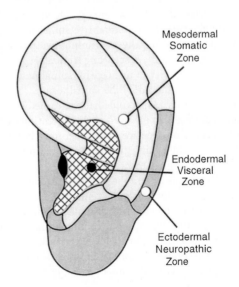

Fig. 4. An inverted somatotopic representation on the
auricle is shown, indicating
that the feet and legs are represented toward the top of the
external ear and the head is
represented toward the lower
antitragus and lobe of the
auricle, with the rest of the
body in between

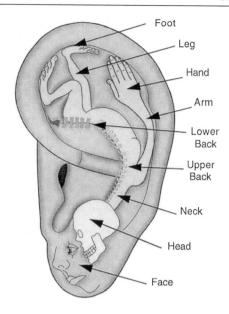

Foot

Leg

Hand

Arm

Lower
Back

Upper
Back

Neck

Head

Face

pain, Melzack and Wall [33] proposed that there was an inhibition of input from nociceptive neurons by input from tactile neurons interacting through spinal cord inter-
neurons. They further allowed that supraspinal gates in the brain could produce
descending inhibition of the ascending pain messages.

Basbaum and Fields [4]showed that lesions in the descending, dorsolateral funicu-
lar tract in the spinal cord blocked behavioral analgesia from deep brain stimulation.
There are both descending pain facilitation and descending pain inhibition systems
in the central nervous system. Destruction of descending, serotonergic, raphe pathways and descending, noradrenergic, locus coeruleus pathways both lead to an
increase in the activity of nociceptive spinal neurons, as measured by increased fos
proteins, indicating that the pain inhibitory pathway has been damaged [55]. Conversely, destruction of descending reticular gigantocellular pathways leads to a
decrease in the activity of nociceptive spinal neurons, suggesting that the pain facilitation system was altered by the spinal lesion.

Liebeskind et al. [30] found that the same areas of the brain which can perceive
pain messages are also involved in the inhibition of pain signals. Deep brain stimulation suppressed nociceptive spinal neurons but not sensory neurons, which only
responded to light tactile stimuli. Multiple unit responses in the midbrain and the
thalamus of rats evoked by noxious stimuli are also attenuated by the activation of the
periaqueductal gray and raphe nuclei of the rat brainstem, whereas neural responses
evoked by non-noxious air puffs remained the same after brain stimulation [40]. The
most potent area for obtaining stimulation-produced analgesia in rats was the midbrain periaqueductal gray, a region containing neurons specifically responsive to noxious stimuli. Research in primates [37] has shown that deep brain stimulation in the
subcortical thalamus is a more potent site for obtaining stimulation-produced analgesia in higher species. Examination of stimulation-produced analgesia in human

patients has shown similar findings [19]. Human research has confirmed that nociceptive pain messages activate positron emission tomography (PET) scan activity in the periaqueductal gray, hypothalamus, somatosensory cortex, and prefrontal cortex [21], which includes the same brainstem and thalamic areas that are able to suppress pain messages. While direct connections between auricular acupuncture points and these antinociceptive brain pathways have not yet been investigated, neurophysiological investigations of body acupuncture points suggest that the regions of the brain related to pain inhibition are also affected by the stimulation of acupoints.

6.3
Neurophysiological Theories of Acupuncture and Microacupuncture Systems

According to Ralph Alan Dale [12], the holographic homunculus pattern shown on the external ear is one of several microacupuncture systems that connect peripheral regions of the body to the central nervous system. Dale suggests that the ear points have remote reflex connections to other parts of the body through neuronal pathways in the central nervous system. Dale has proposed that there are both organocutaneous reflexes, which allow the microsystem to reveal underlying body pathology, and cutaneo-organic reflexes, which enable microacupuncture stimulation to heal the pathological condition. Foot reflexology and hand and scalp acupuncture are other examples of such microacupuncture systems, each serving as peripheral terminals in the body that connect to a central brain computer [36].

Tsun-nin Lee [28, 29] hypothesized a thalamic neuron model to account for reflex connections between acupuncture points and the brain. According to this view, pathological changes in peripheral tissue will eventually lead to dysfunctional neural firing patterns in the correspondent neural microcircuits in the brain and spinal cord. The organization of the connections between peripheral nerves and the CNS is controlled by sites in the sensory thalamus that are arranged like a homunculus. The CNS institutes corrective measures intended to normalize the disordered neural circuits, but strong environmental stressors or intense emotions may cause the CNS circuitry to malfunction. If the neurophysiological programs in the neural circuits are impaired, the peripheral disease may remain chronic. Pain and disease are thus attributed to learned, maladaptive programming of these neural circuits. Stimulation of acupuncture points on the body or the ear can serve to induce reorganization of these pathological brain pathways. The spatial arrangement of these neuronal chains within the thalamic homunculus is said to account for the arrangement of acupuncture meridians in the periphery. The invisible meridians which purportedly run over the surface of the body may actually be due to nerve pathways projected onto neuronal chains in the thalamus. The auricular acupuncture system is more noticeably arranged in a somatotopic pattern on the auricular skin surface.

There have been four main questions in acupuncture research designed to examine these neurophysiological theories:
1. Can the existence of auricular and body acupuncture reflex points be substantiated by electrophysiological measures?
2. Are the areas of the brain associated with stimulation-produced analgesia also affected by the stimulation of acupuncture points?

3. Do changes in the natural opiates, the endorphins and enkephalins, reliably account for the pain relieving effects of auriculotherapy and body acupuncture?
4. Is there evidence that the somatotopic pattern described for the auricle is specifically associated with changes in neural activity in different parts of the brain?

6.4
Electrodermal Determination of Acupuncture Points

A principal area of interest has been the examination of whether the bioelectric properties of auricular acupuncture points correlate with the presence of disease or dysfunction of the corresponding area of the body. The first double blind assessment to validate scientifically the somatotopic pattern of reflex points on the auricle was conducted by Oleson et al. [39]. Forty patients with specific musculoskeletal pain problems were first evaluated by a doctor or nurse to determine the exact body location of their physical pain. They were then draped with a sheet to cover their body so that only their external ear was exposed to view. Crutches and braces were removed from the room in order to prevent any clues as to the nature of their condition. A second medical doctor with extensive training in auricular acupuncture procedures then examined each patient's ear. This second doctor had no prior knowledge of the subject's previously established medical diagnosis and was not allowed to interact verbally with the patient. Auricular diagnosis was determined by numerically rated levels of tenderness to a palpating probe and by the quantified electrical conductivity of the skin. Specific areas of the auricle which corresponded to different musculoskeletal regions of the body were examined. There was a positive correspondence between auricular points identified as reactive, both tender to palpation and exhibiting at least 50 µA of electrical conductivity, and the parts of the body where there was musculoskeletal pain. Nonreactive ear points corresponded to parts of the body from which there was no reported pain. The statistically significant overall correct detection rate was 75.2 %. When the pain was located on only one side of the body, electrical conductivity was significantly greater at the somatotopic ear point on the ipsilateral ear than at the corresponding area of the contralateral ear. These results supported the concept that specific areas of the ear are related to specific areas of the body.

Double blind assessment of auricular points that are related to heart disorders was conducted by Saku et al. in Japan [48]. Reactive electropermeable points on the ear were defined as auricular skin areas with electrical current conductance greater than 50 µA, indicating relatively low skin resistance. There was a significantly higher frequency of reactive ear points at the Chinese heart points in the inferior concha (84 %) and on the tragus (59 %) for patients with myocardial infarctions and angina pain than for a control group of healthy subjects (11 %). There was no difference between the coronary heart disease group and the control group in the electrical reactivity of auricular points that did not represent the heart. The frequency of electropermeable auricular points for the kidney (5 %), stomach (6 %), liver (10 %), elbow (11 %), or eye (3 %), was the same for coronary patients as for individuals without coronary problems. Whereas Oleson et al. [39] had supported the concept that Nogier's mesodermal antihelix zone on the ear corresponds to musculoskeletal pain, Saku et al. established that specific points on the endodermal concha region of the ear were associated with a visceral condition such as heart disease.

Quantified examinations of the electrical properties of the skin have provided the most objective demonstration of the scientific validity of acupuncture points [5, 6, 38, 45]. Observations that acupuncture points exhibit higher levels of skin conductance or lower levels of skin resistance than surrounding skin surface areas were first reported in the 1950s by Nakatani in Japan and Niboyet in France. In the 1970s, Matsumoto showed that 80 % of acupuncture points could be detected as low resistance points. The electrical resistance of acupuncture points was found to range from 100 to 900 kOhm, whereas the electrical resistance of nonacupuncture points ranged from 1100 to 11,700 kOhm. Taking great care to control for electrical resistance variance due to pressure on the skin by the detecting probe, Reichmanis, Becker, and Marino [45] systematically verified that the electrodermal resistance at acupuncture points is significantly lower than in surrounding tissue. In addition, meridian acupuncture points exhibit even lower electrical resistance when there is pathology in the organ they represent. For instance, electrodermal resistance on the lung meridian is lower when one has a respiratory disorder, whereas skin resistance on the liver meridian is lower when one has a liver disorder. The normal, bilateral symmetry of the electrical resistance of acupuncture points is disturbed when there is unilateral pathology in the body. Those acupuncture points that are ipsilateral to the site of body discomfort exhibit a lower electrical resistance than the corresponding meridian point on the contralateral side of the body. Oleson et al. [39] found that auricular points showed a similar ipsilateral pattern.

Xianglong et al. of China examined 68 healthy adults for computerized plotting of low skin resistance points [58]. A silver electrode was continuously moved over a whole area of body surface while a reference electrode was fastened to the hand. Starting from the distal ends of the four limbs, investigators moved the electrode along the known meridians. The resistance of low skin impedance points (LSIP) was approximately 50 kOhm, whereas the impedance at non-LSIP was typically 500 kOhm. The LSIP were distributed over the body, predominantly along the 14 classic acupuncture meridian channels. A total of 64 % of LSIP were located exactly on a channel and 83.3 % were located within 3 mm of a channel. In only a few cases could individual LSIP be found in nonchannel areas. There was not an uninterrupted, continuous line of low skin impedance, but a series of electroactive points distributed along the meridian channel. There was no marked natural fluctuation of skin impedance, and the distribution of LSIP was considerably stable and repeatable from one day to the next.

Chiou et al. [8] examined the topography of low skin resistance points (LSRP) in rats. The moveable search electrode was a polished acupuncture needle applied with uniform pressure which did not pierce the skin, and the reference electrode was a needle inserted into the tail. Specific LSRP loci were distributed symmetrically and bilaterally over the shaved skin of the animal's ventral, dorsal, and lateral surfaces. The arrangement of LSRP corresponded to the acupuncture meridians found in humans and were hypothesized to represent zones of autonomic concentration, the higher electrical conductivity being due to higher neural and vascular elements beneath the points. The LSRP gradually disappeared 30 minutes after the animal's death.

Skin and muscle tissue samples were obtained by Chan et al. [7] from four anesthetized dogs. Acupuncture points, defined by regions of low skin resistance, were compared to control points exhibiting less conductivity. The points were marked for later histological examination. Concentration of substance P was significantly higher at skin acupuncture points (3.33 ng/g) than at control skin points (2.63 ng/g) that did not exhibit low skin resistance. Its concentration was also significantly higher in skin tissue samples (3.33 ng/g) than in the deeper, muscle tissue samples (1.81 ng/g). Substance P is known to be a spinal neurotransmitter found in nociceptive, afferent C-fibers. It plays a role in pain transmission, stimulates contractility of autonomic smooth muscle, induces subcutaneous liberation of histamine, causes peripheral vasodilation, and leads to hypersensitivity of sensory neurons. This neurotransmitter seems to activate a somatoautonomic reflex that could account for the clinical observations of specific acupuncture points that are both electrically active and tender to palpation.

Experimentally induced changes in auricular reflex points in rats were examined by Kawakita et al. [25]. The submucosal tissue of the stomach of anesthetized rats was exposed and acetic acid or saline was injected into the stomach tissue. Skin impedance of the auricular skin was measured by constant voltage square wave pulses. A silver metal ball, the search electrode, was moved over the surface of the rat's ear and a needle inserted into subcutaneous tissue to serve as the reference electrode. Injection of acetic acid led to the gradual development of lowered skin resistance points on central regions of the rats' ears, auricular areas corresponding to the gastrointestinal region of human ears. In normal rats and in experimental rats before the surgical operation, low impedance points were rarely detected on the auricular skin. After experimentally induced peritonitis, there was a significant increase in low impedance points (0–100 kOhm) and moderate impedance points (100–500 kOhm), but a decrease in high impedance points (> 500 kOhm). These results demonstrated a reduction in the electrodermal resistance response to experimentally induced irritation of the internal organ related to that auricular point. Histological investigation could not prove the existence of sweat glands in the rat auricular skin. The authors suggested that the low impedance points are in fact related to sympathetic control of blood vessels. It would have been intriguing if the investigators had conducted further evaluation of the auricular low resistance sites for concentrations of substance P, as Chan et al. had done for body acupoints [7]. Kawakita's study provides objective support for the organocutaneous reflexes described by Dale ([12], wherein low resistance auricular acupuncture points appear in response to pathology of the corresponding internal organ.

6.5
Changes in Brain Activity Following Auricular Acupuncture for Obesity

An intriguing use of auricular acupuncture has been its clinical application for weight control. Sun and Xu [54] treated overweight patients with otoacupoint stimulation, another term for ear acupressure. All patients were also given body acupuncture for the 3-month period of the study. The acupuncture group consisted of 110 patients diagnosed with at least 20 % more than ideal weight. They were compared to 51 obesity patients in a control group given an oral medication for weight control. An electrical point finder was used to determine the following auricular points: mouth, esophagus, stomach, abdomen, hunger, shen men, lung, and endocrine. Pressure pellets made from vaccaria seeds were applied to the appropriate points of both ears. The body acupuncture points needled included St.25, St.36, St.40, Sp.6, and Pe.6. The average 5 kg reduction in body weight by the acupuncture group was significantly greater than the average 2 kg loss shown by the control group. The percentage of body fat was reduced by 3% in the acupuncture group and by 1.54% in the control group, while the triglyceride blood lipid levels were diminished 67 units in the acupuncture group and 38 units in the control group.

A randomized controlled trial by Richards and Marley [47] found that weight loss was significantly greater for women in an auricular acupuncture group than in a control group. Women in the auricular group were given surface electrical stimulation to the ear acupoints for stomach and shen men, whereas women in the control group were given transcutaneous electrical stimulation to the first joint of the thumb. Auricular acupuncture was theorized to suppress appetite by stimulating the auricular branch of the vagus nerve and raising serotonin levels, both of which increase smooth muscle tone in the gastric wall. Rather than examine changes in weight measurements, Choy and Eidenschenk examined the effect of tragus clips on gastric peristalsis in 13 volunteers [9]. The duration of single peristaltic waves was measured before and after the application of ear clips to the tragus. The frequency of peristalsis was reduced by one-third with clips on the ear and returned to normal with the clips off. The ear clips were said to produce inhibition of vagus nerve activity, leading to a delay of gastric emptying, which would then lead to a sense of fullness and early satiety. These obesity studies on human subjects have received potential validation from neurophysiological research in animals.

The areas of the brain classically related to weight control include two regions of the hypothalamus. The ventromedial hypothalamus (VMH) has been referred to as a satiety center; when the VMH is lesioned, animals fail to restrict their food intake. In contrast, the lateral hypothalamus (LH) is referred to as a feeding center, since stimulation of the LH induces animals to start eating food. Asamoto and Takeshige [3] studied selective activation of the hypothalamic satiety center by auricular acupuncture in rats. Electrical stimulation of inner regions of the rat ear which correspond to auricular representation of the gastrointestinal tract produced evoked potentials in the ventromedial hypothalamus (VMH) satiety center but not in the lateral hypothalamic (LH) feeding center. Stimulation of more peripheral regions of the rat ear did not activate hypothalamic evoked potentials, indicating the selectivity of auricular acupoint stimulation. Only the somatotopic auricular areas near the region representing the stomach caused these specific brain responses. Acupuncture needles were subsequently placed into the same auricular sites as those that led to evoked potentials in the VMH. After 16 days, the body weights of rats in the auricular acupuncture group was significantly lower than in a control group of rats that were not needled. The same auricular acupuncture sites that led to hypothalamic activity associated with satiety led to behavioral changes in food intake. Moreover, auricular acupuncture had no effect on a different set of rats that received bilateral lesions of VMH. These results indicate a compelling connection between auricular acupuncture and a part of the brain associated with neurophysiological regulation of feeding behavior. The hypothalamus also regulates visceral activity affected by the autonomic vagus nerve.

In support of this evoked potential research, Shiraishi et al. [49] recorded single unit, neuronal discharge rates in the ventromedial hypothalamus (VMH) and lateral hypothalamus (LH) of rats. The firing pattern of hypothalamic neurons was recorded in response to electrical stimulation of specific areas of the rats' ears. A particular focus was on stimulating low resistance regions of the inferior concha of the ear, areas of the auricle innervated by the vagus nerve and corresponding to the stomach in human ear acupuncture charts. Auricular stimulation tended to facilitate neuronal discharges in the VMH and inhibit neural responses in the LH. Out of 162 neurons recorded in the ventromedial hypothalamus, 44.4 % exhibited increased neuronal discharge rates in response to auricular stimulation, 3.7 % of VMH neurons exhibited decreased activity, and 51.9 % showed no change. Of 224 neurons recorded in the LH feeding center of 21 rats, 22.8 % were inhibited by auricular stimulation, 7.1 % were excited, and 70.1 % were unaffected. When the analysis was limited to 12 rats classified as responding behaviorally to auricular acupuncture stimulation, 49.5 % of LH units were inhibited, 15.5 % were excited, and 35.0 % were unaffected by auricular stimulation. A different set of rats were given lesions of the ventro-medial hypothalamus, which led to significant weight gain. In these hypothalamic obese rats, 53.2 % of 111 LH neurons were inhibited by auricular stimulation, 1.8 % showed increased activity, and 45 % were unchanged. These neurophysiological find-ings suggest that auricular acupuncture can selectively alter hypothalamic brain activity and is more likely to produce sensations of VMH satiety than reduction of LH appetite.

6.6
Reduction of Neurophysiological Nociceptive Responses by Acupuncture Stimulation

A central focus of neurophysiological research on acupuncture treatment has been the assessment of changes in neural responses related to pain. As stated previously, deep brain stimulation of the periaqueductal gray leads to pain reduction in rats, cats, monkeys, and man [30], an analgesic effect which can be reversed by the opiate antagonist naloxone. Such stimulation-produced analgesia by brain electrodes directly elevates endorphin levels in the CSF and blood plasma levels of animals [42] and human patients [2, 19].

Pert et al. [44] showed that 7 Hz electrical auricular stimulation through needles inserted into the concha of the rat produced an elevation of the hot plate threshold which was reversed by naloxone. The behavioral analgesia to auricular electroacu-puncture was accompanied by a 60 % increase in radioreceptor activity in CSF levels of endorphins, a level significantly greater than that found in a rat control group. Concomitant with these CSF changes, auricular electroacupuncture produced deple-tion in beta-endorphin radioreceptor activity in the ventromedial hypothalamus and the medial thalamus but not in the periaqueductal gray. Supportive findings in human back pain patients were obtained by Clement-Jones et al. [11]. Low frequency electrical stimulation of the concha led to relief of pain within 20 minutes of the onset of electroacupuncture and an accompanying elevation of CSF beta-endorphin activity in all ten subjects. Abbate et al. [1] examined endorphin levels in 12 patients under-going thoracic surgery. Six were given 50 % nitrous oxide combined with 50 Hz auric-ular electroacupuncture while six control patients underwent their surgery with 70 % nitrous oxide but no acupuncture. The auricular acupuncture patients not only needed less nitrous oxide than the controls, but the ear acupuncture also led to a significant increase in beta-endorphin immunoreactivity.

A review of the neurophysiological literature by Kho and Robertson [26] provides empirical support for the role of the thalamus in acupuncture analgesia. Afferent acupuncture impulses are thought to activate nociceptive inhibitory pathways and selectively alter specific neurotransmitters. Gao et al. [16] found that after giving 4 Hz electroacupuncture of St.36, the autoradiographic mu-enkephalin receptor binding sites were significantly increased in the following brain areas of rats: caudate, septal nucleus, medial preoptic, amygdala, periaqueductal gray, nucleus raphe magnus, cervical spinal cord, and lumbar spinal cord dorsal horn.

Kalyuzhnyi et al. [24] applied 15 Hz electrostimulation to the auricular lobes of rabbits in an area corresponding to the jaw and teeth in humans. They measured behavioral reflexes and cortical somatosensory evoked potentials in response to tooth pulp stimulation. Auricular electroacupuncture produced a significant decrease in behavioral reflexes and in cortical evoked potentials following electrical stimulation of the teeth. For most animals, the suppression of behavioral and neurophysiological effects was abolished by injection of the opiate antagonist naloxone, suggesting endorphinergic mechanisms. In a few rabbits, however, auriculoacupuncture stimulation did not induce this naloxone reversible effect, and naloxone injections themselves led to an analgesic effect. The authors suggested that this paradoxical effect could be explained by an inhibition of an antiopioid substance in select individuals. Fedoseeva et al. [15] also examined electrical stimulation of auricular acupuncture at earlobe points in rabbits, the auricular area that corresponds to the trigeminal nerve. Auricular electroacupuncture led to a reduction of the amplitude of cortical somatosensory potentials evoked by tooth pulp stimulation. Intravenous injection of the opiate antagonist naloxone diminished the analgesic effect of auricular electroacupuncture at 15 Hz stimulation frequencies but not at 100 Hz stimulation. Conversely, injection of saralasin, an antagonist of angiotensin II, blocked the analgesic effect of 100 Hz auricular acupuncture but not 15 Hz stimulation. The amplitude of cortical potentials evoked by electrical stimulation of the hind limb was not attenuated by stimulation of the auricular area for the trigeminal nerve.

There is a larger body of research which has examined changes in the brain following body acupuncture, often relying on acupuncture needling of the presumed location in animals of St.36 on the lower leg known as zusanli, or LI.4 known as either hegu or hoku. Stimulation of body acupuncture points leads to elevation of pain thresholds in animals [41] and in man [32]. Brain research by Li et al. [31] found that electrical stimulation of the reticularis gigantocellularis nucleus (RGC) of rats could enhance acupuncture analgesia on the tail flick test produced by electroacupuncture at St.36. Lesions of reticularis gigantocellularis nucleus could reduce acupuncture analgesia, while microinjections of naloxone into this same brainstem nucleus could partially block acupuncture analgesia. Radioimmunoassays for opioid peptides released from the RGC revealed that leu-enkephalin and beta-endorphin levels increased after acupuncture stimulation, whereas opioid peptide levels remained stable in a control group. Similar research by Wu et al. [57] showed that electroacupuncture applied to LI.4 led to an increase in pain threshold and in leu-enkephalin and beta-endorphin levels in the preoptic area of rabbits. Norepinephrine release in the preoptic area was decreased by acupuncture and reversed by perfusion with naloxone. Electroacupuncture was also shown to reduce the evoked response to nociceptive input by excitatory preoptic neurons, an effect which was also reversed by naloxone microinjections into the preoptic area.

Renhua et al. [46] examined 24 rabbits anesthetized with urethane and given bilateral stimulation of acupuncture point St.36. Acupuncture was applied with either manual twirling of needles or with electroacupuncture. The volume of microcirculatory blood flow in the cerebral pia mater increased 62 % after electroacupuncture and increased 18 % after manual acupuncture. Sonoda et al. [52] have shown that activation of the brainstem periaqueductal gray can lead to inhibition of palmar galvanic skin reflexes, demonstrating the effect of the pain inhibition pathway on autonomic arousal. This inhibition is eliminated by intravenous administration of naloxone, suggesting that the endorphinergic pathways play a role in acupuncture-induced reductions in autonomic electrodermal activity and autonomic elevations of blood circulation.

Simmons and Oleson [50] examined naloxone reversibility of auricular acupuncture analgesia to acute induced pain. All 40 volunteers were assessed for tooth pain threshold by a dental pulp tester. Dental pain levels were determined before and after auriculotherapy and again after double blind injection of naloxone or placebo. Subjects were assigned to one of four groups: true auricular electrical stimulation (AES) followed by an injection of naloxone, true AES followed by an injection of saline, placebo stimulation of the auricle followed by an injection of naloxone, or placebo stimulation of the auricle followed by an injection of saline. Dental pain thresholds were significantly raised by AES conducted at auricular points appropriate for dental pain. Pain thresholds were not altered by sham stimulation at inappropriate auricular points. Naloxone produced a slight lowering of dental pain threshold in the subjects given true AES, whereas true AES subjects given saline showed a further rise in pain threshold. The minimal changes in dental pain threshold shown by the sham auriculotherapy group were not significantly affected by saline or naloxone. Both Sjolund and Eriksson [51] and Simmons and Oleson noticed that pain threshold levels did not completely return to baseline after administration of naloxone, suggesting nonopioid as well as endorphinergic brain mechanisms.

Hsieh compared manual stimulation of St.36 to 2 Hz electroacupuncture applied at the same point in 13 healthy male subjects [20]. Electrodermal skin responses were recorded from both palms to measure the autonomic arousal response to electric shock stimulation of the median nerve on the right wrist. Somatic cortex evoked potentials were recorded at the hand area of the left somatosensory cortex, consisting of short latency, negative wave potentials (N 13 and N 20), and a long latency, positive wave potential (P 25). The amplitude of evoked electrodermal responses (EDR) was attenuated 50 % by electroacupuncture and reduced 31 % by manual acupuncture. There were no differences in left and right electrodermal responses, indicating a generalized inhibition of the sympathetic nervous system response. The mean amplitude of the N 13 and N 20 wave somatosensory evoked potentials were unaffected by acupuncture, whereas the amplitude of P 25 waves was elevated 13 % by electroacupuncture and 6 % by manual acupuncture. These changes reflected an increase in cortical enhancement of peripheral stimulation but a reduction in sympathetic arousal.

Auricular acupuncture has also been shown to suppress autonomic electrodermal activity associated with the startle reflex to arousing stimuli. Young and McCarthy conducted a controlled clinical trial on 38 healthy volunteers [59]. Forearm electro-dermal recordings to different stimuli were obtained when a needle was inserted into the auricular sympathetic point. In another set of subjects, EDR levels were recorded when a needle was inserted into a placebo auricular point not associated with auto-nomic regulation. Evoked EDR activity was consistently higher when needles were placed in the placebo auricular point than when placed in the sympathetic point. Thus, there was a selective difference between the electrodermal effects of appropri-ate and inappropriate auricular acupuncture stimulation, suggesting that the auricu-lotherapy attenuated the autonomic startle reflex.

6.7
Mechanisms for Withdrawal from Opiate Drugs by Auricular Acupuncture

The discovery by H. L. Wen [56] that auricular acupuncture facilitates withdrawal from narcotic drugs has led to a plethora of studies demonstrating the clinical use of this technique for substance abuse [13, 53]. Auricular electroacupuncture has been shown to raise levels of met-enkephalin in human narcotic addicts [10] and beta-endorphin in mice withdrawn from morphine [18].

Kroening and Oleson [27] examined 14 chronic pain patients switched from their original analgesic medication to an equivalent dose of oral methadone, typically 80 mg per day. An electrodermal point finder was used to determine areas of low skin resistance for the lung point and the shen men point. Needles were bilaterally inserted into these two ear points and electrical stimulation was initiated between two pairs of needles. After 45 minutes of electroacupuncture, these hospitalized pain patients were given periodic injections of small doses of naloxone (0.04 mg every 15 minutes). The daily dose of methadone was cut in half each day, presuming no aver-sive withdrawal effects. All 14 patients were withdrawn from methadone within 2 to 7 days for a mean of 4.5 days. Only a few patients reported minimal side effects of mild nausea and agitation. The authors proposed that occupation of opiate receptor sites by narcotic drugs leads to the inhibition of the activity of natural endorphins, whereas auricular acupuncture facilitates withdrawal from these drugs by activating the release of previously suppressed endorphins. By giving small, incremental doses of naloxone administration after auricular acupuncture, it was theorized that opiate receptor sites can be allowed to return to their normal state.

Other biochemical changes also accompany auricular acupuncture. Debrecini [14] examined changes in plasma adrenocorticotropic hormone (ACTH) and growth hor-mone levels after 20 Hz electrical stimulation through needles inserted into the adre-nal point on the tragus of the ears of 20 healthy females. While growth hormone secretions increased after electroacupuncture, ACTH levels remained the same. Jaung-Geng et al. [23] evaluated lactic acid levels from pressure applied to ear vacca-ria seeds positioned over the liver, lung, san jiao, endocrine, and thalamus (subcor-tex) points. In a within-subjects design, pressure applied to ear points produced sig-nificantly lower levels of lactic acid obtained after physical exercise on a treadmill test than when the seeds were placed over the same auricular points but not pressed. Actual stimulation of these auricular acupressure points seemed to reduce the toxic elevations of lactic acid buildup to a greater extent than did the control condition, perhaps due to improved peripheral blood circulation.

6.8
Conclusions

One is constantly confronted with the need for further scientific studies to verify theoretical mechanisms in many areas of investigation, but this is especially true for neurophysiological studies of auricular acupuncture. Nonetheless, the studies thus far conducted indicate that there is already some support for each of the theoretical issues addressed at the beginning of this chapter. The two controlled studies on auricular diagnosis [39, 48] both support the proposition that specific areas of the auricle are related to specific areas of the body. The neurophysiological evidence for a connection between acupuncture stimulation and brain pathways related to a pain inhibitory system has been better established for body acupuncture than for ear acupuncture, but body points and ear points are both associated with endorphin and enkephalin release. Research in rats and rabbits has shown that stimulation of the vagus nerve via needling of the central concha of the ear selectively activates hypothalamic neurons associated with weight control [3, 49], whereas stimulation of the auricular lobe region representing the trigeminal nerve attenuates cortical evoked potentials to tooth shock [15, 24]. These animal studies suggest that stimulation of auricular points can lead to site-specific elevation of pain thresholds, but the relationship of somatotopic points on the auricle to specific regions of the human brain remains to be determined.

References

1. Abbate D, Santamaria A, Brambilla A, Panerai A, DiGuilio A (1980) Beta-endorphin and electroacupuncture. Lancet 3:1309
2. Akil H, Richardson D, Hughes J, Barachas J (1978) Enkephalin-like material elevated in ventricular cerebrospinal fluid of pain patients after analgetic focal stimulation. Science 209:463–465
3. Asamoto S, Takeshige C (1992) Activation of the satiety center by auricular acupuncture point stimulation. Brain Res Bull 29:157–164
4. Basbaum A, Fields H (1979) Endogenous pain control systems: Brainstem spinal pathway and endorphin circuitry. Annual Rev Neurosci 7:513–532
5. Becker R, Reichmanis M, Marino A, Spadaro J (1976) Electrophysiological correlates of acupuncture and meridians. Psychoenergetic Systems 1:105–112
6. Bergsmann O, Hart A (1973) Differences in electrical skin conductivity between acupuncture points and adjacent skin areas. Am J Acupunct 1:27–32
7. Chan W, Weissensteiner H, Rausch W, Chen K, Wu L, Lin J (1998) Comparison of substance P concentration in acupuncture points in different tissues in dogs. Am J Chin Med 26:13–18
8. Chiou S, Chao C, Yang Y (1998) Topography of low skin resistance points (LSRP) in rats. Am J Chin Med 26:19–27
9. Choy D, Eidenschenk E (1998) Effect of tragus clips on gastric peristalsis: A pilot study. J Altern Complement Med 4:399–403
10. Clement-Jones V, McLoughlin L, Lowery P, Besser G, Rees L, Wen H (1979) Acupuncture in heroin addicts: Changes in met-enkephalin and beta-endorphin in blood and cerebrospinal fluid. Lancet 2:380–383
11. Clement-Jones, V, Mc Loughlin, L, Tomlin, S, Besser, G, Rees, L, Wen H (1980) Increased beta-endorphin but not met-enkephalin levels in human cerebrospinal fluid after acupuncture for recurrent pain. Lancet 3:946–948
12. Dale R (1976) The microacupuncture system. Am J Acupunct 4:7–24
13. Dale R (1993) Addictions and acupuncture: The treatment methods, formulae, effectiveness, and limitations. Am J Acupunct 21:247–266
14. Debrecini L (1991) The effect of electrical stimulation of the ear points on the plasma ACTH and GH level in humans. Acupunct Electrother Res 16:45–51
15. Fedoseeva O, Kalyuzhnyi L, Sudakov K (1990) New peptide mechanisms of auriculoacupuncture electroanalgesia: Role of angiotensin II. Acupunct Electrother Res 15:1–8
16. Gao M, Wang M, Li K, He L (1997) Change of mu opioid receptor binding sites in rat brain following electroacupuncture. Acupunct Electrother Res 22:161–166

17. Helms J (1995) Acupuncture energetics: A clinical approach for physicians. Medical Acupuncture Publishers, Berkeley
18. Ho W, Wen H, Lam S, Li A (1978) The influence of electroacupuncture on naloxone-induced morphine withdrawal in mice: Elevation of brain opiate-like activity. Eur J Pharmacol 49:197–199
19. Hosobuchi Y, Rossier J, Bloom FE, Guillemin R (1979) Stimulation of human periaqueductal gray for pain relief increases immunoreactive beta-endorphin in ventricular fluid. Science 203:279–281
20. Hsieh C (1998) Modulation of cerebral cortex in acupuncture stimulation: A study using sympathetic skin response and somatosensory evoked potentials. Am J Chin Med 26:1–11
21. Hsieh J, Stahle-Backdahl M, Hagermark O, Stone-Elander S (1995) Traumatic nociceptive pain activates the hypothalamus and the periaqueductal gray: A positron emission tomography study. Pain 64:303–314
22. Huang, H (1974) Ear acupuncture. Rodale Press, New York
23. Jaung-Geng L, Salahin H, Jung-Chang L (1995) Investigation on the effects of ear acupressure on exercise-induced lactic acid levels and the implications for athletic training. Am J Acupunct 23:309–313
24. Kalyuzhnyi L (1990) Analgetic naloxone's effect on acupuncture-resistant, acupuncture-tolerant, and acupuncture-sensitive rabbits. Acupunct Electrother Res 15:259
25. Kawakita K, Kawamura H, Keino H, Hongo T, Kitakohji H (1991) Development of the low impedance points in the auricular skin of experimental peritonitis rats. Am J Chin Med 19:199–205
26. Kho H, Robertson E (1997) The mechanisms of acupuncture analgesia: Review and update. Am J Acupunct 25:261–281
27. Kroening R, Oleson T (1985) Rapid narcotic detoxification in chronic pain patients treated with auricular electroacupuncture and naloxone. Int J Addictions 20(9):1347–1360
28. Lee TN (1977) Thalamic neuron theory: A hypothesis concerning pain and acupuncture. Med Hypotheses 3:113–121
29. Lee TN (1994) Thalamic neuron theory: Theoretical basis for the role played by the central nervous system (CNS) in the causes and cures of all disease. Med Hypotheses 43:285–302
30. Liebeskind J, Mayer D, Akil H (1995) Central mechanisms of pain inhibition: Studies of analgesia from focal brain stimulation. In: JJ Bonica (ed) Advances in neurology, vol 4. Raven Press, New York
31. Li Z, Gen-Cheng W, Xiao-Ding C (1995) Role of opioid peptides of rat's nucleus reticularis paragigantocellularis lateralis in acupuncture analgesia. Acupunct Electrother Res 20:89–100
32. Mayer D, Price D, Rafii A (1977) Antagonism of acupuncture analgesia in man by the narcotic antagonist naloxone. Brain Res. 121:368–372
33. Melzack R, Wall P (1965) Pain mechanisms: A new theory. Science 150:197
34. Nogier P (1972) Treatise of auriculotherapy. Maisonneuve, Moulins-les-Metz
35. Nogier P (1983) From auriculotherapy to auriculomedicine. Maisonneuve, Moulins-les-Metz
36. Oleson T (1996) Auriculotherapy manual: Chinese and Western systems of ear acupuncture, 2nd edn. Health Care Alternatives, Los Angeles
37. Oleson T, Kirkpatrick D, Goodman S (1980) Elevation of pain threshold to tooth shock by brain stimulation in primates. Brain Res 194:79–95
38. Oleson T, Kroening R (1983) Electroacupuncture and auricular electrical stimulation. IEEE Eng Med Biol Mag 2:22–26
39. Oleson T, Kroening R, Bresler D (1980) An experimental evaluation of auricular diagnosis: The somatotopic mapping of musculoskeletal pain at ear acupuncture points. Pain 8:217–229
40. Oleson T, Liebeskind J (1978) Effect of pain-attenuating brain stimulation and morphine on electrical activity in the raphe nuclei of the awake rat. Pain 4:211–230
41. Pomeranz B, Chiu D (1976) Naloxone blockade of acupuncture analgesia: Endorphin implicated. Life Sci 19:1757–1763
42. Pomeranz B (1996) Scientific research into acupuncture for the relief of pain. J Compl Alt Med 2:53–60
43. Penfield W, Rasmussen T (1950) The cerebral cortex of man. Macmillan, New York
44. Pert A, Dionne R, Ng L, Bragin E, Moody T, Pert C (1981) Alterations in rat central nervous system endorphins following transauricular electroacupuncture. Brain Res 224:83–93
45. Reichmanis M, Marino A, Becker R (1975) Electrical correlates of acupuncture. IEEE Trans Biomed Eng 22:533–535
46. Renhua S, Guangchen J, Luming Z, Shijun W (1998) Effects of electroacupuncture and twirling reinforcing-reducing manipulations on volume of microcirculatory blood flow in cerebral pia mater. J Trad Chin Med 18:220–224
47. Richards D, Marley J (1998) Stimulation of auricular acupuncture points in weight loss. Austr Fam Physician 27 [Suppl 2]:S73–S77

48. Saku K, Mukaino Y, Ying H, Arakwa K (1993) Characteristics of reactive electropermeable points on the auricles of coronary heart disease patients. Clin Cardiol 16:415–419
49. Shiraishi T, Onoe M, Kojima T, Sameshima Y, Kageyama T (1995) Effects of auricular stimulation on feeding-related hypothalamic neuronal activity in normal and obese rats. Brain Res Bull 36:141–148
50. Simmons M, Oleson T (1993) Auricular electrical stimulation and dental pain threshold. Anesthesia Progress 40:14–19
51. Sjolund B, Eriksson M (1976) Electroacupuncture and endogenous morphines. Lancet 2:1985
52. Sonoda H, Ikenoue K, Yokota T (1986) Periaqueductal gray inhibition of viscerointercostal and galvanic skin reflexes. Brain Res. 369:91–102
53. Smith M (1988) Acupuncture treatment for crack: Clinical survey of 1500 patients treated. Am J Acupunct 16:241–246
54. Sun Q, Xu Y (1993) Simple obesity and obesity hyperlipema treated with otoacupoint pressure and body acupuncture. J Trad Chin Med 13:22–26
55. Wei F, Dubner R, Ren K (1999) Nucleus reticularis gigantocellularis and nucleus raphe magnus in the brain stem exert opposite effects on behavioral hyperalgia and spinal fos protein expression after peripheral inflammation. Pain 80:127–141
56. Wen H, Cheung S (1973) Treatment of drug addiction by acupuncture and electrical stimulation. Am J Acupunct 1:71–75
57. Wu G, Zhu J, Cao X (1995) Involvement of opioid peptides of the preoptic area during electroacupuncture analgesia. Acupunct Electrother Res 20:1–6
58. Xianglong H, Baohua W, Xiaoqing H, Jinsen X (1992) Computerized plotting of low skin impedance points. J Trad Chin Med 12:277–282
59. Young M, McCarthy P (1998) Effect of acupuncture stimulation of the auricular sympathetic point on evoked sudomotor response. J Altern Complement Med 4:29–38

Suggested Reading

Chen B-Y (1997) Acupuncture normalizes dysfunction of hypothalamic-pituitary-ovarian axis. Acupunct Electrother Res 22:97–108
Chen, H (1993) Recent studies on auriculoacupuncture and its mechanism. J Tradit Chin Med 13:129–143
Hyvarinen J, Karlsson M (1977) Low skin resistance skin points that may coincide with acupuncture loci. Med Biol 55:88–94
Ionescu-Tirgoviste C, Pruan S, Bajenaru P (1991) The participation of the autonomic nervous system in the mechanism of action of acupuncture. Am J Acupunct 19:21–28
Kashiba H, Ueda Y (1991) Acupuncture to the skin induces release of substance P and calcitonin gene-related peptide from peripheral terminals of primary sensory neurons in the rat. Am J Chin Med 19:189–197
Kumar A, Tandon O, Bhattacharya A, Gupta R, Dhar D (1995) Somatosensory evoked potential changes following electroacupuncture therapy in chronic pain patients. Anaesthesia 50:411–414
Lin X, Liang J, Ren J, Mu F, Zhang M, Chen J (1997) Electrical stimulation of acupuncture points enhances gastric myoelectrical activity in humans. Am J Gastroenterol 92:1527–1530
Ng L, Douthitt T, Thoa N, Albert C (1975) Modification of morphine withdrawal in rats following transauricular electrostimulation: An experimental paradigm for auricular electroacupuncture. Biol Psychiatr 10:575–580
Ng L (1996) Auricular acupuncture in animals: Effects of opiate withdrawal and involvement of endorphins. J. Compl Alt Med 2:61–64
Reichmanis M, Marino A, Becker R (1976) D. C. skin conductive variation at acupuncture loci. Am J Chin Med 4:69–72
Sjolund B, Terenius L, Eriksson M (1977) Increased cerebrospinal fluid levels of endorphins after electroacupuncture. Acta Physiol Scand 100:382–384
Takeshige C, Sato T, Mera T, Hisamitu T, Fang J (1992) Descending pain inhibitory system involved in acupuncture analgesia. Brain Res Bull 29:617–634
Wang Y, Wang S, Zhang W (1991) Effects of naloxone on the changes of pain threshold and contents of monoamine neurotransmitters in rat brain induced by electroacupuncture. J Trad Chin Med 11:286–290
Wen H, Ho K, Ling N, Ma L, Choa G (1979) The influence of electroacupuncture on naloxone-induced morphine withdrawal. II. Elevation of immunoassayable beta-endorphin activity in the brain but not the blood. Am J Chin Med 7:237–240
Wheeler A, Beitz D, Swift C (1976) Mapping of acupuncture points of the goat. Am J Acupunct 4:57–65
Zhu Z (1981) Research advances in the electrical specificity of meridians and acupuncture points. Am J Acupunct 9:203–213

Assessing Clinical Efficacy of Acupuncture: What Has Been Learned from Systematic Reviews of Acupuncture?

J. Ezzo · L. Lao · B. M. Berman

7.1
Introduction

This chapter summarizes the evidence of the clinical efficacy of acupuncture. Treatment efficacy pertains to the differential effect observed from a treatment as compared to a placebo or another treatment using a rigorous methodological design. Efficacy is often assessed using a double blind controlled trial design [1]. While some chapters in this book focus primarily on animal studies, the question of clinical efficacy can only be addressed in human studies. Therefore, this chapter will focus on summarizing the evidence from human acupuncture trials. It is divided into two major sections. The first presents an overview of evidence-based medicine and explains why the systematic review is the most reliable and valid method for assessing efficacy. The second section summarizes the current evidence from systematic reviews on acupuncture for specific conditions and, when applicable, presents results of trials published subsequently to each systematic review.

7.2
The Role of Systematic Reviews in Evidence-Based Medicine

Although there are many experimental designs in research, the gold standards for assessing efficacy are large, well-designed, randomized controlled trials (RCTs) and systematic reviews (Table 1) [2], because these designs are less likely to mislead than other study designs [3]. To date, trials of acupuncture are notably small [4–6], and few fulfill the description of a large RCT. Therefore, the most comprehensive assessment of acupuncture efficacy will be found in the existing systematic reviews on the topic.

Until about the mid-1990s, the terms "systematic review" and "meta-analysis" were used interchangeably. That is why the review by ter Reit and colleagues [4] is termed a "meta-analysis." More recently, these terms have been clarified: A systematic review is the whole process of conducting a comprehensive evidence synthesis from search strategy, evaluation of trial quality, and analysis, whereas a meta-analysis is a specific statistical technique of pooling data. By today's definition the ter Reit chronic pain review is actually a systematic review without a meta-analysis. Examples of acupuncture systematic reviews which have used meta-analysis are the reviews of acupuncture for chronic pain by Patel and colleagues [30] and on acupuncture for smoking cessation by White and Rampes [31].

Table 1. Type and strength of efficacy evidence [2]

1. Strong evidence from at least one systematic review of multiple well-designed randomized controlled trials
2. Strong evidence from at least one properly designed randomized controlled trial of appropriate size
3. Evidence from well designed trials without randomization, single group pre-post, cohort, time series or matched case-controlled studies
4. Evidence from well designed nonexperimental studies from more than one center or research group
5. Opinions of respected authorities, based on clinical evidence, descriptive studies or reports of expert committees

Evidence-based medicine is the "conscientious, explicit, and judicious use of the current best evidence in making decisions about the care of individual patients" [2]. This requires that clinicians combine their best clinical wisdom and experience with the best systematically researched clinical evidence available. It is not, as some have suggested [7], a reliance on abstract clinical evidence to the exclusion of clinicians' experiences and common sense. In essence, by applying their best clinical experience while keeping abreast of new research, clinicians have always striven to practice evidence-based medicine, which is why some have called it "old wine with a new label" [8].

What is new about evidence-based medicine is the systematic review method, which is an explicit methodology designed to summarize and synthesize evidence [3]. In the past, traditional literature reviews, commonly called narrative reviews, have been used to summarize evidence. One major difference between narrative reviews and systematic reviews is that systematic review methodology requires all trials which meet specified criteria to be included in the review, regardless of the trial results. By contrast, narrative reviews may exclude trials with findings that did not match the writer's point of view or had simply been inadvertently haphazard and noncomprehensive and therefore prone to bias [9]. Experience has demonstrated that a treatment which appears promising according to a narrative review can appear less promising when the systematic review methodology is applied [10]. Because systematic reviews follow an explicit methodology designed to minimize bias, they are becoming increasingly preferred over narrative reviews. For example, policy makers are growing increasingly partial to them as a way of summarizing evidence [11]. And, in the midst of the information explosion, clinicians rank reviews as their most preferred source of new information [12] while ranking individual RCTs close to the bottom of the list. Consumers, too, can use reviews to guide health decisions [13].

Finally, because systematic reviews comprehensively summarize research already completed, they are valuable tools for guiding the design of proposed clinical research. Systematic reviews can prevent the inadvertent duplication of work already done, underscore where knowledge gaps exist, and generate hypotheses for future research. For these reasons, trialists advocate conducting a systematic review and meta-analysis in the planning stages of a trial [14, 15], and funding agencies are increasingly inquiring on grant applications whether a systematic review has been conducted on the topic for which funding is sought [16].

7.2.1
Validity of the Study Design: How Systematic Reviews Limit Bias

It is important to understand the systematic review process in order to appreciate how this type of data analysis can limit bias. McQuay and Moore [2] describe the following as key steps of any systematic review: finding, appraising, and combining the evidence. Bias, a systematic error which can make a treatment appear less or more effective than it really is, can occur in any stage of this process. Although the examples presented here pertain to acupuncture, the potential biases discussed below apply to all systematic reviews for any treatment of any condition.

7.2.1.1
Finding the Evidence

One of the most striking ways that systematic reviews differ from narrative summaries is the comprehensiveness of the search for relevant trials. A trials search should be both comprehensive and replicable. MEDLINE is the most obvious place to begin searching for relevant acupuncture trials, but a search should not stop there. MEDLINE sensitivity, which is the proportion of relevant RCTs found by MEDLINE divided by the total of known trials on the topic, is estimated to be only about 58 % for acupuncture [17]. Obviously, this suggests that a universe of acupuncture trials exist that are not listed in MEDLINE. Additional sources can include other electronic databases [18], articles in journals not indexed by any database, conference abstracts that never become fully published articles, and trials which are completed but remain in researchers' file drawer or diskette and never reach print at all [19].

Publication bias is "the tendency of investigators, reviewers, and editors to submit or accept manuscripts for publication differentially, based on the direction or strength of the findings" [20]. Therefore, articles which are the most easily accessible because they are published may not be representative of the results of all the trials done. To the extent that publication bias exists, systematic reviews that omit unpublished studies risk overestimating treatment effects. Bias has been demonstrated both in what investigators submit to journals [21] and in what editors accept [22].

The recent findings by Egger and colleagues [23] raise the question of whether trials published in English are representative of the available trials. They observed that authors publishing in both German and English tend to report nonsignificant findings in German and significant findings in English. This suggests that one must search not only beyond the published literature, but also beyond the English language.

7.2.1.2
Appraising the Evidence

It may seem obvious that evidence is only as good as the trials upon which it is based, but the concept of assessing the methodological quality of the trials included in a systematic review is a relatively recent practice. A validated, user friendly scale (Jadad scale) for assessing methodological quality did not exist until 1996 (Table 2) [24]. Therefore, many reviews exist which form conclusions about the efficacy of a treat-

Table 2. Validated Jadad scale
for assessing trial quality [24]

1. Was the study described as randomized?
2. Was the randomization scheme described and appropriate?
3. Was the study described as double blind?
4. Was the method of double blinding appropriate?
5. Was there a description of drop outs and withdrawals ?

ment without taking into consideration the quality of the individual trials. The Jadad scale asks two questions pertaining to double blinding (defined as blinding both the patients and the outcomes assessor). Because it is not possible to blind the patients in most acupuncture trials, some reviewers have used a slightly different scale [6] which asks two separate questions: (1) Were the patients blinded? and (2) Was the outcomes assessor blinded? However, even if double blinding did not occur, it is still possible for a trial to earn a high quality score on the Jadad scale if the trial quality was satisfactory in other areas.

When trial quality is taken into account, results show that all RCTs are not created equal and, in general, low quality RCTs can bias trial results by exaggerating the positive effects of a treatment [25, 26]. Relative to acupuncture in particular, low quality RCTs have been associated with results favoring acupuncture for chronic pain [4, 27], asthma [5], and tobacco addiction [28].

Previously, many also assumed that RCTs not published in English were likely to be inferior methodologically compared to those in English, and therefore non-English language studies were often omitted from systematic reviews. Recently, Moher and colleagues [29] have demonstrated that the quality of studies in French, German, Spanish, and Italian is comparable with those published in English and, therefore, excluding these trials from a systematic review cannot be justified.

7.2.1.3
Combining the Evidence

Meta-analysis, the statistical pooling of results, is a preferred way to combine data from several trials when the data permit [2]. When the data are not conducive to pooling, an alternative method known as best evidence synthesis [32], which gives more weight to the high quality trials and less weight to low quality trials, is preferred over a simple one-trial, one-vote method. The latter method is discouraged because low quality trials should not be given the same weight as high quality trials. The reviews on acupuncture for low back pain by Tulder and colleagues [33] and for chronic pain by Berman and colleagues [27], demonstrate this approach.

As has already been noted, bias can occur if high quality studies are combined with low quality studies. One way to assess whether low quality studies may be biasing results is to perform a sensitivity analysis. This method combines the results of both high and low quality trials and compares these results to those of the high quality trials alone. If the combined low and high results appear more optimistic than the high quality results alone, then bias may be at work.

Bias can also occur if the reviewers inadvertently count the same trial twice (duplicate bias). Duplicate bias occurs when two articles appear sufficiently different so that the reviewers fail to realize that they actually represent the same trial. If the duplicate trial has a positive result, it biases results towards the positive side, whereas, if the trial has a negative or nonsignificant result, it biases results the other way. Duplicate bias is no small problem in systematic reviews and can exaggerate a treatment effect by as much as 20 % [34].

7.2.2
Validity of the Acupuncture Procedure:
Assessing the Quality of the Acupuncture Treatment

So far, most of the discussion about trial validity has concerned how the methodological quality of trial design can bias trial outcome. However, inadequate acupuncture treatment can also jeopardize trial validity and bias outcome. Basing conclusions about acupuncture efficacy on suboptimal or inadequate acupuncture procedures is analogous to pharmaceutical trials formulating conclusions about the efficacy of drugs based on inadequate dose. While some conditions such as nausea and vomiting have a straightforward, commonly accepted acupuncture procedure (i.e., the stimulation of P6), other conditions such as chronic pain have tremendously different treatment approaches. Therefore, the question of acupuncture treatment adequacy is more urgent for some conditions than for others. Although it is an issue to be addressed and defined in primary studies (e.g., cohort studies or RCTs), systematic reviews must have a method for assessing whether treatments meet basic criteria. Three methods have been used to assess the adequacy of acupuncture procedures retrospectively.

One way that reviewers have retrospectively assessed acupuncture treatment adequacy was first proposed by Linde et al. [6]. An acupuncturist was presented with the inclusion criteria and acupuncture methods in the papers, blinded to trial results, and asked to rate whether the acupuncture treatment was adequate to treat the condition under investigation based on five aspects: (1) points selected, (2) total number of treatments, (3) number of times per week the patient was treated, (4) duration of each session, and (5) whether or not "de qi" was elicited.

A second way of assessing acupuncture treatment quality retrospectively is to specify a minimally acceptable treatment. This approach, used by Molsberger and Bowing [35], defined a minimally adequate acupuncture treatment as consisting of at least ten total treatments of at least 15 minutes each and a description of the points used. Only 16 of 88 studies on musculoskeletal and/or neurological conditions met the minimal criteria and, of those, only two were controlled trials. What was learned from this method is that most studies do not meet the minimal criteria of an acceptable acupuncture procedure.

A third, less efficacious approach to quantifying acupuncture procedure is to identify those aspects of the acupuncture procedure that are associated with positive outcomes. Although this cannot answer the question of whether the treatment is adequate, it can provide important information for guiding future clinical trials. Patel and colleagues [30] used this approach with their pooled data. They noted that individualized treatments significantly favored acupuncture, whereas formulaic approaches, in which all the patients received the same treatment, fared less positively. They proposed that individualized acupuncture treatments might produce better outcomes than cookbook approaches but that these findings could be confounded by the methodological quality of the trials.

This third approach was also used in a recent acupuncture and chronic pain review [27]. The specific aspects of the acupuncture treatment which were hypothesized as associated with positive outcomes were based on findings reported in a doctoral thesis [36]. The thesis analyzed the acupuncture procedures in textbooks from China, Japan, and Korea seeking recommendations which could be generalized for treating certain pain conditions. No generalized recommendation could be made on the specific acupuncture points, because they varied so much from textbook to textbook. On the other hand, generalizations could be made pertaining to the recommended number of needles used and the number of total treatments administered: 6 points per treatment were probably adequate but 10 were better, and six total treatments were probably adequate but ten were better. When these hypotheses were tested in the chronic pain review [27], no association was observed between the number of points used and positive outcome, but a statistically significant association ($p <$ 0.05) was found between the total number of treatments given and the outcome, even when controlling for methodological quality of the trials. Interestingly, virtually no trial administering fewer than six acupuncture treatments achieved a positive outcome.

Although these significant findings merely show an association and not a causal relationship between six or more treatments and positive outcome, like Patel's observation about individualized treatments, they may be able to guide future studies. Given the paucity of information as to what constitutes an adequate acupuncture treatment, it is advisable to compare the effectiveness of various acupuncture protocols in a small pilot study to ascertain the preferred procedure before conducting a larger RCT. One common problem in assessing an acupuncture procedure retrospectively is that very few trials present sufficient information about the acupuncture procedure to assess its adequacy. For example, data on the various aspects of the acupuncture treatment were extracted for one chronic pain review [27] but found to be insufficient for assessment. The problem of missing information was also encountered by ter Reit and colleagues [4] when they attempted to use a proxy measure for treatment adequacy by assessing whether the papers reported on the extent of training and experience of the acupuncturist. What has been learned from this method is that reporting on the details of the acupuncture procedure needs to be improved in trials.

7.2.3
Summary

In conclusion, summarizing evidence can be likened to Aesop's story of the blind men and the elephant:

Each of five blind men is asked to touch an elephant and describe what the animal looks like. One blind man feels the tail and claims the animal is long and thin like a rope. Another, feeling the elephant's leg, insists that the animal is round, thick, and solid like a tree trunk. And so on.

As children hearing this story, we were amused at the obvious foolishness of each man forming an opinion of the elephant based on one small study. Now, as researchers and clinicians, we are challenged to transcend the mistaken assumption that one small study represents the whole reality. Small RCTs, which are typical of current acu-

Table 3. Eight reasons to use systematic reviews [9]

1. Large quantities of information must be reduced to palatable pieces for digestion
2. Various decision makers need to integrate the critical pieces of available biomedical information
3. It is an efficient scientific technique
4. The generalisability of scientific findings can be established
5. The consistency of relationships can be assessed
6. Inconsistencies and conflicts in data can be examined
7. When meta-analysis is performed, they increase power and precision
8. They offer an improved reflection of reality over traditional reviews

puncture trials, seldom answer efficacy questions definitively. A trial may lack sufficient power to detect a difference that exists in reality (known as a type II or false negative error), it may be biased, or the results may be applicable only to a certain group of people or patients but not to all. There are many advantages to using the systematic reviews method (Table 3). In short, this offers the most comprehensive way to describe "the elephant."

7.3
A Summary of the Results of Systematic Reviews of Acupuncture

This section summarizes the results of systematic acupuncture reviews. The first part of this section will summarize the systematic reviews which have been done for painful conditions. The remaining part will summarize the results of systematic reviews for other conditions, such as acupuncture for nausea and vomiting or for asthma (Table 4).

7.3.1
Acupuncture for Painful Conditions

7.3.1.1
Is Acupuncture Effective for Chronic Pain?

Patel and colleagues [30] published the first systematic review on chronic pain, observing that few of the 14 acupuncture trials included had statistically significant results. However, the pooled results favored acupuncture. Furthermore, pooled subgroup analyses by site of pain significantly favored acupuncture for low back pain and head/neck pain. However, statistical pooling produced another interesting finding: when trials with some degree of blinding (of patients and/or outcomes assessors) were compared to trials with no blinding, the unblinded trials significantly favored acupuncture, whereas the blinded trials did not. One interpretation for this is that lack of blinding may have biased the results to favor acupuncture. Other methodological deficiencies were also noted, and the more methodologically rigorous trials tended to yield less favorable results. Because of this, the authors stated that, although the pooled results favoring acupuncture were statistically significant, the various sources of bias prevented this finding from being a definitive conclusion.

Ter Reit and colleagues [4] published a more extensive systematic review on chronic pain the following year, including an extensive search strategy and a way of

Table 4. A summary of acupuncture systematic reviews

First author	Condition	Objective	Inclusion criteria	N studies included	Major outcomes	Results[a]
Patel 1989 [30]	Chronic pain	Investigate whether individually inconclusive trials would yield a definitive result when results were pooled	All RCTs published in English and listed in Index Medicus from 1970 onwards	14	Pain relief	Inconclusive
ter Reit 1990 [4]	Chronic pain	Assess whether acupuncture is efficacious in chronic pain	Needles used, "chronic" mentioned in title or abstract or patient selection criteria stated that pain had existed for at least 6 months, a reference group	51	Pain relief	Inconclusive
Ezzo 2000 [27]	Chronic pain	Assess the efficacy of acupuncture for chronic pain within the context of the studies' methodological quality	RCTs published in English, pain greater than 3 months	51	Pain relief	Limited evidence that acupuncture is better than waiting list; inconclusive evidence for acupuncture vs placebo, sham acupuncture, or standard care
Tulder, 1999 (33)	Low back pain	Assess the effectiveness of acupuncture for acute and chronic low back pain	RCTs with an acupuncture treatment for acute or chronic low back pain	11	Pain relief	Inconclusive
Ernst 1997 (39)	Osteoarthritis	Evaluate the effectiveness of acupuncture for osteoarthritis	Controlled trials on human patients symptomatic with osteoarthritis	13	Pain relief	Inconclusive
Berman 1999 [42]	Fibromyalgia	Assess the effectiveness of acupuncture for fibromyalgia, report adverse effects, and generate hypotheses for future investigation	All RCTs or cohort studies of fibromyalgia patients treated with acupuncture	7	Pain reduction, increased pain threshold, sleep quality, depression, morning stiffness	Positive with reservations
Ernst 1997 [45]	Acute dental pain	Assess the effectiveness of acupuncture in dental pain	Controlled trials testing acupuncture as a treatment of dental pain in humans	16	Pain	Positive

Table 4. (Cont.)

First author	Condition	Objective	Inclusion criteria	N studies included	Major outcomes	Results[a]
Melchart 1999 [47]	Headache	Evaluate whether acupuncture is effective in relief of recurrent headache	Randomized or quasirandomized trials comparing acupuncture to any type of control intervention	22	One clinical outcome related to headache (e.g., pain intensity, global assessment)	Positive trend toward real vs. sham acupuncture; inconclusive for real acupuncture vs. other forms of treatment
Vickers 1996 [50]	Nausea and vomiting	Evaluate the effectiveness of stimulating P6 for treating nausea and/or vomiting associated with chemotherapy, pregnancy or surgery	Trials in which P6 acupoint stimulation by needling, manual pressure, or electricity was compared with intervention, placebo or nonacupuncture intervention	33	Number and duration of vomiting episodes, symptom-free patient days, nausea score	Positive
White 1997 [31]	Tobacco addiction	Evaluate whether acupuncture has a specific effect in smoking cessation beyond placebo effects	All RCTs comparing a form of acupuncture with either sham acupuncture, another intervention, or no intervention	16	Complete abstinence from smoking after first treatment and at 6 and 12 months	Negative
Kleijnen 1991 [5]	Asthma	Ascertain whether clear conclusions could be obtained by assessing as many studies as possible according to methodological criteria	Trials in which a needle and a reference group were used. (not necessarily RCTs)	13	Measures of lung capacity (FEV, forced vital capacity, peak expiratory flow rate), or subjective improvement	Inconclusive
Linde 1996 [6]	Asthma	Evaluate the effectiveness of acupuncture for the treatment of asthma bronchiale	RCTs of acupuncture for the treatment of asthma or asthma-like symptoms	7	Objective measures of lung function (FEV, forced vital capacity, peak expiratory flow rate); subjective measures of improvement, global rating, quality of life	Inconclusive
Hammerschlag 1997 [51]	Various	Examine the design and reporting of trials comparing acupuncture to standard medical care	All clinical trials comparing acupuncture with standard medical care	23	Methodological quality scores	Only three of the studies were rated as adequate

[a] Results: positive, significantly favors acupuncture; inconclusive, no conclusions can be made at this time; negative, evidence convincingly shows no benefit from acupuncture; limited evidence, based on several low quality positive trials.

Table 5. Levels of evidence in best evidence synthesis [33]. Generally consistent outcomes mean that three fourths or more of the studies should have the same results (either positive or negative)

Strong evidence	Multiple, relevant, high quality RCTs with generally consistent outcomes
Moderate evidence	One relevant, high quality RCT and one or more relevant, low quality RCTs with generally consistent outcomes
Limited evidence	One relevant, high quality RCT or multiple relevant low quality RCTs with generally consistent outcomes
No evidence	Only one relevant, low quality RCT, no relevant high quality RCTs, or RCTs with inconsistent outcomes

scoring trial methodology. Their findings were inconclusive, noting that no studies emerged as high quality, making it impossible to draw definitive conclusions.

In the decade since the ter Reit review was published, a validated quality assessment scale has been developed (Table 2) [24], a notable number of high quality randomized trials of acupuncture for chronic pain have been published, and, due to the formation of the Cochrane Collaboration [52], systematic review methodology has become more explicit. Therefore, the question of acupuncture for chronic pain was recently revisited in another systematic review which used the best evidence synthesis method (Table 5) [27]. There, a slightly different efficacy question is asked depending on the comparison group used in an acupuncture trial. In the best evidence synthesis review [27], the comparison groups were therefore categorized according to the similarity of the question being answered. The results by type of comparison group were: limited evidence that acupuncture is more effective than no treatment (waiting list) and inconclusive evidence that acupuncture is more effective than inert placebo (sham TENS or sugar pills), sham acupuncture, or standard medical care.

7.3.1.2
Is Acupuncture Effective in the Treatment of Low Back Pain?

Although Patel and colleagues [30] found acupuncture to be effective in low back pain in meta-analysis, they warned that the results should be interpreted with caution because of design flaws. Tulder and colleagues [33] recently revisited the question of acupuncture for chronic low back pain using the best evidence synthesis method (Table 5). Nine of the 11 trials included were of low quality and had small sample sizes. The contradictory results and few high quality RCTs were the reasons given that the authors classified the evidence as level 4 (Table 5), concluding there is no evidence that acupuncture is an effective treatment for chronic low back pain.

Since the systematic review was published, Molsberger and colleagues [38] have completed a large, methodologically rigorous trial assessing two questions: (1) Can acupuncture contribute as an adjunctive therapy to the conservative management of LBP? and (2) Is real acupuncture superior to sham acupuncture? In a three-arm parallel group design, 186 low back pain patients with pain for more than 6 weeks and a pain intensity score greater than 50 on the visual analogue scale (VAS) were randomly assigned to one of three groups. Patients in all groups received a baseline treatment consisting of conservative orthopedic therapy everyday.

Real acupuncture, consisting of 12 acupuncture treatments at 30 minutes each, was added to this baseline treatment in group 1. Sham acupuncture consisting of 12 sham treatments at 30 minutes each was added to the baseline treatment in group 2. Group 3 received baseline treatment only. Patients in both acupuncture groups were blinded and the outcomes assessor for all three groups was also blinded. The primary outcome was a pain reduction of 50 % or more on the VAS at 3 months after the end of treatment. Achievement of the primary outcome by group, based on intention-to-treat analysis, was: real acupuncture 76.6 %, sham acupuncture 29.3 %, and conservative orthopedic therapy 13.9 %. Additionally, for low back pain patients with pain over more than 5 years, the relative probability of experiencing 50 % or greater pain reduction was 10 times higher in real acupuncture than sham. The investigators concluded that real acupuncture is an important supplement in the management of chronic low back pain.

7.3.1.3
Is Acupuncture Effective in the Treatment of Osteoarthritis?

Of the 13 trials included in a recent systematic review [39], results were equivocal, with seven demonstrating positive results and six demonstrating nonsignificant results. Design flaws noted in the trials with positive findings included failure to control for placebo effects and lack of randomization. When RCTs were considered separately, results were still equivocal, with five trials having positive results and five having nonsignificant results. Ernst observed that four of the five trials comparing real acupuncture to sham acupuncture yielded nonsignificant findings.

Two large trials, both with positive findings, were not included in this systematic review [40, 41]. In a comparison of real vs. sham acupuncture ($n = 97$), Molsberger and colleagues [40] found that real acupuncture significantly outperformed sham acupuncture for pain relief at 3 months following the end of the acupuncture treatment ($p < 0.05$). However, functional improvement did not differ significantly between groups.

A second trial [41] comparing acupuncture as an adjunct to standard medical care vs. standard medical care alone, showed significantly more improvement in the acupuncture group ($p < 0.05$) in both pain and functional indices. These significant differences continued to be observed at both 4 and 8 weeks follow-up.

The results of these two trials, which were notably larger than the trials included in the systematic review, raise the question of whether the nonsignificant results of the earlier trials were a result of small sample size (type II error) rather than the equivocacy of the two treatments.

7.3.1.4
Is Acupuncture Effective in the Treatment of Fibromyalgia?

A recent systematic review of acupuncture for fibromyalgia syndrome (FMS) included both RCTs and cohort studies [42]. It was decided a priori that high quality RCTs would be used for hypothesis (efficacy) testing, whereas low quality RCTs and cohort studies would be used for hypothesis generation. Quality assessment revealed only one high quality RCT. Scoring a perfect quality score, the one high quality RCT

[43] demonstrated that real acupuncture is more effective than sham acupuncture in relieving pain, increasing pain thresholds, and improving global ratings. However, because long-term follow-up was not performed, the duration of benefit following completion of the acupuncture series could not be ascertained.

Based on the outcomes in the studies used for hypothesis generation, three important questions were raised:

1. Can booster doses sustain benefit in responders? The use of periodic booster doses of acupuncture was anecdotally described in two cohort studies as an effective way to sustain benefit in responders, once regular sessions ceased, but remains to be tested in an RCT.

2. What is the optimal acupuncture treatment for FMS? The high quality RCT used a combination of low and high electrical frequencies, which is consistent with acupuncture analgesia literature suggesting that optimal pain relief can be achieved by combining low (2–4 Hz) and high (50–100 Hz) frequencies [43]. However, comparing the combined frequencies approach to other approaches remains to be tested in the same fibromyalgia population.

3. Does acupuncture work synergistically with antidepressant medication? One study noted that the combined use of acupuncture and antidepressants appeared to be more globally effective across the many dimensions of pain, depression, and sleep than either acupuncture or antidepressants alone, suggesting synergistic benefits of acupuncture plus medication [44]. However, due to methodological shortcomings of the study, the synergism remains to be tested under rigorous conditions.

7.3.1.5
Is Acupuncture Effective in the Treatment of Acute Dental Pain?

Ernst and Pittler concluded in a systematic review that acupuncture is effective in alleviating pain during or after dental operations [45]. This is consistent with the NIH consensus panel opinion that "there is evidence of efficacy for postoperative dental pain [1]." Mechanisms of action for the analgesic effects may be endorphin release, afferent pathway blockade, and/or efferent pathway inhibition. They noted that the methodological details and quality varied among studies, which limited the generalizations that could be made. Among the most common methodological shortcomings cited were nonrandomization, lack of control for placebo effects, and small sample sizes. The wide variation in types of acupuncture used precluded generalizations about which procedure was superior.

Since this systematic review was published, an additional RCT ($n = 39$) comparing real vs. placebo acupuncture has been published which further substantiates the efficacy of acupuncture for dental pain [46]. Outcomes included were patients' self-reports of duration until moderate pain, time until use of medication, total pain relief, pain half gone, and total pain medication consumption over 7 days. Results demonstrated that the mean pain-free postoperative time was significantly longer in the acupuncture group than in the placebo acupuncture group ($p = 0.01$), as was duration of time until moderate pain ($p = 0.008$). The time until use of medication was significantly longer in the acupuncture group ($p = 0.01$).

In addition to giving more evidence that acupuncture is effective in the treatment of dental pain, this recent RCT makes three other important observations:

1. Acupuncture was significantly superior to placebo acupuncture in preventing pain before it began but was not more effective than placebo acupuncture after the pain had reached moderate intensity. This observation may suggest that acupuncture is most effective when administered preemptively rather than once the pain begins.
2. When compared to real acupuncture, placebo acupuncture was associated with more adverse effects directly related to the tooth excision procedure. This may suggest that real acupuncture is protective against some of the adverse effects of surgery.
3. The dental pain technique used in this study is a commonly accepted acute pain model used to assess analgesic drugs. The favorable findings of acupuncture using this model suggest that acupuncture may be valuable as an analgesic for other types of acute pain besides dental pain.

7.3.1.6
Is Acupuncture Effective in the Treatment of Headache?

Melchart and colleagues [47] conducted a systematic review assessing the efficacy of acupuncture in the treatment of tension headache and migraine. To score the results for each included trial, at least two reviewers voted on each trial using the following five categories as the classifications: (1) control significantly better than acupuncture, (2) trend towards control group, (3) no difference, (4) trend towards acupuncture, and (5) acupuncture significantly better than control.

The overall results using this method in trials comparing true vs. sham acupuncture in migraine and tension headache patients showed a trend in favor of true acupuncture. A more definitive statement could not be made, because most trials were small with either methodological or reporting limitations. Furthermore, due to variations in patients, trial quality, and types of acupuncture procedures used, a clear recommendation as to what constitutes the best acupuncture treatment could not be made. The trials comparing acupuncture to other headache treatments yielded insufficient evidence to assess whether acupuncture is as effective as standard medical care.

The reviewers concluded that acupuncture might have a role in the treatment of recurrent headaches, stating that although acupuncture is not completely risk-free, it is generally safe in the hands of adequately trained practitioners and, therefore, there is no reason to discourage headache sufferers interested in trying acupuncture. The reviewers also concluded that the data are not conclusive enough to justify recommending acupuncture nor can the data ascertain what kind of acupuncture is most effective for headache.

7.3.2
Acupuncture for Other Conditions

7.3.2.1
Is Acupuncture Effective in the Treatment of Asthma?

One proposed mechanism of action by which acupuncture intervenes in asthma is through the release of adrenocorticotropic hormone by the pituitary gland, which in turn results in the release of adrenal corticosteroids, a natural anti-inflammatory agent. In 1991, Kleijnen and colleagues [5] first explored the clinical evidence by assessing both randomized and nonrandomized trials. The results were inconclusive and, in 1996, Linde and colleagues [6] revisited the question, looking at only RCTs. The overall trends were similar in both reviews: the benefits of acupuncture for asthmatic attacks were inconsistent among studies. Benefits measured in long-term follow-up were characterized more by subjective reports of improvement than by objective improvements in pulmonary function.

Although the findings were equivocal, their interpretation varied. Linde and colleagues concluded that "up to now, there is insufficient data from randomized clinical trials to assess reliably the efficacy and effectiveness of acupuncture in the treatment of asthma [6]." In a narrative review, Jobst offered a more generous interpretation, saying that there is "no reason to withhold acupuncture as a safe and potentially effective treatment in patients with bronchial asthma and chronic obstructive lung disease" [48].

The most important issue raised by the review by Linde et al. is that only one trial compared acupuncture to standard care or as an adjunct to standard care. The authors emphasized that trials comparing sham vs. real acupuncture are not clinically useful and do not assess acupuncture as it is actually used in practice. Because standard care is already quite effective for asthma, the choice to use acupuncture should not be made in place of standard care, but rather as an adjunct to it. In fact, avoidable deaths from asthma have been reported when patients have refused conventional care in preference for acupuncture [49]. The best recommendation based on the available evidence comes from the NIH consensus panel: "acupuncture treatment for asthma should be part of a comprehensive management program" [1]. Whether acupuncture has some adjunctive benefit as part of a comprehensive asthma treatment program remains to be seen. What is certain is that trials comparing real and sham acupuncture or a placebo offer little of substantial clinical relevance. Furthermore, it is also unethical to withhold treatment when effective standard care exists.

7.3.2.2
Is Acupuncture Effective in the Treatment of Nausea and Vomiting?

Perhaps the most compelling and consistent evidence for the efficacy of acupuncture is in the treatment of nausea and vomiting [50]. Of the 29 trials in which acupuncture was used while the patient was fully awake (not under anesthesia), 27 favored acupuncture. When only trials of the highest methodological quality were examined, 11 out of these 12 trials, representing nearly 2000 patients, showed positive results. The positive results are strikingly consistent, although the high quality trials represent different investigators, patients, and an assortment of ways in which P6 was stimulated. These findings are summarized by the NIH consensus panel in its affirmative statement that "there is clear evidence that needle acupuncture is efficacious for adult postoperative and chemotherapy nausea and vomiting and probably for the nausea of pregnancy" [1].

Interestingly, the four trials in which P6 was stimulated while the patients were under anesthesia all demonstrated acupuncture to be ineffective in preventing nausea and vomiting. The reason for this is not clear. However, Vickers offers three possibilities: (1) P6 stimulation may behave like conventional antiemetic drugs and must be administered preemptively, before the emetic stimulus occurs, (2) the mechanism of action may require an intact nervous system, or (3) acupuncture may work by psychological mechanisms. This last possibility is unlikely, however, because stimulation of a fake point consistently has a lower antiemetic effect than P6, even though the fake points are credible to patients. That inappropriately high levels of P6 stimulation can increase nausea and vomiting also argues against the effects of P6 as a purely psychological phenomenon.

7.3.2.3
Is Acupuncture Effective in Smoking Cessation?

The 16 studies included in a systematic review [31] were methodologically inadequate in that they seldom reported details of randomization or used biochemical indicators to validate self-reports of smoking cessation. Variations in trial quality made it difficult to ascertain whether one type of acupuncture (e.g., auricular vs. body acupuncture) was superior.

The pooled results demonstrated that real acupuncture provided no statistically significant benefit compared to sham acupuncture or other antismoking treatments at any time point (less than 6 weeks, at 6 or 12 months). This is consistent with the NIH consensus opinion that "there is evidence that acupuncture does *not* demonstrate efficacy for cessation of smoking" [1]. In the short run, acupuncture appeared to be better than doing nothing (no intervention). However, this benefit attenuated over time and had disappeared by 6-month follow-up. The negative conclusion of this review suggests that research should focus on whether acupuncture can ameliorate the adverse symptoms of acute withdrawal rather than provide long lasting cessation of tobacco use. One question not addressed in this review is whether long lasting cessation may have been achieved, had acupuncture treatments been continued.

7.3.2.4
What Can Be Learned in Trials Comparing Acupuncture
to Standard Medical Care?

Generally, systematic reviews address a specific clinical question. However, systematic review methodology can also be used to answer methodological questions. For example, it is of great interest to the scientific community to know how acupuncture compares to standard medical care. Hammerschlag and Morris recently examined how well this type of important trial has been performed and presented [51]. They included only trials for which standard care was either cited or computer-search identified as previously having outperformed placebo in an RCT. Trials were selected independently of outcome. Only three of the 23 studies were rated as adequate on at least 60 % of the evaluation criteria. Two of the most important elements of a trial showed very different scores: randomization was reported in 20 (87 %) of the trials, whereas blinding of the outcomes assessor was reported in only four (17 %).

Their summary also highlights what can be learned from the highest quality studies: "By reviewing those studies that were scored adequate for each criterion, informative examples can be gleaned: acupuncture had a more rapid analgesic onset than Avafortan for relieving renal colic; when used as adjunctive treatment to physical therapy, acupuncture enabled a significantly greater percent of low back pain patients to return to their original or equivalent jobs relative to those treated with physical therapy alone; and while acupuncture was as effective as the beta blocker metoprolol for reducing the frequency and duration of migraine attacks, it had fewer side effects but was patient-rated as less effective than metoprolol in global effect on headaches [51].

7.4
Looking to the Future: The Role of the Cochrane Collaboration in Conducting and Maintaining Systematic Reviews

The Cochrane Collaboration was formed in 1993 with the explicit and sole purpose of conducting, maintaining, and disseminating systematic reviews relevant to all aspects of health care [52]. For systematic reviews to be optimally valuable to users, reviews must be widely disseminated and regularly updated to accommodate new information as it becomes available. To meet the growing need for systematic literature reviews as a way of synthesizing evidence and contributing to evidence-based medicine, Cochrane reviews have an explicit and transparent methodology, are peer reviewed, use an electronic format conducive to regular updates, are consumer reviewed to ensure readability, and have been available on MEDLINE in abstract form as of 1999. Therefore, the Cochrane Collaboration offers health care a forum of international and interdisciplinary cooperation and an important vehicle for timely and accessible dissemination of evidence.

The complementary medicine field within the Cochrane Collaboration [53, 54] specializes in producing systematic reviews related to complementary medicine, including acupuncture. In the future, we believe that the Cochrane Collaboration will be one of the most important vehicles serving clinicians, consumers, researchers, and policy makers who want timely and comprehensive summaries on the clinical effectiveness of acupuncture[1].

Acknowledgement. We would like to express our appreciation to Victoria Hadhazy, MA, for her kind assistance in preparing this manuscript.

References

1. NIH Consensus Conference (1998) Acupuncture. JAMA 280:1518–1524
2. McQuay H, Moore A (1998) An evidence-based resource for pain relief. Oxford Medical Publications, Oxford, p 3
3. Sackett DL, Richardson WS, Rosenberg W, Haynes RB (1997) Evidence-based medicine: How to practice and teach EBM. Churchill Livingstone, NewYork, pp. 4–5
4. ter Reit GK, Kleijnen J, Knipschild P (1990) Acupuncture and chronic pain: A criteria-based meta-analysis. J Clin Epidemiol 43:1191–1200
5. Kleijnen J, ter Reit G, Knipschild P (1991) Acupuncture and asthma: A review of controlled trials. Thorax 46:799–802
6. Linde K, Worku F, Stor W, Wiesner-Zechmeister M, Pothmann R, Weinschutz T, Melchart D (1996) Randomized clinical trials of acupuncture for asthma – a systematic review. Forsch Komplementarmed 3:148–155

---

[1] To subscribe to the Cochrane Collaboration library, contact Update Software, 936 La Rueda, Vista CA 92084, USA

7. Jacobson LD, Edwards AG, Granier SK, Butler CC (1997) Evidence-based medicine and general practice. Br J Gen Pract 47:449–452
8. Rangachari PK (1997) Evidence-based medicine: Old French wine with a new Canadian label? J R Soc Med 90:280–284
9. Mulrow C (1994) Rationale for systematic reviews. BMJ 309:597–599
10. Knipschild P (1994) Systematic reviews: Some examples. BMJ 309:719–721
11. Dickersin K, Manheimer E (1998) The Cochrane Collaboration: Evaluation of health care and services using systematic reviews of the results of randomized controlled trials. Clin Obstet Gynecol 41:315–331
12. Lehmann HP, Goodman SN (1995) Specifications for formalizing clinical significance. Med Decision Making 15:424
13. Bero LA, Jadad AR (1997) How consumers and policymakers can use systematic reviews for decision making. Ann Intern Med 127:37–42
14. Baussell RB (1993) After the meta-analytic revolution. Evaluation and the Health Profession 1993;16:2–12
15. Meinert C (1989) Meta-analysis: Science or religion. Controlled Clin Trials 10:257S–263S
16. O'Toole LB (1998) Using systematically synthesized evidence to inform the funding of new clinical trials – the UK Medical Research Council approach. Paper presented at Sixth International Cochrane Colloquium, Baltimore
17. Dickersin K, Scherer L, Lefevbre C (1997) Identifying relevant studies for systematic reviews. In: Chalmers I and Altman D (eds) Systematic reviews. BMJ Press, London
18. Hofmans EA (1990) Acupuncture and MEDLINE. Lancet 336:357
19. Knipschild P(1993) Searching for alternatives: Loser pays. Lancet 341:1135–1136
20. Cook DJ, Guyatt GH, Ryan G et al (1993) Should unpublished data be included in meta-analyses? JAMA 269:2749–2753
21. Dickersin K, Min Y, Meinert CL (1992) Factors influencing publication of research results. JAMA 267:374–378
22. Callaham ML, Wears RL, Weber EJ, Barton C, Young G (1998) Positive-outcome bias and other limitations in the outcome of research abstracts submitted to a scientific meeting. JAMA 280:254–257
23. Egger M, Zellweger-Zahner T, Schneider M, Junker C, Lengeler C, Antes G (1997) Language bias in randomized controlled trials published in English and German. Lancet 350:326–329
24. Jadad AR (1996) Blind assessment of the quality of trial reports. Controlled Clin Trials 17:1–12
25. Schultz KF, Chalmers I, Hayes RJ, Altman DG (1995) Empirical evidence of bias: Dimensions of methodological quality associated with estimate of treatment effects in controlled trials. JAMA 273:408–412
26. Khan KS, Daya S, Jadad A (1996) The importance of quality of primary studies in producing unbiased systematic reviews. Arch Intern Med 156:661–666
27. Ezzo J, Berman B, Hadhazy V, Jadad A, Lao L, Singh B (2000) Is acupuncture effective for the treatment of chronic pain? A systematic review. Pain 86:217–225
28. ter Riet G, Kleijnen J, Knipschild P (1990) A meta-analysis of studies into the effect of acupuncture on addiction. Br J Gen Pract 40:379–382
29. Moher D, Fortin R, Jadad AR, et al. (1996) Completeness of reporting of trials published in languages other than English. Lancet 347:363–366
30. Patel M, Gutzwiller F, Paccaud F, Marazzi A (1989) A meta-analysis of acupuncture for chronic pain. Int J Epidemiol 18:900–906
31. White AR, Rampes H (1998) Acupuncture for smoking cessation (Cochrane review). In: The Cochrane Library, Issue 3. Update Software, Oxford
32. Slavin R (1995) Best evidence synthesis: An intelligent alternative to meta-analysis. J Clin Epidemiol 48:9–18
33. van Tulder MW, Cherkin DC, Berman B, Lao L, Koes BW (1999) The effectiveness of acupuncture in the treatment of low back pain (Cochrane review). In: The Cochrane Library, Issue 1. Update Software, Oxford
34. Tramer MR, Reynolds DJ, Moore RA, McQuay HJ (1997) Impact of covert duplicate publication on meta-analysis: A case study. BMJ 315:635–640
35. Molsberger A, Bowing G (1997) Acupuncture for pain in locomotive disorders. Critical analysis of clinical studies with respect to the quality of acupuncture in particular. Der Schmerz 11:24–29
36. Birch S (1997) An exploration with proposed solutions of the problems and issues in conducting clinical research in acupuncture. University of Exeter; Exeter
37. Chalmers I, Altman D (eds) (1997) Systematic reviews. BMJ Press, London
38. Molsberger A (1998) Acupuncture in chronic low back pain. Paper presented at the International Society for the Study of the Lumbar Spine, Brussels

39. Ernst E (1997) Acupuncture as a symptomatic treatment of osteoarthritis: A systematic review. Scand J Rheumatol 26:444–447
40. Molsberger A, Bowing G, Jensen KU, Lorek M (1994) Schmerztherapie mit Akupunktur bei Gonarthrose: eine kontrollierte Studie zur analgetischen Wirkung der Akupunktur bei Gonarthrose. Der Schmerz 8:37–42
41. Berman B, Singh BB, Lao L, Langenberg P, Li H, Hadhazy V, Bareta J, Hochberg M (1999) A randomized trial of acupuncture as an adjunctive therapy in osteoarthritis of the knee. Rheumatol 39:346–354
42. Berman B, Ezzo J, Hadhazy V, Swyers J (1999) Is acupuncture an effective treatment for fibromyalgia? A clinical review. J Fam Pract 48:213–218
43. Deluze C, Bosia L, Zirbs A, Chantraine A, Vischer TL (1992) Electroacupuncture in fibromyalgia: Results of a controlled trial. BMJ 305:1249–1252
44. Cassisi G, Roncaglione A, Ceccherelli F, Donolato C, Gagliardi G, Todesco S (1995) Trattamento agopunturale dell fibromyalgia primaria. Confronto con mianserena. G Ital Reflessot Agopunt 7:33–36
45. Ernst E, Pittler MH (1998) The effectiveness of acupuncture in treating acute dental pain: A systematic review. Br Dent J 184:443–447
46. Lao L, Bergman S, Hamilton GR, Langenberg P, Berman B (1999) Evaluation of acupuncture for pain control after oral surgery: A placebo-controlled trial. Arch Otolaryngol Head Neck Surg 125:567–572
47. Melchart K, Linde K, Fischer P, Berman B, White A, Vickers A, Allais G (1999) Acupuncture for recurrent headaches (Cochrane review). In: The Cochrane Library, Issue 3. Update Software, Oxford
48. Jobst KA (1995) A critical analysis of acupuncture in pulmonary disease: Efficacy and safety of the acupuncture needle. J Altern Comp Med 1:57–84
49. O'Mathuna DP (1998) Acupuncture for quick relief of asthmatic exacerbation. Alternative Med Alert 1:109–113
50. Vickers AJ (1996) Can acupuncture have specific effects on health? A systematic review of acupuncture antiemesis trials. J R Soc Med 89:303–311
51. Hammerschlag R, Morris MM (1997) Clinical trials comparing acupuncture with biomedical standard care: A criteria-based evaluation of research design and reporting. Complement Ther Med 5:133–140
52. Bero L, Rennie D (1995) The Cochrane Collaboration: preparing, maintaining, and disseminating systematic reviews of the effects of health care. JAMA 274(24):1935–1938
53. (1998) The complementary medicine field module. The Cochrane Library [database on disk and CD-ROM]. Vol. 4 Update Software, Oxford
54. Ezzo J, Berman B, Vickers A, Linde K (1998) Complementary medicine and the Cochrane Collaboration. JAMA 280:1628–1630

An Overview of Acupuncture in the Treatment of Stroke, Addiction, and Other Health Problems

S. Birch

8.1
Introduction

Acupuncture has been used and tested in a wide range of health problems [16]. Often there are only one or two studies in a particular area and systematic reviews have thus not yet been possible. This chapter will focus on a number of areas with at least two controlled clinical trials or at least one controlled and one noncontrolled clinical trial. This is not a systematic review; rather it is an overview of the quality of the clinical trials in these areas. It is also not intended to be an exhaustive review but more as an introduction and overview of important areas where as yet limited research has been done. The chapter is thus an overview of potentially promising areas where acupuncture is used and further clinical and scientific work should be focused.

The central theme of this chapter, the quality of research, was chosen in part because there are not enough studies in each area to draw clear conclusions about efficacy and in part because reviewers have found a wide range of methodological problems in clinical trials of acupuncture [2, 4, 14, 15, 19, 27, 31, 34, 35, 37, 38, 49, 50, 52, 55, 58, 60, 76, 81, 83–85]. Key problems we found are inadequate sample size, inadequate treatment, inappropriate control treatment, inadequate follow-up, inadequate control of nonspecific effects, inadequate reporting of side effects, and a few studies' failure to replicate results. These problems make it very difficult to draw clear conclusions about efficacy in most areas where acupuncture has been tested, including those covered in this chapter. Some studies clearly show good or very promising results [1, 22, 43, 70], but much better quality research is needed [4]. A recent U. S. National Institutes of Health consensus development conference on acupuncture listed stroke rehabilitation and addiction among a number of clinical conditions as "disorders for which the research evidence is less convincing but for which there are some positive clinical trials" [4]. There has been enough good research for discussion but not yet enough to draw clear conclusions.

8.2
Preliminary Analysis

A wide range of control groups has been used in these studies. Acupuncture has been compared to various forms of control acupuncture, to standard care, placebo medication, placebo transcutaneous electrical nerve stimulation (TENS), no treatment, and historical controls, i.e., in retrospective comparisons with results from other studies.

This diversity of models makes the task of designing and performing systematic reviews or meta-analyses more difficult. For example, the fact that acupuncture does not outperform a standard therapy is not necessarily a negative result. As long as it has the same or less cost and the same or fewer side effects, it remains a viable treatment option, and thus results could be interpreted positively. But if acupuncture does not significantly outperform in comparisons with control acupuncture, this tends to indicate that the acupuncture is not effective. It becomes difficult to make a straight comparison of these two models. Also, in studies where the efficacy of acupuncture was examined in something like ease and pain of childbirth, it is not necessary to make long-term assessments to find clinically significant results. But in other studies it is essential that long-term results be examined to achieve clinical significance. Thus, not all studies are comparable on the criterion of length of follow-up.

In general, there has been a major problem with the inadequate treatment often administered in acupuncture studies [15, 73]. If a control acupuncture model is used, it is important that the control treatment is appropriate. A study using a needling treatment as valid as the test acupuncture treatment is not appropriate for controls [15]. In studies that use control acupuncture or placebo control design, some researchers have suggested that it is not enough simply to state that the study was placebo-controlled but that the nonspecific effects must also be assessed using, for example, the credibility scale [14, 82, 84]. Studies using placebo or control acupuncture designs without these assessments can be difficult to interpret. In many, the treatments are also inadequately described, so that the studies become nonreproducible and are therefore less useful [15]. Further, to avoid bias, studies comparing acupuncture to standard care generally need larger sample sizes, as it is more likely that the treatment effects will appear similar with smaller numbers. Some analyses have found that the quality of acupuncture research appears to be improving over time [38]; thus it is useful to consider whether later studies are better than earlier ones. These general issues are all important in an examination of the areas covered in this review.

This review will not prejudge which methodology to use. There has been a wide range of research models applied in acupuncture studies [4, 37, 50], each with advantages and disadvantages. Each answers different questions and has specific study design needs. Some of the needs to be met are dependent upon the research design; some are independent. For example, adequate acupuncture treatment needs to be applied, regardless of the study design. Researchers have shown that this is a major problem in acupuncture studies, with suboptimal or completely inadequate treatments often being administered [14, 15, 73]. There is also a need for the treatment to be properly described so as to allow readers to assess what was done. This, too, has been a frequent problem [15].

Different reviewers have used varied criteria to rate or judge the quality of clinical trials [27, 34, 38, 50, 52, 60, 65, 68, 76]. Since the present review is also intended as an assessment of the quality of acupuncture trials, the author has chosen the following design criteria.

8.3
Primary Evaluative Criteria

The 33 studies were examined according to the following criteria:
1. Was the study randomized?
2. Was there an adequate description of the acupuncture treatment (possible answers: yes/no)?
3. Was the acupuncture treatment adequate (yes/possibly/no/unclear)?
4. Was the training of the acupuncturist mentioned (yes/no/not applicable)?
5. Was the control treatment (CT) adequately described (yes/no/not applicable)?
6. Was the CT appropriate (yes/no/unclear/not applicable)?
7. Was a sample size calculation presented (yes/no/not applicable)?
8. Were the evaluators blinded (yes/no/not applicable)?
9. Was there follow-up after 3 or more months (yes/no/not applicable)?
10. Were side effects monitored and presented (yes/no)?

Items 2–6 relate to important design issues of controlled acupuncture trials. Items 1 and 7–10 are relevant for virtually any controlled clinical trial.

8.4
General Findings

In Tables 1–8, one can see the following: the 33 studies were published in the period from 1985 to 1999, inclusively. The majority used a prospective active (noninert) control treatment (26/33). Overall, 29 studies found results favoring acupuncture. Dividing the studies in half, 16 were published in the period 1985–1993 and 17 in 1994–1999. Taking this arbitrary division, one can see a general trend toward less use of the control acupuncture model and more use of the standard care model. Sample sizes in the 1994–1999 trials increased considerably compared to the earlier, 1985–1993 trials: the range increased from 16–100 to 24–878, the median increased from 35 to 49, and the mean increased from 41.8 to 129.2.

Tables 9–11 present the results of the analysis for each of the 33 papers. Table 12 summarizes these results in relation to the ten criteria. With regard to issues particularly relevant to acupuncture trials: the majority of the studies (31) had an adequate description of the treatment. The treatment was clearly adequate in only 17. The qualifications of the acupuncturist were mentioned in only eight. The majority of the studies that needed to describe the control treatment gave an adequate description (20/27). The majority appeared to use an appropriate control treatment (17/28). With regard to general study design, one can see that the majority of the studies were randomized (25/30) and used blinded evaluators (19/28), only 13 of 25 included follow-up of 3 months or more, and only 16 of 33 mentioned side effects.

Table 12 also presents a summary comparison of the results of the 16 studies published in 1985–1993 and the 17 studies published in 1994–1999. One can see that studies in both time periods are comparable on all the criteria. Surprisingly, many studies in the latter period did not follow the methodology recommendations made in a number of important review papers published in the former period [55, 60, 65, 68, 76, 81, 83, 85]. For example, only 5/17 studies mentioned the qualifications of the acupuncturist, only 8/17 studies mentioned side effects, and only 9/15 used blinded evaluators. Additionally, definitely two and possibly seven more of the 17 studies still applied inadequate acupuncture treatments. However, later studies tended to use larger sample sizes and were more likely to use longer-term follow-up.

8.5
Possible Roles of Acupuncture

It is useful to examine briefly each of the major areas included in this review. Since stroke rehabilitation and addiction treatment were covered in the National Institutes of Health Consensus Development Conference and mentioned in their final report [4], it is useful to start with these.

8.5.1
Stroke Rehabilitation

Tables 1 and 9 summarize four reasonably well designed studies of adjunctive acupuncture in stroke rehabilitation. The results show consistently that if acupuncture is added to a standard care treatment regimen, the outcome is significantly better than the standard care treatment regimen alone, sometimes with significant cost reduction. This suggests a potential use of adjunctive acupuncture in the rehabilitation of stroke patients. Reviews of the use of acupuncture in stroke rehabilitation generally agree with these conclusions [33, 41, 61]. For additional studies see [63, 64].

Table 1. Controlled clinical trials in stroke rehabilitation

Condition	n	AT	CT	Primary assessments	Results
Stroke in last 3 months [62]	16	MA, EA, SC: 20 sessions in 1 month	CA, SC: 20 sessions in 1 month	Range of motion tests by blinded evaluators (pre- and post-therapy) and CT scan	AT sig > CT in patients with lesions in less than half of motor pathways
Stroke in last 10 days [43]	78	MA, EA, SC: 20 sessions AT over 10 weeks	SC only	ADL, motor function, and QOL pretherapy and at 1-, 3-, 6-, and 12-month follow-up	AT sig >CT with faster, more complete recovery; average costs AT<CT by $26,000 per patient
Stroke in last 36 hours [42]	30	MA, EA, SC: 14 sessions AT	SC only	Neurological and functional tests at 7, 14, 21, 28, and 90 days postonset	AT sig > CT in neuro-logical and functional tests at 28 and 90 days in low baseline score patients
Stroke in last 15–71 days [71]	49	MA, EA, SC: 18–24 sessions AT over 6 weeks	SC only, 6 weeks	Motor function ADL plus QOL at pre- and post-therapy	QOL: only AT sig better; motor function and ADL: sig better AT and CT but AT sig > CT

AT, acupuncture therapy; CT, control therapy; MA, manual acupuncture; EA, electroacupuncture; CA, sham acupuncture; SC, standard care; ADL, activities of daily living; QOL, quality of life; sig, significantly.

8.5.2
Addiction – Drug Dependence

Tables 2 and 9 summarize four reasonably well designed studies of adjunctive acupuncture in the treatment of addiction. The studies included focus on alcohol, cocaine, and opiate dependence. The evidence in these three areas is variable and there are contradictory results in each. However, the treatment of drug dependence is a huge and very complex problem. To date, there are few effective standard care treatment options in each of these areas, making the use of adjunctive acupuncture treatment a viable option in many drug rehabilitation programs in the U. S. and Europe [16, 20]. There are also a number of large-scale studies underway or near completion in the U. S. The author worked on a large study for cocaine addiction in methadone-maintained patients at Yale University and was a scientific advisor to a larger six-center multisite study for cocaine addiction through Columbia University [59]. Preliminary results from the Yale study are very promising (Arthur Margolin, personal communication). Looking at the evidence so far, we can see quite promising results in the area of alcohol dependence, with some promising but contradictory evidence in the areas of cocaine and opiate dependence. The results suggest there is potential for the use of acupuncture in drug rehabilitation programs, but more research is needed. For additional studies

Table 2. Controlled clinical trials in addiction

Condition	n	AT	CT	Primary assessments	Results
Severe recidivist alcoholics [22]	80	MA and SC: 15 sessions AT in 5 weeks	CA, SC: 15 sessions CT in 5 weeks	Therapy completion plus follow-up interviews at 1, 3, and 6 months post-therapy plus readmission to detoxification centers	Sig more AT than CT patients completed therapy, at 3- and 6-month follow-up AT sig>CT abstinence; AT: sig lower readmission rates
Cocaine addiction in methadone-maintained patients [57]	32	MA, SC: up to 40 sessions AT in 8 weeks	Historical controls: two medications and placebo	Urine testing for cocaine metabolites, abstinence rates, cocaine craving, study completion rates, psychosocial tests	50 % completed study, of these 88 % abstinent by end of study Depression and craving sig less AT sig better abstinence rate than amantidine, desipramine, and placebo
Crack-cocaine addiction [53]	192	MA (no counseling): up to 30 sessions AT	CA (no counseling): up to 30 sessions CT	Urine testing for cocaine metabolites plus craving and study completion rates	Reduced cocaine use in first 2 weeks, then CT group>AT group in rate of cocaine use
Heroin withdrawal [86]	100	MA and SC: up to 21 sessions AT	CA and SC: up to 21 sessions CT	Urine drug testing, withdrawal symptoms, treatment attendance, and self-reported use	Treatment attendance: AT>CT Urine testing: AT similar to CT self-reported use: AT<CT

AT, acupuncture therapy; CT, control therapy; MA, manual acupuncture; CA, sham acupuncture; SC, standard care; sig, significantly.

see [7, 21, 46, 47, 67, 87, 88]. It is important to remember that acupuncture alone is not effective in treating drug dependence. The use of acupuncture should always be as an adjunct to a standard drug rehabilitation program with individual and group counseling [20]. It should also be noted that addiction treatment research is a particularly difficult area. There are many problems to be overcome before research can be performed successfully [27].

8.5.3
Angina Pectoris

Tables 3 and 9 summarize four controlled studies on the use of acupuncture in the treatment of angina pectoris. The results of the first two are contradictory [9, 13], but the possible benefits found in the first of these studies are reinforced by the results of Richter et al. [69]. Perhaps the most interesting results are those of the fourth, larger study [10]. Here, acupuncture was added into a novel treatment plan for patients with angina pectoris. While the comparison group was only a historical control (retrospective comparison of published data for a similar patient population) so that nonspecific effects were not at all controlled, the significant benefits found suggest that it may be undesirable or unnecessary to conduct only controlled studies with appropriate nonspecific controls in the treatment of angina pectoris. Subjective and objective

Table 3. Controlled clinical trials in angina pectoris

Condition	n	AT	CT	Primary assessments	Results
Angina pectoris [9]	26	MA: 7 sessions over 3 weeks	CA: 7 sessions over 3 weeks	Diaries, exercise tests, subjective evaluation	AT sig>CT on several exercise variables but not in angina attacks More subjective evaluation items improved with AT than CT
Angina pectoris [13]	49	MA: 10 sessions over 3 weeks	CA: 10 sessions over 3 weeks	Diaries, exercise tests, subjective evaluation	AT group: sig improved exercise tolerance and delay to pain onset, but no sig differences between groups
Angina pectoris [69]	21	MA: 12 sessions over 4 weeks	Placebo medicine for 4 weeks	Exercise tests, life quality questionnaire, number angina attacks	Angina attacks: AT sig < placebo Some exercise parameters sig better with AT Some self-rating items better with AT
Angina pectoris [10]	105	MA: 12 sessions in 4 weeks plus self-care education	Retrospective comparison to drug and surgical therapies plus population survey	Rates of heart attacks and deaths, exercise tests, need for medication, costs over 5-year follow-up	AT outperformed other groups Estimated savings = $ 32,000 per AT patient Exercise tests, medication use, cardiac risk, and QOL better for AT group

AT, acupunture therapy; CT, control therapy; MA, manual acupuncture; CA, sham acupuncture; QOL, quality of life.

improvements as well as cost reduction were very significant. It may be best to consider the use of acupuncture in the treatment of angina pectoris as part of an overall treatment plan, especially one that uses self-help procedures such as those recommended in the study (acupressure, stress reduction measures, relaxation-inducing measures, exercise recommendations, and dietary recommendations.) The results suggest a potential use of adjuvant acupuncture in the treatment of angina pectoris. For additional studies see [11, 12].

8.5.4
Urology

Tables 4 and 10 summarize four controlled studies on the use of acupuncture in the treatment of various urological problems, including lower urinary tract infection, kidney stone pain, incontinence in the elderly, and urgent incontinence with frequent urination and nocturia. There have also been a number of uncontrolled studies suggesting positive effects of acupuncture on bladder function and urinary problems [26, 66]. While the data regarding the efficacy of acupuncture in urology is not yet sufficient for clear conclusions, the few controlled studies in this area are suggestive of positive effects of acupuncture in urology, even in cases of recurrent lower urinary tract infections and kidney stone pain, notoriously one of the most painful conditions which may present to the emergency room of a hospital. Two of these studies used an acupuncture treatment versus standard treatment design and found that, while the acupuncture generally had similar, possibly somewhat better treatment effects, the side effects were markedly less in acupuncture treatment groups than in standard drug therapy groups [45, 48]. Clearly, more studies are necessary before conclusions

Table 4. Controlled clinical trials in urology

Condition	N	AT	CT	Primary assessments	Results
Recurrent lower urinary tract infection [6]	67	MA: 8 sessions for 4 weeks	Group 1: CA, 8 sessions for 4 weeks; Group 2: no therapy	UTI plus self-report (monthly for 6 months)	Rate of UTI: AT < CT-1, AT sig < CT-2
Acute renal colic from kidney stone [48]	38	MA, EA: 1 session	SC: 1 dose avafortan	Intensity and onset of pain	Pain relief: AT sig>SC, onset of pain relief: AT > SC Side effects: AT < SC
Nocturia and incontinence in the elderly [29]	20	MA: 10 sessions over 2 weeks	Placebo: mock TENS, 10 sessions over 2 weeks	Number nocturnal bladder voidings from baseline through therapy	Bladder voidings: AT sig < placebo
Noncompliant, urgent incontinence, frequent urination, and nocturia [45]	39	MA: 6 weekly sessions	SC: oxybutyrin	Urinary symptom diary, symptom VAS scale, urodynamic investigations	Urgency and frequency: AT sig > SC Nocturia: AT > SC Side effects: AT sig < SC

AT, acupuncture therapy; CT, control therapy; MA, manual acupuncture; CA, sham acupuncture; UTI, urinary tract infection; SC, standard care; TENS, transcutaneous electrical nerve stimulation.

can be drawn, but at present the current evidence is quite promising for the use of acupuncture in the treatment of urinary frequency, incontinence, and urgency, recurrent lower urinary tract infection, and renal colic.

8.5.5
Obstetrics

Tables 5 and 10 summarize five controlled clinical trials on the use of acupuncture during pregnancy and labor. In particular, the studies examined the efficacy of acupuncture on breech presentation and the duration of and preparation for labor. In general, one may conclude that these studies show a clear effect of acupuncture on the rate of turning of breech babies [25] and in the duration of labor and maturation of the uterus for labor [70]. The latter study by Romer et al. is particularly impressive. The sample size was very large, the methodology good, the assessments very good, and the results very clear for acupuncture, compared both to control acupuncture and to a "no additional treatment" group. This study will stimulate much more research in acupuncture and pregnancy. While more research needs to be done in these areas to confirm the findings, the results so far are very encouraging for the use of acupuncture on pregnant women with breech presentation around the 33rd week

Table 5. Controlled clinical trials in obstetrics

Condition	n	AT	Control therapy	Primary assessments	Results
Breech version [25]	260	MT: 7–14 sessions	SC	Fetal movements, rate of turning	Fetal movements: MT sig > SC Rate of turning: MT sig > SC
Breech version [24]	23	MT: 5–40 sessions	HC	Rate of turning, birthweight, neonatal APGAR score	Rate of turning: AT 70 %, HC 39 % Birth weight and APGAR score: AT>HC
Pain relief during labor [77]	180	AT: 1 session during labor	SC	Use of pain therapy during labor	Analgesic use: AT sig < SC
Duration of labor [92]	120	AT: 4 sessions, 1 per week	SC	Time of first stage labor, time of second stage labor, oxytocin use during labor	Time of first stage: AT sig < SC Time of second stage: AT = SC Oxytocin use: AT sig<SC
Duration of labor [70]	878	AT started at week 36, (n = 329)	Group 1: CA therapy begun at week 36, (n = 224); Group 2: SC (n = 329)	Duration of labor, change of cervical length, Bishop score[a]	Duration of labor: AT sig < controls Cervical length and Bishop score: AT sig>controls

AT, acupuncture therapy; MT, moxibustion therapy; HC, historical control; SC, standard care; sig, significantly.
[a] Shortening of the cervix and Bishop score are signs of ripening of the uterus in preparation for labor.

of pregnancy and in general for women around week 36 to improve preparation for labor and make the labor easier and quicker. Acupuncture is clearly indicated in these two areas. For additional studies see [23, 30, 51, 75, 80, 91].

8.5.6
Gynecology

Tables 6 and 10 summarize three controlled studies on the use of acupuncture for the gynecological problems of dysmenorrhea, female infertility, and menopausal hot flashes. There are clearly not enough studies in this area, but the results to date are somewhat promising. Acupuncture seems to be helpful for dysmenorrhea, which is supported by other, less well designed studies [79]. The results of acupuncture for female infertility are interesting but need replication. The study for menopausal hot flashes is excellent in many regards, with the exception that the so-called placebo acupuncture treatment, i.e., superficial needling at the same acupoints as those used in the treatment group, was actually a better form of therapy for this symptom than the "real acupuncture" [15]. The application of inadequate acupuncture treatment and/or inappropriate control acupuncture treatment is a common and major problem in the design and interpretation of clinical trials [14, 15, 73]. Overall, we see suggestive evidence for the use of acupuncture in gynecological problems.

Table 6. Controlled clinical trials in gynecology

Condition	n	AT	CT	Primary assessments	Results
Dysmenor-rhea [40]	43	MA: 12 weekly sessions	Group 1: CA 12 sessions; Group 2: office visit only; CT-Group 3: no therapy	Pain and medication diary, 1 year	AT sig better than controls for pain reduction Similar trend in medication consumption
Infertility: amenorrhea and luteal insufficiency [36]	45	MA: up to 12 sessions with optional additional 12 sessions	HC: hormone therapy	Pregnancy, hormone levels	Successful pregnancies: AT 14, HC 16 Side effects: AT<HC
Menopausal hot flashes [89]	24	MA, EA: 10 sessions	CA: 10 sessions	Daily diary, QOL, urinary excretion of endogenous opioid-related peptides	Sig decrease of hot flashes in both groups No sig difference between groups Effects persisted in AT group but not in CA group

AT, acupuncture therapy; MA, manual acupuncture; EA, electroacupuncture; CA, sham acupuncture; HC, historical control; QOL, quality of life; sig, significantly.

8.5.7
Mental Health

Tables 7 and 11 summarize four controlled studies of the use of acupuncture in the treatment of mental health problems, three for depression and one for schizophrenia. The study by Allen et al. [1] is perhaps the most interesting. It was a very well designed study, with clear results favoring acupuncture for depression. While the evidence for the three studies examining efficacy of acupuncture for depression is still not very large, it is important to note that Allen and colleagues are in the middle of a larger study exploring acupuncture for depression, and other research teams are examining this use of acupuncture, notably one in Australia (Im Quah-Smith, personal communication). Further, possible physiological mechanisms have been put forward that support the use of acupuncture in affective disorders such as depression [39]. The evidence for the use of acupuncture in schizophrenia is still scant but raises interesting questions in this very difficult problem. Some supportive evidence can be found in uncontrolled case study reports [44]. Further evidence of possible efficacy can be found in the area of drug dependence treatment, where acupuncture has shown promising results in the treatment of schizophrenic patients (Michael Smith, personal communication).

Table 7. Controlled clinical trials in mental health

Condition	n	AT	CT	Primary assessments	Results
Major depression in women [1]	38	MA: 12 sessions over 8 weeks	Group 1 CA: 12 sessions over 8 weeks, then AT for 12 sessions; Group 2: waiting list 8 weeks, then AT for 12 sessions	Hamilton and Beck depression inventories, Beck hopelessness scale, completed weekly	First 8 weeks: AT sig < control group 1, AT not sig < control group 2 After 16 weeks: all groups showed major improvement 64 % of patients remitted
Depression [54]	47	EA: 30 sessions over 5 weeks	SC: amitriptyline	Hamilton depression scale, clinical global impressions, clinical ratings	Good improvement: 70 % AT group vs. 65 % CT group Side effects: AT < CT
Depression [90]	41	MA, EA: 36 sessions over 6 weeks	SC: amitriptyline	Hamilton depression scale, clinical assessments	AT showed similar degree of improvement as CT
Schizophrenia [93]	40	EA 36 sessions over 6 weeks, reduced level antipsychotic medication	SC: normal level antipsychotic medication	Clinical assessments, clinical global impressions, brief psychiatric rating, lab exams	AT showed similar effects as SC on psychotic symptoms AT faster onset of therapy effects Side effects: AT < CT

AT, acupuncture therapy; CT, control therapy; CA, sham acupuncture; EA, electroacupuncture; SC, standard care.

8.5.8
Male Sexual Problems

Tables 8 and 11 summarize two studies on the use of acupuncture for sexual problems in men. Very little research has been done in this area. While neither study was well-designed, both provide sufficient evidence to warrant further studies of higher quality in the areas of acupuncture for impotence and low sperm quality.

8.5.9
Xerostomia

Tables 8 and 11 summarize two studies on the use of acupuncture for xerostomia, or dry mouth. Xerostomia can result secondary to problems like Sjögren's syndrome and radiation therapy for certain cancers. The two studies were performed by the same research team and provide some evidence of the efficacy of acupuncture in this difficult problem. However, the second trial has been criticized for a number of problems, including overuse of statistical tests, poor hypothesis testing, and possible problems with randomization [3]. Taking the two studies together, promising evidence can be seen indicating the possible use of acupuncture for the difficult problem of xerostomia. Further clinical research would be useful in this area.

Table 8. Miscellaneous controlled clinical trials

Condition	n	AT	CT	Primary assessments	Results
Nonorganic male sexual dysfunction [8]	60	MA, EA: 12 sessions in 6 weeks	Group 1: CA (MA, EA) 12 sessions; Group 2: hypnotic suggestion (HY); Group 3: vitamin supplements (SU)	Standard objective tests, medical and sexual history, physical exam	AT and HY>CA and SU, but not at sig levels
Male subfertility [72]	32	MA: 10 sessions in 5 weeks	No treatment	Standard objective semen analysis methods	AT: sig better on 3 parameters. CT: no sig changes
Xerostomia [17]	21	MA: 12 sessions in 6 weeks	CA: 12 sessions in 6 weeks	Standard objective salivary flow rates	AT sig > CT, especially at long-term follow-up
Xerostomia [18]	38	MA: 12 sessions in 6 weeks	CA: 12 sessions in 6 weeks	Standard objective salivary flow rates	Both groups improved, AT more than CT
Raynaud's syndrome [5]	33	MA: 7 sessions in 2 weeks	No treatment	Symptom diary, nailbed capillary examination	AT: sig capillary and subjective improvement. CT: no sig changes

AT, acupuncture therapy; CT control therapy, MA, manual acupuncture; EA, electroacupuncture; CA, sham acupuncture; sig, significant.

8.5.10
Raynaud's Syndrome

Tables 8 and 11 also summarize one controlled study examining the effects of acupuncture on Raynaud's syndrome. Since the sample size is small and the study used only a "no treatment control" group, it should be considered only as a useful pilot study. The results suggest a possible benefit of acupuncture in the treatment of Raynaud's syndrome, but a larger, well-designed, controlled clinical trial is needed to answer the question of its efficacy.

Table 9. Criteria scoring and comments on controlled clinical trials

Condition/ study	1	2	3	4	5	6	7	8	9	10	Comments
Stroke [62]	Y	Y	Y	N	Y	Y	N	Y	N	N	Small sample size but well-designed study. Lack of nonspecific assessments weakens study
Stroke [43]	Y	Y	Y	N	Y	Y	N	Y	Y	N	Well-designed study. Impressive results argue for use of standard care controls in serious problems such as stroke
Stroke [42]	Y	Y	Y	N	Y	Y	N	Y	Y	N	Well-designed study supports findings of last two studies
Stroke [71]	Y	N	Y	Y	Y	Y	N	N	N	N	Reasonably well designed study supports last three studies
Alcohol recidivism [22]	Y	Y	Y	N	Y	U	Y	Y	Y	N	Good study weakened by high dropout rate in control group but which itself is an indicator of treatment efficacy
Cocaine [57]	N	Y	Y	Y	NA	Y	NA	NA	N	Y	Small sample size and lack of prospective controls weaken the study
Crack cocaine [53]	Y	Y	Y[a]	N	Y	U	N	Y	Y	N	High dropout rates, inadequate intervention, and lack of nonspecific assessments weaken the study
Heroin detoxification [86]	Y	Y	Y	Y	Y	U	N	N	NA	Y	Lack of nonspecific assessments weakens study
Angina pectoris [9]	Y	N	N	N	N	Y	N	Y	N	Y	Despite small sample size and inadequate treatment, results favored acupuncture, but lack of nonspecific controls weakens the study
Angina pectoris [13]	Y	N	U	N	N	Y	N	Y	N	N	Inadequate treatment and lack of nonspecific controls undermine the study
Angina pectoris [69]	Y	Y	Y	Y	Y	U	N	N	NA	N	Small sample size and lack of nonspecific controls weaken the study
Angina pectoris [10]	N	Y	P	N	Y	Y	NA	NA	Y	N	Interesting study. Raises question of whether control group is appropriate in serious diseases with few treatment side effects

Y, yes; N, no; U, unclear; P, possibly; NA, not applicable.
[a] Acupuncture therapy was adequate but acupuncture is an adjunctive therapy in treatment for addiction. Since standard therapy (counseling) was omitted in this study, the therapy intervention was inadequate.

Table 10. Criteria scoring and comments on controlled clinical trials

Condition/ study	1	2	3	4	5	6	7	8	9	10	Comments
Urinary tract infection [6]	Y	Y	P	N	N	U	N	Y	Y	Y	Reasonably well designed study. Inadequate control therapy makes overall interpretation of results difficult
Renal colic [48]	Y	Y	P	N	Y	Y	N	Y	NA	Y	Reasonably well designed study. Needs replicating
Urinary incontinence [29]	Y	Y	N	N	Y	U	N	Y	N	N	Small study. Suffers from inadequate controls and inadequate therapy
Frequent urination [45]	Y	Y	Y	Y	Y	Y	N	Y	Y	Y	Reasonably well designed study. Needs replicating
Breech version [25]	Y	Y	Y	NA	Y	Y	Y	N	NA	Y	Well-designed study. Shows clear effect of treatment
Breech version [24]	N	Y	Y	NA	NA	NA	NA	NA	NA	Y	A preliminary study, with problems corrected in larger follow-on study [25]
Labor pain [77]	N	Y	P	N	NA	NA	N	N	NA	Y	Not very well designed study. Suffers from lack of prospective comparison
Duration of labor [92]	N	Y	N	N	NA	NA	N	NA	NA	N	Lack of randomization and inadequate treatment undermine study
Duration, preparation labor [70]	Y	Y	Y	Y	Y	Y	N	Y	NA	N	Well-designed study. Clear results. Would benefit from assessment of non-specific effects
Dysmenorrhea [40]	Y	Y	Y	N	N	U	N	N	Y	N	Reasonably well designed study but small sample size in each group. Needs larger-scale replication
Female infertility [36]	N	Y	P	N	Y	Y	N	NA	N	Y	Lack of prospective control undermines otherwise reasonably well designed study
Menopausal symptoms [89]	Y	Y	N	Y	Y	N	N	Y	Y	N	Well-designed study except that control treatment is a better treatment than acupuncture [15]

Y, yes; N, no; U, unclear; P, possibly; NA, not applicable.

There are a number of other areas where research has been done and reviews have concluded that treatment efficacy is doubtful. These are not included in the tables but are briefly discussed here.

8.5.11
Weight Loss

Edzard Ernst conducted a systematic review of controlled studies examining the effects of acupuncture/acupressure on weight loss [32]. His review concluded: "On balance, no clear picture emerges to show that acupuncture/acupressure is effective in reducing appetite or body weight." This conclusion generally agrees with that of Vincent and Richardson in 1987 [85]. The weight of evidence suggests that acupuncture is not effective as an appetite suppressant or for weight loss.

Table 11. Criteria scoring and comments on controlled clinical trials

Condition/ study	1	2	3	4	5	6	7	8	9	10	Comments
Depression [1]	Y	N[a]	Y	Y	Y	Y	N	Y	N	N	Very well designed pilot study. A full scale RCT is underway. Would benefit from addressing criteria 9 and 10
Depression [54]	Y	Y	P	N	Y	Y	N	Y	N	Y	Reasonably well-designed, but problems with assessment scale undermine interpretation of results
Depression [90]	Y	Y	Y	N	Y	Y	N	N	N	Y	Reasonably well-designed, but problems with assessment scale undermine interpretation of results
Schizophrenia [93]	Y	Y	Y	N	Y	Y	N	Y	N	Y	Reasonably well-designed, but problems with assessment scale undermine interpretation of results
Nonorganic male sexual dysfunction [8]	N	Y	P	N	N	N	N	N	N	N	Lack of randomization, problems with "placebo" controls, and small sample size make interpretation of results difficult
Low sperm quality [72]	N	Y	P	N	NA	NA	N	Y	Y	N	Small sample size and lack of randomization weaken the study
Xerostomia [17]	Y	Y	P	N	N	N	N	Y	Y	Y	Small sample size and confusion over nonspecific controls with lack of nonspecific evaluations weaken the study
Xerostomia [18]	Y	Y	P	N	N	N	N	Y	Y/ NA	Y	Usefullness of long-term follow-up doubtful in light of crossover design. Lack of nonspecific controls also weakens study
Raynaud's syndrome [5]	Y	Y	Y	N	NA	NA	N	N	Y	Y	Small sample size and lack of treatment controls weaken the study, but there is useful pilot data

Y, yes; N, no; U, unclear; P, possibly; NA, not applicable.
[a] Treatment protocol was referenced but not described.

8.5.12
Hearing Problems

Acupuncture has been used for chronic auditory problems such as sensorineural deafness and tinnitus. A few studies have been done in this area, but results have been quite inconsistent, with at best only temporary improvement. In 1975, Taub reviewed the literature and concluded that acupuncture made no contribution for sensorineural deafness [74]. In 1987, Vincent and Richardson also reviewed the studies in this area and concluded that there appear to be some short-term benefits but no long-term benefit [85]. There have been significant problems in study design in this area. A more recent study investigating acupuncture for tinnitus found some transient effects but no positive long-term effects [78]. The weight of evidence suggests that acupuncture is not very effective for hearing problems such as those described here.

Table 12. Scoring by criterion

Criterion	Scoring and Comments	Test answers 1985–1993	Test answers 1994–1999
1	25/30 randomized (three historical control studies did not need randomization)	13/14	12/16
2	31/33 presented adequate treatment descriptions	15/16	16/17
3	17/33 clearly provided adequate treatment (4 did not, 11 possibly, 1 unclear)	Y = 9, N = 2, P = 4, U = 1	Y = 8, N = 2, P = 7
4	8/31 mentioned training of the acupuncturist (2 NA)	3	5
5	20/27 adequately described the control treatment (6 NA)	10/14	10/13
6	17/28 gave an appropriate control treatment (4 did not, 7 unclear)	Y = 9, N = 1, U = 5	Y = 8, N = 3, U = 2
7	2/30 presented sample size calculation (historical control studies were rated as not needed)	1/14	1/16
8	19/28 used blinded evaluators	10/13	9/15
9	13/25 performed long-term follow-up	5/12	8/13
10	16/33 reported adverse effects	8/16	8/17

Y, yes; N, no; U, unclear; P, possibly; NA, not applicable.

8.6
Conclusions

Acupuncture has been tested in a relatively broad range of medical problems. This brief review has examined a number of areas where research can be found but, in most cases, there is insufficient evidence to perform systematic reviews. We found either good or promising evidence of the efficacy of acupuncture in most of these areas but, at the same time, methodological problems that undermine interpretation of the results.

The evidence for the use of acupuncture as an adjunctive therapy for stroke rehabilitation is increasing. While there are conflicting data about the use of acupuncture as an adjunctive treatment for addictions, the existing evidence shows enough promise to warrant continued examination. Evidence for the adjunctive use of acupuncture for angina pectoris is also quite promising, as it is in various urological and gynecological problems. Evidence for acupuncture in breech version and to prepare for and assist in labor is already strong, especially with the 1998 studies of Cardini and Weixin for breech version [25] and Romer et al. for labor [70]. Evidence that acupuncture can be used to treat depression is also mounting and quite promising. In the case of male sexual problems, xerostomia, and Raynaud's syndrome, the results are somewhat promising, but much more data is needed. Acupuncture's efficacy in weight loss and hearing problems is less convincing. Each of the areas examined needs more research, usually with better methodology. In some areas such as angina pectoris, stroke, and addiction, it appears useful to focus study design more on the use of acupuncture as an adjunctive therapy in comparison to standard therapy alone, rather than only the gold standard of placebo-controlled double blind research. It appears necessary to continue the debate about the selection of appropriate research methodologies for future acupuncture studies.

References

1. Allen JJB, Schnyer RN, Hitt SK (1998) The efficacy of acupuncture in the treatment of major depression in women. Psychol Sci 9:397–401
2. Alpert S, FDA (1996) Letter – reclassification order, Docket No. 94P-0443, Acupuncture needles for the practice of acupuncture. In: Birch S, Hammerschlag R (eds) Acupuncture efficacy: A compendium of controlled clinical trials. National Academy of Acupuncture and Oriental Medicine, New York, pp 76–78
3. Andersen SW, Machin D (1997) Acupuncture treatment of patients with radiation-induced xerostomia. Oral Oncol 33:146–147
4. Anon (1998) Acupuncture: NIH consensus development panel on acupuncture. JAMA 280:1518–1524
5. Appiah R, Hiller S, Caspary L, Alexander K, Creutzig A (1997) Treatment of primary Raynaud's syndrome with traditional Chinese acupuncture. J Inter Med 241:119–124
6. Aune A, Alraek T, Huo LH, Baerheim A (1998) Acupuncture in the prophylaxis of recurrent lower urinary tract infection in adult women. Scand J Prim Health Care 16:37–39
7. Avants SK, Margolin A, Chang P, Kosten TR, Birch S (1995) Acupuncture for the treatment of cocaine addiction in methadone-maintained patients: Investigation of a needle puncture control. J Subst Abuse Treat 12:195–205
8. Aydin S, Ercan M, Caskurlu T, Tasci AI, Karaman I, Odabas O, Yilmaz Y, Agargun MY, Kara H, Sevin G (1997) Acupuncture and hypnotic suggestions in the treatment of nonorganic male sexual dysfunction. Scand J Urol Nephrol 31:271–274
9. Ballegaard S, Jansen G (1986) Acupuncture in severe, stable angina pectoris: A randomized trial. Acta Med Scand 220:307–313
10. Ballegaard S, Johanssen A, Karpatschof B, Nyhoe J (1999) Addition of acupuncture and self-care education in the treatment of patients with severe angina pectoris may be cost beneficial – an open prospective study. J Alt Complem Med 5:405–413
11. Ballegaard S, Meyer CN, Trojaborg W (1991) Acupuncture in angina pectoris: Does acupuncture have a specific effect? J Int Med 229:357–362
12. Ballegaard S, Norrelund S (1996) Cost-benefit of combined use of acupuncture, shiatsu, and lifestyle adjustments for treatment of patients with severe angina pectoris. Acupunct Electrother Res 21:187–197
13. Ballegaard S, Pedersen F, Pietersen A, Nissen VH, Olsen NV (1990) Effects of acupuncture in moderate, stable angina pectoris: A controlled study. J Int Med 227:25–30
14. Birch S (1995) Testing the clinical specificity of needle sites in controlled clinical trials of acupuncture. Proceedings of the Second Symposium of the Society for Acupuncture Research, pp 274–294
15. Birch S (1997) Issues to consider in determining an adequate treatment in a clinical trial of acupuncture. Complem Ther Med 5: 8–12
16. Birch S, Felt R (1999) Understanding acupuncture. Churchill Livingstone, London
17. Blom M, Dawidson I, Angmar-Mansson B (1992) The effect of acupuncture on salivary flow rates in patients with xerostomia. Oral Surg Oral Med Oral Pathol Oral Radiol Endod 73:293–298
18. Blom M, Dawidson I, Fernberg J-O, Johnson G, Angmar-Mansson B (1996) Acupuncture treatment of patients with radiation-induced xerostomia. Oral Oncol Eur J Cancer 328:182–190
19. Brewington V, Smith M, Lipton D (1994) Acupuncture as a detoxification treatment: An analysis of controlled research. J Subst Abuse Treat 11:289–307
20. Brumbaugh A (1994) Transformation and recovery: A guide to the design and development of acupuncture-based chemical dependency treatment programs. Stillpoint Press, Santa Barbara
21. Bullock ML, Umen AJ, Culliton PD, Olander RT (1987) Acupuncture treatment of alcoholic recidivism: A pilot study. Alcohol Clin Exper Res 11:292–295
22. Bullock ML, Culliton PD, Olander RT (1989) Controlled trial of acupuncture for severe recidivist alcoholism. Lancet 2:1435–1439
23. Cardini F, Basevi V, Valentini A, Martellato A (1991) Moxibustion and breech presentation: preliminary results. Am J Chin Med 19:105–114
24. Cardini F, Marcolongo A (1993) Moxibustion for correction of breech presentation: A clinical study with retrospective control. Am J Chin Med 21:133–138

25. Cardini F, Weixin H (1998) Moxibustion for correction of breech presentation. JAMA 280:1580–1584
26. Chang PL (1988) Urodynamic studies in acupuncture for women with frequency, urgency, and dysuria. J Urol 140:563–66
27. Culliton PD, Kiresuk TJ (1996) Overview of substance abuse acupuncture treatment research. J Alt Complem Med 2:149–159
28. Dunn PA, Rogers D, Halford K (1989) Transcutaneous electrical nerve stimulation at acupuncture points in the induction of uterine contractions Obstet Gynecol 73:286–90
29. Ellis N, Briggs R, Dowson D (1990) The effect of acupuncture on nocturnal urinary frequency and incontinence in the elderly. Complem Med Res 4:16–17
30. Engel K, Gerke-Engel G, Gerhard I, Bastert G (1992) Foetomaternal macrotransfusion after succesful internal cephalic version from breech presentation by moxibustion. Geburtsh U Frauenheilk 52:241–243
31. Ernst E (1994) Acupuncture research: Where are the problems? Acup Med 12:93–97
32. Ernst E (1997) Acupuncture/acupressure for weight reduction? A systematic review. Wien Klin Wochenschr 109:60–62
33. Ernst E, White AR (1996) Acupuncture as an adjuvant therapy in stroke rehabilitation? Wien Med Wochenschr 146:556–558
34. Ernst E, White AR (1997) A review of problems in clinical acupuncture research. Amer J Chin Med 25:3–11
35. Filshie J, White A (1998) Medical Acupuncture. Churchill Livingstone, Edinburgh
36. Gerhard I, Postneek F (1992) Auricular acupuncture in the treatment of female infertility. Gynecol Endocrinol 15:114–117
37. Hammerschlag R (1998) Methodological and ethical issues in clinical trials of acupuncture. J Alt Complem Med 4:159–171
38. Hammerschlag R, Morris MM (1997) Clinical trials comparing acupuncture with biomedical standard care: A criteria-based evaluation of research design and reporting. Complem Ther Med 5:133–140
39. Han JS (1986) Electroacupuncture: An alternative to antidepressants for treating affective diseases? Int J Neurosci 29:79–92
40. Helms JM (1987) Acupuncture for the management of primary dysmenorrhea. Obstet Gynecol 69:51–56
41. Hopwood V (1996) Acupuncture in stroke recovery: A literature review. Complem Ther Med 4:258–263
42. Hu HH, Chung C, Liu TJ, Chen RC, Chen CH, Chou P, Huang WS, Lin JCT, Tsuei JJ (1993) A randomized controlled trial on the treatment for acute partial ischemic stroke with acupuncture. Neuroepidemiol 12:106–113
43. Johansson K, Lindgren I, Widner H, Wiklung I, Johansson BB (1993) Can sensory stimulation improve the functional outcome in stroke patients? Neurology 43:2189–2192
44. Kane J, Di Scipio WJ (1979) Acupuncture treatment of schizophrenia: A report on three cases. Amer J Psychiat 136:297–302
45. Kelleher CJ, Filshie J, Burton G, Khullar V, Cardozo LD (1994) Acupuncture and the treatment of irritative bladder symptoms. Acup in Med 12:9–12
46. Konefal J, Duncan R, Clemence C (1994) The impact of the addition of an acupuncture treatment program to an existing Metro-Dade County outpatient substance abuse treatment facility. J Addict Dis 13:71–99
47. Konefal J, Duncan R, Clemence C (1995) Comparison of three levels of auricular acupuncture in an outpatient substance abuse treatment program. Alt Med J Sept-Oct:8–17
48. Lee YH, Lee WC, Chen MT, Huang JK, Chung C, Chang LS (1992) Acupuncture in the treatment of renal colic. J Urol 147:16–18
49. Lewith GT, Machin D (1983) On the evaluation of the clinical effects of acupuncture. Pain 16:111–127
50. Lewith G, Vincent C (1996) On the evaluation of the clinical effects of acupuncture: A problem reassessed and a framework for future research. J Alt Complem Med 2:79–90
51. Li QH, Wang L (1996) Clinical observation on correcting malposition of fetus by electroacupuncture. J Trad Chin Med 16:260–262
52. Linde K, Worku F, Stor W, Wiesner-Zechmeister M, Pothmann R, Weinschutz T, Melchart D (1996) Randomized clinical trials of acupuncture for asthma – a systematic review. Forsch Kompl 3:148–155
53. Lipton DS, Brewington V, Smith M (1994) Acupuncture for crack cocaine detoxification: Experimental evaluation of efficacy. J Subst Abuse Treat 11:205–215

54. Luo H, Jia Y, Zhan L (1985) Electroacupuncture vs. amitriptyline in the treatment of depressive states. J Trad Chin Med 5:3–8
55. Lytle CD (1993) An overview of acupuncture. U. S. Department of Health and Human Services, Public Health Service, Food and Drug Administration, Center for Devices and Radiological Health
56. Magnusson M, Johansson K, Johansson BB (1994) Sensory stimulation promotes normalization of postural control after stroke. Stroke 25:1176–1180
57. Margolin A, Avants SK, Chang P, Kosten TR (1993) Auricular acupuncture for the treatment of cocaine dependence in methadone-maintained patients. Am J Addict 2:194–200
58. Margolin A, Avants SK, Birch S, Falk CX, Kleber HD (1997) Methodological investigations for a multisite trial of auricular acupuncture for cocaine addiction. A study of active and control auricular zones. J Subst Abuse Treat 13:471–481
59. Margolin A, Avants SK, Kleber HD (1998) Rationale and design of the cocaine alternative treatments study (CATS): A randomized, controlled trial of acupuncture. J Alt Complem Med 4:405–418
60. McLellan AT, Grossman DS, Blain JD, Haverkos HW (1993) Acupuncture treatment for drug abuse: A technical review. J Subst Abuse Treat 10:569–576
61. Naeser MA (1996) Acupuncture in the treatment of paralysis due to central nervous system damage. J Alt Complem Med 2:211–248
62. Naeser MA, Alexander MP Stiassny-Eder D, Galler V, Hobbs J, Bachman D (1992) Real vs. sham acupuncture in the treatment of paralysis in acute stroke patients: A CT scan lesion site study. J Neurol Rehab 6:163–173
63. Naeser MA, Alexander MP Stiassny-Eder D, Galler V, Hobbs J, Bachman D (1994) Acupuncture in the treatment of paralysis in chronic and acute stroke patients: Improvement correlated with specific CT scan lesion sites. Acup Electrother Res Int J 19:227–250
64. Naeser MA, Alexander MP Stiassny-Eder D, Lannin LN, Bachman D (1994) Acupuncture in the treatment of hand paresis in chronic and acute stroke patients: Improvement observed in all cases. Clin Rehab 8:127–141
65. Patel M, Gutzwiller F, Paccaud F, Marazzi A (1989) A meta-analysis of acupuncture for chronic pain. Int J Epidem 18:900–906
66. Philp T, Shah PJR, Worth PHL (1988) Acupuncture in the treatment of bladder instability. Brit J Urol 61:490–493
67. Rampes H, Pereira S, Mortimer A, Manoharan S, Knowles M (1997) Does electroacupuncture reduce craving for alcohol? A randomized controlled study. Complem Ther Med 5:19–26
68. Richardson PH, Vincent CA (1986) Acupuncture for the treatment of pain: A review of evaluative research. Pain 24:15–40
69. Richter A, Herlitz J, Hjalmarson A (1991) Effect of acupuncture in patients with angina pectoris. Euro Heart J 12:175–178
70. Romer A, Weigel M, Zieger W, Melchert F (1998) Veränderungen von Cervixreife und Geburtsdauer nach geburtsvorbereitender Akupunkturherapie. In: Romer A (ed) Acupunkturtherapie in der Geburtshilfe und Frauenheilkunde. Hippocrates, Stuttgart
71. Sallstrom S, Kjendahl A, Osten PE, Stanghelle JH, Borchgrevink CF (1996) Acupuncture in the treatment of stroke patients in the subacute stage: A randomized, controlled study. Complem Ther Med 4:193–197
72. Siterman S, Eltes F, Wolfson V, Zabludovsky N, Bartoov B (1997) Effect of acupuncture on sperm parameters of males suffering from subfertility related to low sperm quality. Arch Androl 39:155–161
73. Stux G, Birch S (2000) Proposed standards of acupuncture treatment in clinical studies. In: Stux G, Hammerschlag R (eds) Scientific bases of acupuncture in basic and clinical research. Springer-Verlag, Berlin
74. Taub HA (1975) Acupuncture and sensorineural hearing loss: A review. J Speech Hearing Disord 40:427–433
75. Tempfer C, Zeisler H, Heinzl H, Hefler L, Husslein P, Kainz CH (1998) Influence of acupuncture on maternal serum levels of interleukin-8, prostaglandin F (2-alpha), and beta-endorphin: A matched pair study. Obstet Gynecol 92:245–248
76. Ter Riet, G, Kleijnen J, Knipschild P (1990) A meta-analysis of studies into the effect of acupuncture on addiction. Brit J Gen Pract 40:379–382
77. Ternov K, Nilsson M, Lofberg L, Algotsson L, Akeson J (1998) Acupuncture for pain relief during childbirth. Acup Electrother Res Int J 23:19–26
78. Thomas M, Laurell G, Lundeberg T, (1988) Acupuncture for the alleviation of tinnitus. Laryngoscope 1988:664–667

79. Thomas M, Lundeberg T, Bjork G, Lundstrom-Lindstedt V (1995) Pain and discomfort in primary dysmenorrhea is reduced by preemptive acupuncture or low frequency TENS. Eur J Phys Med Rehab 5:71–76

80. Tsuei JJ, Lai YF, Sharma SD (1977) The influence of acupuncture during pregnancy: The induction and inhibition of labor. Obstet Gynecol 50,4:479–88

81. Vincent CA (1989) The methodology of controlled trials of acupuncture. Acup Med 6:9–13

82. Vincent CA (1990) Credibility assessment in trials of acupuncture. Compl Med Res 4:8–11

83. Vincent CA (1993) Acupuncture as a treatment for chronic pain. In: GT Lewith, D Aldridge (eds) Clinical research methodology for complementary therapies. Hodder and Stoughton, London, pp 289–308

84. Vincent C, Lewith G (1995) Placebo controls for acupuncture studies. J Royal Soc Med 88:199–202

85. Vincent CA, Richardson PH (1987) Acupuncture for some common disorders: A review of evaluative research. J Royal Coll Gen Pract 37:77–81

86. Washburn AM, Fullilove RE, Fullilove MT, Keenan PA, McGee B, Morris KA, Sorensen JL, Clark WW (1993) Acupuncture heroin detoxification: A single blind clinical trial. J Subst Abuse Treat 10:345–351

87. Wells EA, Jackson R, Diaz OR, Stanton V, Saxon AJ, Krupski A (1995) Acupuncture as an adjunct to methadone treatment services. Am J Addict 4:198–214

88. Worner TM, Zeller B, Schwartz H, Zwas F, Lyon D (1992) Acupuncture fails to improve treatment outcome in alcoholics. Drug Alcohol Depend 30:169–173

89. Wyon Y, Lindgren R, Lundeberg T, Hammar M (1995) Effects of acupuncture on climacteric vasomotor symptoms, quality of life, and urinary excretion of neuropeptides among postmenopausal women. Menopause 2:3–12

90. Yang X, Liu X, Luo H, Jia Y (1994) Clinical observation on needling extra channel points in treating mental depression. J Trad Chin Med 14:14–18

91. Ying YK, Lin JT, Robins J (1985) Acupuncture for the induction of cervical dilation in preparation for first-trimester abortion and its influence on HCG. J Reprod Med 30:530–534

92. Zeisler H, Tempfer C, Mayerhofer K, Barrada M, Husslein P (1998) Influence of acupuncture on duration of labor. Gynecol Obstet Invest 46:22–25

93. Zhou G, Jin SB, Zhang LD (1997) Comparative clinical study on the treatment of schizophrenia with electroacupuncture and reduced doses of antipsychotic drugs. Am J Acup 25:25–31

CHAPTER 9

Beyond Numbers: Qualitative Research Methods for Oriental Medicine

C. M. Cassidy

9.1
Introduction

Qualitative research is the term given to the branch of scientific research that emphasizes the collection and study of perceptions and experiences – the "stories" – of living people. Stories are powerful. Some years ago, I was sitting in the treatment trailer at a city jail listening to women receiving acupuncture detoxification (detox) talk about their lives, their addictions, and their experiences of acupuncture care. All of it was interesting. But near the end of the visit, one woman uttered a few poignant words that encapsulated everyone's hopes and reminded the practitioners of their deep task: "I chose acupuncture because I figured if a needle got me into this mess in the first place, maybe a needle could get me out."

Words can be needles, too. By gathering the thoughts and feelings of people – patients, practitioners, lawmakers, teachers, students – one can learn more about the "why" and "how" of people's preferences and decisions, the images that compel and the emotions that propel, than by any other method. Qualitative research encourages people to speak their lives, beliefs, dreams, and visions, their experiences and interpretations of events, their motivations. From their words comes a better understanding of "what matters" to those who speak. This is information that those who listen can put to work usefully to solve problems.

This chapter introduces the basic ideas and methods of qualitative research for practitioners of oriental medicine. Because some qualitative techniques use skills already familiar to clinicians, office-based practitioners can easily adapt them to use in assessing elements of their own practice and in planning for survey research.

9.2
Qualitative Research Is Scientific

There is a tendency among quantitative researchers to view "stories" as anecdotes – minor if interesting sidelights on the "real" stuff, that is, distributions expressed as statistical probabilities. Qualitative researchers take a rather different view, one which we must understand from the outset.

The "anecdote" is a single story without context. It is used to make a specific point. The quotation that appears in the first paragraph above is anecdotal because it is segregated from the other data gathered that same day, on subsequent days in the same locale, and from other settings in which jailed women received detox acupuncture.

Anecdotes are not scientific; at the same time, they are not worthless: they draw one's attention, help memory, provide imagery, succinctly summarize complexities, and often serve to "put a human face" on medicine. The fact is, everyone relishes a good anecdote.

However, the focus of qualitative research is not on anecdote. Instead, like quantitative researchers, qualitative researchers apply the usual rules of science:
- To gather and analyze information systematically
- To do so with attention to minimizing bias
- To achieve data that is accurate, valid, credible, and usable to answer questions, predict behaviors, and plan for the future.

Qualitative research is as scientific as quantitative research, but it starts from different premises and demands different techniques for both data gathering and data analysis [1–3, 5, 7, 16, 20]. Frequently, qualitative and quantitative methods are applied in the same research task. As might be expected, this is called "mixed qualitative-quantitative" research.

9.3
Gathering Qualitative Data

9.3.1
Identifying the Research Question

As in all research, the qualitative researcher first must identify an appropriate study question. The best uses of qualitative research are in finding out the parameters of a new subject (exploratory research) and gathering detail about the *meanings* of events. Table 1 compares the kinds of questions best asked of quantitative and qualitative research. Note that only qualitative and experimental laboratory research can answer the questions "why?" and "how?" – that is, provide *explanations*. Other research – archival, survey, clinical outcomes, and clinical trials research – provides rich descriptive data, including statistical distributions that define "who, what, where, when, how many, and how much" but cannot detail the linkages that explain behaviors. Therefore, if you are interested in why people do what they do – their perceptions and motivations – use qualitative research methods.

Table 1. Questions that research can answer

Scientific function	Questions asked	Research types
Description	Who? What? When? Where? How many? How much?	All types of scientific research produce descriptive data: archival, qualitative, quantitative (survey, clinical outcomes and trials, laboratory experiment)
Prediction	If (a), then does (b)?	Some types of scientific research produce data that can be used for prediction: qualitative, quantitative (clinical outcomes and trials, laboratory experiment)
Explanation	Why? How?	Few types of research produce data that can explain: qualitative, laboratory experiment

When very little is known about a topic, qualitative research is time and cost effective for finding out generally what people think is going on. Oriental medicine is full of such areas of mystery:

– Does needle depth matter?
– Do the patients of practitioners of TCM, Worsley Five Element, French Energetic, and *Toyo Hari* styles have significantly different experiences with acupuncture?
– Are students at schools that provide a cultural context for Chinese medicine more secure in their knowledge afterwards than students from schools that do not?
– What does it mean when practitioners claim to be "holistic" healers?
– Are the concepts of "energy" and "qi" combined for American practitioners?
– What factors help make for successful practitioners 5 years out of school?
– What do *qi gong* practitioners experience when they "throw" *qi*?
– What do patients understand about the theory of oriental medicine after a course of treatment?

There are also many situations where it is useful simply to know what people perceive and interpret and what experiences they take away from an event, for example, acupuncture care. Such information can be used immediately to remedy fault lines in the design of an office or in the delivery of care, or it can be used to help create survey and clinical trials designs that accurately reflect the wants, values, and needs of research participants.

To illustrate the latter use, suppose a group of practitioners in a large private clinic suspected that many of their clients were dissatisfied with their clinic experiences and wanted to identify points of strain in their receipt of oriental medical care. The practitioners could sit down and create a survey questionnaire containing questions concerning the waiting room, practitioners' behavior, attitudes toward needles, quality of parking, and so forth. Once a sufficiency of clients had ticked off answers on this survey form, the practitioners would receive data – quantitative data. But would these really answer the core question they hoped to ask? Perhaps not, for the questions the practitioners thought to ask might not cover the whole range of issues important to the patients. Something crucial might have been left out. In order to get at the *clients'* issues – which are after all what matter most if clients are showing signs of discomfort and distress – these practitioners must make it possible for the clients to tell them what is right and not so right with their clinic. How? – Ask them directly.

To ask people directly is at the core of the qualitative method. It sounds so simple, but it is surprising how often research is designed in accord with researchers' assumptions, without direct knowledge of the client population. The classic approach is via in-depth interviews with a sample of the patients, the gathering of qualitative data. In our example, the practitioners could use the analyzed results of a series of interviews either to make immediate modifications in their office procedures or, if they wanted more data on a larger sample, to construct a high quality survey form that both reflected the clients' issues and phrased them in the clients' language. The quantitative data from this new questionnaire would more accurately report client issues (the technical term is "be more valid") and therefore could be more safely applied to making effective changes in clinic arrangements.

A similar procedure is appropriate when, for example, an oriental medicine professional organization wants to survey members or a school wants to survey alumni:

Table 2. Qualitative data collection techniques discussed in this chapter

Direct techniques	In-depth interview
	Focus-group interview
	Diary
	Open-ended written response on questionnaire
	Case study/series
Indirect techniques	Card-sort

first collect a detailed, small scale qualitative sample and use the qualitative data later to create a large scale survey questionnaire to sample the whole membership. A questionnaire designed this way – with a firm understanding of the importance of knowing respondents' issues and reflecting their language habits – has (another technical term) *high model fit validity*. Validity is a measure of whether a piece of research gathers data that *actually answers the research question asked*[1]. The model one wishes to fit, in this case, is the model of reality held by the respondent population. This is partly conscious and expressible, partly unconscious, which brings us to the next issue: how do you actually collect experiential data from people?

9.3.2
Direct Data Collection Techniques

There are two ways to gather qualitative data, direct and indirect (Table 2). Direct methods help respondents talk about what they know "at the top of the mind." Indirect methods allow respondents to reveal what they don't realize they know – such as attitudes, assumptions, and logical structures that can markedly affect their responses to treatment, teaching, or practice.

Although there are many other qualitative techniques, for our purposes only those listed in Table 1 will be described. The most popular direct methods are the oral interview, the written diary, and the case study. The focus group and written techniques are frequently used in mixed qualitative-quantitative research.

9.3.2.1
In-Depth Interviews

The most important direct research method in qualitative research is the in-depth interview [12, 17]. One interviewer (researcher) talks with one respondent about a fairly broad topic such as (with a patient) what experiences they have had with acupuncture or (with a practitioner or student) why they chose to study oriental medicine and how it is or is not rewarding. The interviewer prepares a short list of *open-ended questions* intended to allow respondents to describe their experiences and reflect on them. An open-ended question is one which sets a topic but does not lead

---

[1] Validity (also called credibility) is the most important of several mechanisms – called criteria of soundness – that are designed to minimize bias in scientific research [15, 16]. There are many subtypes of validity. Other mechanisms that will not be discussed in this paper include precision, reliability, and transferability. The exception is model fit validity, which is a form of validity identified by this author [4, 5]

the respondent to answer in any particular direction. For example, one might ask: "What made you decide to study acupuncture?" Because no answer is implied, respondents are free to "tell their story" as they wish.

Besides using open-ended questions, in-depth interviewers must develop another skill, which is to listen attentively, so-called active listening. After asking a main question, the interviewer tries not to interrupt. At most, he or she uses affirmative "hmmm" and "mm" or very short *probe* questions – "Yes?" "Oh?...," or "What happened next?" – to keep the respondent talking. Another technique is to *reflect* the respondent's words back to him. To illustrate these points, here are two brief excerpts taken from interviews with acupuncture patients at a school clinic:

Interviewer: *What helped you make the final decision to come [for acupuncture care]?*
Respondent: *Honestly?*
I: *Honestly.*
R: *It was the discount on the money.*
I: *Can you tell me about some of the bad stuff?*
R: *Well, the very first treatment they did on me, I cried through the whole thing. I didn't really want to come back. But [practitioner's name] assured me the next one wouldn't be as bad [respondent laughs] – and it wasn't. It was better. The next one, better. And each time I came, I felt different.*
I: *In what way?*
R: *In a good way. I felt better in a good way.*
I: *What was that? What's your "better in a good way?"*
R: *I guess the best way to describe it is I feel more grounded and, before, I didn't.*

Practitioners will recognize that many of the skills of the clinical interview are transferable to the informational interview. However, there is a mistake clinicians can easily make and must avoid: transforming an informational interview into a medical interview. Note that this may be especially troublesome if the respondent is in fact one of the interviewer's patients. Thus, clinicians must keep very clear throughout research interviews that they are "wearing a researcher hat," not a practitioner hat. The following excerpt illustrates this mistake. As we begin, the interviewer functions as researcher, but by the second question he has stepped into practitioner mode. Rather than gathering detail on the concepts broached by the respondent – the idea that all things are interrelated – he is gathering detail on the patient's pain:

I: *What is your expectation of acupuncture?*
R: *I learned from physical therapy that everything can affect everything else...so I'm open to the idea that just tension or stress in one part of the body can trigger something somewhere else and bring down a whole raft of symptoms. For example, my teeth ache, but [the dentist] says there's nothing wrong with my teeth.*
I: *When you talk about them aching, what is the sensation in your body?*
R: *It's just the teeth themselves ache. It's not like a toothache from decay.*
I: *It's ongoing and you feel it all different times of the day?*
R: *All different times of the day. And then also, my life's gone down the drain, emotionally, socially, everything else.*
I: *Due to these complications?*
R: *Yes. Too many times you find out who your friends really are–*
I: *Has that been hard, giving up the relationship?*

This excerpt also illustrates another common error in interviews, that of putting words into the respondent's mouth. This occurs in this interview in the third interviewer remark. Here he *suggests* to the respondent that the pain is ongoing and his teeth ache at all times of the day. These are not ideas that the respondent has previously stated. As clinicians, we can understand that this interviewer (functioning as clinician) is searching for symptom patterns that matter in oriental medicine; in the process, however, he is preventing the respondent from telling his own story in his own words. *Qualitative interviewers must allow respondents to speak for themselves.* Indeed, as far as possible, the qualitative interviewer should become virtually invisible to the respondent.

This idea of "invisibility" implies one more extremely important feature of the in-depth interview: it must be *nonjudgmental* in tone. The interviewer's task is to gather information, *not* to guide, correct, or offer advice to the respondent. This point is extremely important: the informational interview is not a clinical interview. The qualitative interviewer stands in a position of open listening, of learning; he or she must not stand in the position of expert. Sometimes this requirement may be difficult for a clinician to heed, but it is necessary if one wishes to do research rather than practice one's medicine.

Is this unfair, unfeeling? Does it sound like the bogey of the manipulative scientist in the white coat? It shouldn't. The fact is, when people volunteer to be interviewed, there is no expectation that the quality of their beliefs or health will be called into question. The interviewer and respondent establish a bond of trust, but it is a different bond than that between clinician and patient. In the qualitative interview, the researcher's task is to pay attention, listen, and be an open well into which the respondent can pour the water of his/her life. Interestingly, most respondents report that they thoroughly enjoy being the focus of in-depth interviews. In many cases, an interview is the first time that they have felt really heard, the first time they could "tell it like it is" to someone who would not interrupt and correct and advise. This is rewarding to the respondent; it is also rewarding to the interviewer!

In-depth interviews are long – 45 to 90 minutes is not unusual – and repeated interviews with the same respondent may be arranged. It is wise to audiotape all lengthy interviews. You must receive the respondent's permission to interview and to tape-record. Use a brief written consent form to explain the uses that will be made of the data. Additionally, after you turn on the tape recorder, ask the respondent to answer out loud with a clear "yes" to your first question, "Is it all right with you if I tape-record this interview?" Assure the respondent that you will turn off the tape recorder if he or she wishes to discuss something private. You may take notes during the interview – as long as you keep good eye contact with your interviewee – but stop writing if the respondent indicates a wish to speak privately.

Needless to say, a single interview does not a research project make! In order to understand a topic thoroughly, the researcher must perform in-depth interviews with a number of people. As in quantitative research, qualitative researchers develop an appropriate *sampling frame* to select the interviewees, for example, by sex, age, location, specialty, length of experience – whatever is most relevant to the research issue.

They are also concerned with *sample size*. However, in contrast to quantitative research, the goal is not "large" samples, but samples that best reveal all facets of the issue. Therefore, qualitative researchers typically do not set the sample size before beginning research. Instead, they let the research itself guide sample size. Suppose the task were to find out the experiences of practitioners in treating migraine-type headaches in the Portland, Oregon region. The researcher would begin by identifying as many practitioners as possible who are known to emphasize the care of headaches. When interviewing these specialists, the researcher would ask if the respondent can recommend anyone else who is well-known for treating migraine headaches. By this method, the researcher would gradually locate all the people regionally who have special interest or expertise with headaches.

The researcher might interview all these people or might sample among them. For example, one might wish to know the various explanations practitioners give for the causes of migraine-type headaches. In this case, one would continue interviewing until explanations kept recurring and could then say with some certitude that there are, for example, ten explanations of cause for migraine-type headaches among the study population, of which four are widely shared (mentioned by nearly everyone in the sample), four are shared by several respondents, and two are mentioned by only one respondent each. This information is interesting in itself. It could also be used secondarily to help guide the design of a survey instrument, if the researcher wished to expand his research but knew that he could not do nationwide in-depth interviews. In this case, he would be sure to include the four most popular options on the survey instrument and would add a space labeled "other" so respondents could write in other explanations which might or might not be the same as those mentioned in Portland.

Note that with in-depth interviews, the rules of science listed above are followed. Data collection is systematic: there are a specific research question, sampling frame, and sample size, and there are formal parameters to the interview process. There is attention to minimizing bias: the interviewer adopts a special stance and uses special techniques to ensure that the ideas and experiences of the respondent are revealed as accurately and completely as possible – that is, validly and credibly. Once analyzed, such data can be used to offer interpretation and explanation, predict behaviors, and plan for the future.

9.3.2.2
Focus-Group Interview

In this form of interview, several people are interviewed at once [12, 20]. A main interviewer asks the questions and an assistant runs tapes, observes people as they answer, and "spells" the main interviewer when necessary. This approach is appropriate when the topic under study is broad and the answers needed are relatively easy for people to discuss publicly. Groups are formed that share important characteristics – such as age and sex – plus the focus issue. The group of jailed women receiving acupuncture detox mentioned at the beginning of this paper were interviewed in an informal focus-group manner.

Focus-group interviewing can be carried out as a qualitative *or* a quantitative procedure. As a qualitative procedure, the interviewing goals – and most of the methods – are the same as for in-depth interviews: researchers want to find out what meanings are contained in an issue. In the quantitative procedure, interviewers use a predetermined closed-ended set of questions and carry out what is essentially an oral opinion survey. This approach is popular with those who measure attitudes to new products, politicians, or public issues.

Some differences are introduced by having many people involved at once. For example, trust must now be established not merely between two people but among many. This is best achieved by being sure the sample membership shares similarities and by a lead interviewer who is skilled at helping people establish rapport. It is also important to establish ground rules for the respondents from the outset – for example, that although they may respond to others' comments and should express their opinions, they must not be harshly judgmental nor should they give advice.

9.3.2.3
Keeping a Diary or Journal

In this method, participants in research track their attitudes and experiences by writing about them every day, generally at home [8, 20]. In its simplest form, the diary is completely open-ended, with respondents simply asked to describe "whatever" about their lives with regard to, say, receiving or studying acupuncture care. Commonly, diaries are added to clinical trials or outcome studies of specific topics and used to gauge participant perception and interpretation of test interventions. In this case, respondents still talk about their lives, but this time with a focus on the test issue. For example, if one were comparing the recovery of stroke patients, some of whom received standard care and some of whom received standard care plus acupuncture, one might use the diary method to find out how participants perceive their progress. One could also use in-depth interviews in this situation, but the diary has the advantage of tracking change over time and not requiring as much time investment by the researchers.

Note that the word "diary" is applied in two very different situations. The true diary is a qualitative method in which the writer is simply asked to report "what is happening" with regard to some issue. A quantitative procedure version of the diary is not open-ended and instead resembles a survey form that one must fill out repeatedly at specified intervals.

9.3.2.4
Open-Ended Response on a Survey Questionnaire

In this example of mixed quantitative-qualitative research, a quantitative survey questionnaire includes space for personal responses. This can be done by adding *white space* at the end of forced-choice survey questions or it can be done by providing space at the end of the survey and inviting respondents to add their own comments. Here's an example of the first type, adding white space after a forced-choice question:

Many different methods of paying for acupuncture care have been considered. Which of the following payment options would you prefer, if you could choose any of them? (Select one).

Insurance that covers 80 % of my bill and does not limit my choice of acupuncturists but does limit the number of times I can visit my acupuncturist.

Membership in a preferred provider organization that limits my choice of acupuncturists but covers all costs except for a small copayment.

Membership in a referral organization that offers a select group of acupuncturists and a 20 % discount on care.

The way it is for most of us right now. I choose my acupuncturist and pay directly for my care.

Please use the space below to explain briefly your choice from the above list.

9.3.2.5
Case Study, Case Series

In a case study, the researcher examines a single example of the issue in extreme detail [22]. This form of study is very popular in medicine, where it is often called a case history; it is a relatively easy entree to research for clinicians. Case studies usually describe and analyze puzzling clinical situations and report how the practitioners handled and often solved them [18]. In the sense that they describe single events, case studies are like extended anecdotes. However, when well-done, case studies can meet scientific criteria for systematic collection and analysis of data. They are useful to other practitioners and may even spur focused research.

At the same time, the danger always exists in case studies that the practitioner misinterprets the event or his part in it. Thus, when careful practitioners think they've found a novel way to help people with a distinct pattern of malfunction, they will attempt to collect a whole series of similar cases. Each must be collected in much the same way – reporting the symptomatology, previous care, test care, response of the patient, and how long the improvement lasted. The researcher then tries to draw conclusions from the massed data and tries to make generalizations linking the specific cases. When convincing, case series serve two important functions: they allow a researchable hypothesis to emerge from clinical data and they provide pilot data for writing proposals to examine the hypothesis via a quantitative design, such as a clinical trials design. Thus, case series – a qualitative technique – are often used to fuel subsequent quantitative research.

9.3.3
Indirect Data Collection Techniques

The techniques summarized above emphasize the collection of information that the respondent can fairly easily think about and verbalize, that is, information that is consciously known. It is also possible to gather information that respondents do not know consciously or do not realize they know. Suppose you want to know what factors in patient beliefs affect the probability that they will recover from illness. Asking a direct question such as: "Do you want to get well?" is likely to provoke a knee-jerk response: "Of course!" However, you observe that some people who answer this way do get well while others linger in illness. Supposing you have already deleted "easy" causes such as different degrees of severity, what explains such differences? Research has shown that it is often differences in unconscious values, beliefs, and logical structures [21].

To gather information on unconscious knowledge, researchers have developed a set of techniques called *projective tests*. There are many. In this chapter, I will describe just one which is simple enough for office-based practitioners to use in concert with in-depth interviews. This is called the *card-sort method* [20]. Most people respond to it as a game and enjoy it.

In this method, the researcher prepares a set of cards on each of which is printed a single word or short phrase; each card is also numbered. The respondent is asked to sort the cards into stacks that "make sense." The researcher records the content of each stack by recording the numbers and then asks the respondent to "name" the stack and to explain why the cards that are in it go together. The respondent may also be asked to sort within a stack, for example, to sort disorders by severity. Once such data has been gathered from a sample of respondents, the researcher can analyze it by frequency (a quantitative function) and by content (a qualitative function).

Here is a simple example. Suppose a researcher wrote the names of acupuncture points on cards and asked practitioners to sort them "in any way that makes most sense to you."

– The set: SI.16, SI.17, Du15, Du16, Du26, Lu.11, Sp.1, Sp.6.
– Respondent 1 sorts by meridians: SI.16, 17; Du 15, 16, 26; Lu.11; Sp.1, 6.
– Respondent 2 sorts by location: shoulder and neck SI.16, 17, Du 15, 16; face Du 26; arm Lu.11; leg Sp.1, 6.
– Respondent 3 sorts by specialty: window of the sky point SI.16, 17, Du 15, 16; ghost point Du 26, Lu.11, Sp.1; three yin leg point Sp.6.

Note that all these sorts are "correct," although correctness is not the issue. Instead, we are interested in the different ways that people choose to organize data. Such differences could have clinical or other significance.

In a real example that was part of a team effort to remedy inadequacies in a national questionnaire, I wrote terms descriptive of "mental illness" on a set of 50 cards and asked respondents to a survey of "attitudes to mental illness" to sort them into stacks. They were given no further guidance, although the task I'd been given as researcher was to assess public attitudes to five common conditions including "depression." All respondents did, in fact, create stacks of cards containing words like "blue," "down," "depressed," "sad," and so forth. The fact that they selected the same words out of 50 means that all respondents perceived certain sensations as belonging together, forming a pattern. However, only one of 16 respondents used the psychologists' term and named the stack "depression." All the others used different descriptors such as "this is a person who doesn't feel too good about himself."

When respondents were asked to sort within the stack for severity, they revealed unconscious beliefs that were novel to psychology: that most words relating to the psychologists' construct "depression" were *not* considered pathological by respondents (although they were by psychologists) and that the adjective "depressed" was considered much less serious a condition than the noun "depression." No one could have verbalized these points individually, but the card-sort method allowed unconscious knowledge to "speak" and (in this case) showed that it is similarly framed among the people sampled. Additionally – and here we arrive at an example of qualitative research providing explanations that quantitative methods cannot provide – the data helped explain the rather large gap between public behavior around "depression" symptoms and the perception by psychologists that "people don't come for treatment soon enough." According to the card-sort data, this is at least partly because they do not interpret the symptoms as pathological nearly as soon as psychologists do.

These data also illustrate how the language of questions may inadvertently mislead researchers: a change such as that from adjective to noun in the questions below may mean that questions are interpreted very differently by respondents:

In the last 3 weeks, how often have you experienced a depressed mood?
In the last 3 weeks, how often have you been depressed?

The card-sort technique is relatively easy to develop and respondents are often surprised and fascinated by the decisions they find themselves making. If they are encouraged to verbalize their processing of the card sort, the researcher may gain rich additional material for an in-depth interview.

9.3.4
Data Analysis Techniques

In all research, one must first gather data, then analyze and interpret it. In quantitative research, the data collection process is usually more time-consuming than analysis; the reverse is true of qualitative research.

In quantitative research, a limited number of possible answers are provided. This means that computer programs can easily manage them and statistical programs can easily count responses and show distributions of the data points. With qualitative research, in contrast, respondents use their own words to talk about issues in ways that are generally not predictable ahead of time. The analytic task, then, is not to count responses but to study the words so as to identify distinctive themes and shared perceptions among the respondents [2, 11, 19]. For example, when some people say "acupuncture makes me feel more grounded," do they mean much the same thing as those who say "acupuncture makes me feel more centered?" This process of analyzing the verbal, metaphorical, thematic, and other content of qualitative data is formally called *content analysis*. Content analysis often suggests that there are other issues worth pursuing; in this case, one may apply other analytic methods such as cognitive mapping, an illustration of which is given below.

9.3.4.1
Content Analysis

Content analysis can often be done by hand. This is appropriate if the data set is quite small – for example, 30 or fewer respondents. However, if one is working with a large data set, nowadays it is much easier to use one of several qualitative analysis software packages on the market. In either case, the first step is to transcribe the interview tapes or written material from survey questionnaires or diaries into typed or word processed form so that they can be printed out and made easy to read. This unanalyzed data is called *raw data*.

In the next step, the researcher reads the material – usually several times – to "get a feel" for its overall content. At this point, he is trying to find ways to analyze the data that will accurately reflect what has been said. For example, when people are asked "What has acupuncture been like for you?" they may answer by describing:

1. How their health has changed
2. What their practitioner is like

3. What they think about the health care they received before acupuncture
4. How their relationship to their spouse, children, job, or school has changed
5. How their attitudes to life have changed

A given person may discuss several of these themes; others may focus on just one. Some people speak poetically, using many metaphors and much imagery; others speak emotionally, yet others analytically. Some laugh while they describe their experiences, others weep. Some use strong language. As the researcher studies the raw data, he must decide which of the many issues and values are actually relevant to the research. Is it worth studying the metaphors people use? Does it matter if one person cries and another laughs? Additionally, the researcher must decide how to "cut" the data – one type of cut is shown by the five categories above.

Supposing our researcher decides to use these five categories. He can now use a software program to help with the analysis. Most of the programs work more or less in the same fashion:

The researcher moves the raw data from the word processing program into the qualitative analysis program, using identifiers as specified by the program. He then reads through the material, marking the themes as they appear, again according to the format of the particular software program. Once the themes are marked, the program can capture each theme with identifiers and print them out together. Now every instance of any theme, such as "practitioner description," is centralized in one file and can be printed out for further study.

Such a treated theme is now much easier to study. Usually it rewards further subdivision, for example, descriptions featuring particular words or images: practitioner as genuine, caring or loving, skilled, knowledgeable, insightful, or trustworthy. In each case, negative descriptors are also recorded, that is: practitioner as untrustworthy, uncaring, and so forth.

Now notice that one can make a count of images at this point – one can say, for example, how many times practitioners are described as genuine. However, the resulting number is *not* a valid indicator of how often acupuncture practitioners are viewed as genuine by patients, because *this was not the question asked*. What it actually measures is how often respondents *thought to use the word "genuine"* when describing their practitioner. And the reasons for thinking to use this word are potentially legion. For example, it could be a popular word in a particular region, while in other regions people prefer other terms such as "trustworthy." In a real case, I found that patients in two sites referred to their acupuncturist as "doctor," while in other sites patients used terms like "guide," "friend," and "partner." Was there a major difference in perception of practitioners going on between sites? The answer was no; in the two sites where "doctor" was used, the practitioner held a doctoral degree; in the other sites, the practitioners did not [6].

In sum, when reporting frequencies of themes or imagery in qualitative research, researchers must avoid statistical formulations ("10 % of respondents said..."), and instead use appropriate relativistic language: *many, a minority, frequently, generally, rarely*. In the context of qualitative research, such terms are not vague; they are accurate because the research set out to find patterns and perceptions, not frequencies.

9.3.4.2
Interpretation

Notice that qualitative, similar to quantitative, research is heavily dependent on researcher interpretation. This means that the researcher must know as much as possible about the vagaries of interpretation and his or her own assumptive habits. This topic is developed in many methods texts, e.g., Bernard 1998 [2]. An example of (almost) letting one's own issues or hypotheses color the interpretation was mentioned above ("I wonder if practitioners called 'doctor' are authoritarian?"). The solution was also mentioned: first try to find an explanation within the data by going back to the source.

This example signposts an important "rule" of scientific method (often called Occam's Razor): seek the simpler answer, because it is likely to be more trustworthy. In short, do not develop unnecessarily complex interpretations.

9.3.5
Data from a Qualitative Study of Oriental Medicine Patients

Several qualitative studies of oriental medicine patients have been published. For example, Martha Hare studied the design of acupuncture health care delivery in private and public (including detox) clinics in New York City [13, 14]. Mitra Emad richly analyzed patient and practitioner experiences and perceptions [10] and discussed the meaning of pain during acupuncture needling [9]. Several similar studies are ongoing as of this writing.

To provide readers with an on-the-ground example of qualitative research, I will describe data and details of the logic of data collection and analysis from my own survey of Chinese medicine patients in six private acupuncture clinics in five states (for the complete report, see [6]). As we move through this section, notice that raw data become increasingly refined and abstracted – the proper process of science – and that, at the end, some highly practical generalizations emerge, each of which is based solidly on data from the survey.

9.3.6
Developing the Survey Questionnaire

With the intention of developing a quantitative survey questionnaire with high model fit validity, the study began with a preliminary qualitative research step: we performed in-depth interviews with 60 present and former patients of Chinese medicine. Each was asked six open-ended questions; all interviews were audiotaped. The tapes were transcribed and their content analyzed to identify issues important to respondents. These were used to develop questions about, for example, reasons for selecting acupuncture, attitudes to practitioners, presenting or chief complaints, changes in health in the presence of acupuncture, how relevant they thought acupuncture was in explaining their health improvements, how cost effective they thought acupuncture was, and so on. Practitioners and selected patients were invited to critique the questionnaire that emerged from this qualitative analytic process. (Normally, during this phase of questionnaire development, one would also study existing questionnaires designed to survey similar populations; but with Chinese medicine this is rarely possible, since so little survey research has been performed.)

After developing a questionnaire that reflected the language and issues of patients and also satisfied practitioners, we performed two pilot tests. These test not only the questionnaire but the survey process; they are used to identify weaknesses in design. Adjustments were made in response to the pilot results and finally the pretested, mixed qualitative-quantitative questionnaire survey was run in six clinics that met predefined criteria for "large client population size." The survey received 575 responses, including 460 questionnaires that contained written or qualitative material.

9.3.7
Analyzing the Qualitative Data

The quantitative and qualitative data from this survey were separately analyzed using statistical, word processing, and qualitative analysis software, as appropriate. Here I will discuss only the qualitative survey segment, specifically the search for themes in the handwritten responses to an open-ended final question inviting respondents to discuss their experiences with Chinese medicine.

1. After transcribing the handwritten responses into the word processor, I printed them out and began to read and reread them, the first step in content analysis. The task is to know the material well enough to identify which themes best describe the material. I chose to list two types of themes separately, those that the respondents themselves identified and those that I felt emerged organically from their responses, such as popular metaphors about the body or being.
2. Eventually, I identified five respondent-identified themes. Chinese medicine (as practiced in these clinics):
   a. Relieves symptoms and improves function.
   b. Improves physiological coping or adaptive ability.
   c. Improves psychosocial coping or adaptive ability.
   d. Involves a close patient-practitioner relationship.
   e. Treats the "whole" body/mind/spirit/social person.

As you see, these themes are abstract: no respondents used exactly these words in writing about their experiences nor, had I asked directly, would anyone have said: "Oh yes, my experience can be broken down into the following themes...."

In short, I used the specific – stories – to abstract and study larger issues. I used individual accounts to identify commonalities that matter in the delivery of health care. No statistical analysis was involved, but the result is similar to what one would receive from quantitative analysis: general findings that can be applied to describe why American patients select and appreciate acupuncture care. In addition, the analysis allowed me to examine some broader issues, especially why Chinese medicine as framed in the U. S. fulfills many of the characteristics of the low-tech, low-cost, high-relational "new" medicine that health care planners wish to see emerge.

Within each of the major themes were subthemes for which I could adduce evidence – that is, provide the words of respondents. For example, one subtheme within Theme 1 was "decreases the frequency, intensity, or duration of chronic complaints."

Comments that sounded this message were frequent; one example reads: "Acupuncture makes the pain go away part of the time and each time staves it off for longer amounts of time. Soon I hope to be pain-free." No other respondent, of course, spoke exactly like this; qualitative researchers must pay attention to the content of each sentence to identify when respondents are sounding a particular analytic theme. Notice how different this situation is from that in quantitative research, where a forced-choice question might ask respondents to say how much they agreed with a set phrase, such as "With acupuncture my pain is less severe." In the latter case, respondents can reveal degrees of acceptance of a question put to them by researchers, but they cannot reveal their own issues, put their own "spin" on issues, or talk about their hopes and fears ("Soon I hope to be pain-free").

9.3.8
Cognitive Mapping

Certain words appeared in so many respondents' stories that it was obvious that these words were especially important to people in trying to express their relationship to Chinese medicine. I decided to follow up on these words to explore whether the ideas behind Chinese medicine had penetrated to patients. For example, Theme 3 – Chinese medicine improves psychosocial coping or adaptive ability – contained a popular subtheme which I called "engenders a sense of wholeness, balance, centeredness, well-being." Were these words and similar ones like "calm" and "grounded" all describing much the same response to Chinese medicine? With what other terms were these words associated? Specifically, were they associated with Chinese medicine terms like *qi* or its popular transfiguration as "energy"?

To find out, I carried out an analytic procedure – not very difficult – called *cognitive mapping* [19]. In this procedure, you identify *cue words* that appear in many responses. You then use a simple "find" function in a word processing program to count how often these words occur. Using a qualitative analysis program, you can also print out the cue words with the two preceding and succeeding lines of type. You now begin to map: for example, how often does a "self-awareness/wholeness" word (calm, peaceful, centered, grounded, whole...) occur within two lines of a "Chinese medicine" word (*qi, shen, yang*, deficiency, sedate...), an "energy" cue word, or a "stress" cue word? Basically, you simply find all instances in which categories of cue words occur together and count them. (Notice that quantitative data is emerging from this qualitative analytic method.) The map consists of stating how close one set is to the next.

In the present case, I found some surprising results: the strongest association was between self-awareness/holism words and stress words – when cue words occurred together, 40 % of the time it was these two kinds together; the second strongest link was between "energy" and "self-awareness" (21.5 % of sample). There were, however, very few links between "Chinese medicine" and any other category, including "energy."

What was I to make of this map? First of all, it was clear that respondents were not using the language of Chinese medicine to describe their experiences. In fact, only seven used any language relating to Chinese medicine theory and not even one of the 460 respondents used the cue word *qi*. On the other hand, a majority of respondents used words redolent of the language and concepts of holism. In fact, what they were saying was "this thing called Chinese medicine delivers holistic care and allows me to convert stress to self-awareness/wholeness."

Based on such information, one could argue that acupuncturists and herbalists are doing a poor job of teaching their clients the explanatory model of oriental medicine. Other qualitative data – specifically, the fact that respondents claimed that their practitioners were good teachers – suggested this is not the best explanation. Another possibility was that practitioners have successfully translated the oriental medicine idiom into an acceptable English language idiom featuring words such as stress, energy, and balance. This is the interpretation I chose. Such words are also used by practitioners of other alternative medical practices and are abroad in the society whenever people discuss the construct called "holism." Thus, based on story content, word use and cognitive mapping, I concluded that it appears that many consumers of Chinese medicine are purchasing not an exotic Chinese philosophy or theory but a home-grown holism.

From this example, readers can understand not only the technique of cognitive mapping but also see how words and their patterns and the contents of handwritten or oral "stories" can be studied and abstracted to create generalizations. But of what use is it to know that American consumers are purchasing holism more than Chinese medicine *per se*? Actually, it has several practical applications. Let me quote from the end of the article:

"...the present study is important not only because it reveals patient perceptions and values, but also because it defines theoretical components of holism, shows how these might be actualized in practice, and then goes on to show that, in at least one case, a large sample of patients are receiving care that they experience and define as holistic. This is all the more remarkable as these patients are located in clinics that are geographically remote from each other. What links the clinics, then, is not location or experience, but a construct called 'Chinese medicine' – and this medicine, whatever the case elsewhere in the world, or even in other American settings, emerges in this setting as holistic."

"This study, then, can serve as a model not only of what holism feels like to patients, but also of what it might look like in practice. And what it 'looks like' is very much what health care philosophers and planners are seeking: a low-tech, high-relationship practice with users experiencing both relief of presenting complaints and expanded effects of care including improved self-reliance, plus high satisfaction with the care and the experience."

9.4
Qualitative Research Needs in Oriental Medicine

I hope that this discussion and the illustrations have piqued the interest of readers. Clearly, some aspects of qualitative research lend themselves to use by acupuncture practitioners, even if they are not formally trained in research methods. I particularly recommend the in-depth interview, the card-sort technique, using initial qualitative research to develop quantitative survey questionnaires, and using qualitative diaries during clinical outcomes and trials research.

Anyone deciding to do such research is also well-advised to consult a specialist to check whether his or her plans meet the formal criteria for good qualitative research. If you don't know a qualitative researcher, contact a nearby university or college for help. Look for qualitative specialists especially in anthropology, sociology, and nursing departments.

Here is a sampling of appropriate questions that will reward qualitative research – it's easy to add many more – and notice that all are pragmatic:

1. What is most meaningful to experienced practitioners about their work?
2. What features of their education reaffirm student decisions to stay in school and which make them want to drop out of the field?
3. What characteristics of acupuncture practitioners are most valued by acupuncture patients?
4. What messages from practitioners are most rewarding to patients and which are least rewarding?
5. How can practitioners speak so as best to motivate their patients to make needed changes in lifestyle?
6. What easily identifiable features make patients most or least likely to respond to acupuncture care?
7. How would patients like most to pay for their care? What is the reasoning behind their choice?
8. What practitioner characteristics are most common in those who have rewarding full-time practices 5 and 10 years after graduating from school, respectively? Can success of incoming students be predicted by these parameters?
9. Does needle depth matter?
10. Do the patients of practitioners of TCM, Worsley Five Element, French Energetic, and *Toyo Hari* styles have significantly different experiences with acupuncture?
11. Are students at schools that provide a cultural context for Chinese medicine more secure in their knowledge afterwards than students from schools that do not?
12. What does it mean when practitioners claim to be "holistic" healers?
13. What is the relationship between the concepts of "energy" and "*qi*" for American practitioners?
14. What do *qi gong* practitioners experience when they "throw" *qi*?
15. What do patients understand about the theory of oriental medicine after a course of treatment?
16. What do practitioners say about the "intentionality" of their care?

9.5
Uses of Qualitative Research

In this chapter, I have defined qualitative research and given examples of its use and advantages in a number of situations. Still, qualitative research remains the "mystery stepchild" in the minds of many researchers and in the public mind. Why is this? A full answer is too complicated for this chapter, but it is worth mentioning that the issue is partly one of cultural values and perception.

When asking "Does oriental medicine work?" it is common for people to focus on comparative clinical questions such as "Is acupuncture as effective as standard care in the treatment of a given condition?" This is the familiar biomedical formulation and the sort of topic most likely to receive funding since the biomedical framework remains sociopolitically dominant. However, this kind of question addresses only a fraction of what needs attention in the field of oriental medicine and it can provide only a fraction of the information needed to answer the "Does it work?" question. Other issues that help answer the question include those concerning (a) within-the-field issues such as the significance of differing needle depths, (b) physiological mechanisms, (c) demographic and epidemiological distributions, and d) people's motivations for seeking and continuing the use or practice of oriental medicine. Each of these issues is right for research and it is in the last field listed where qualitative research will reap its greatest harvest. This is because, no matter how much we may know about the mechanism or comparative effectiveness of oriental medical care, *if people won't buy it*, the other information becomes insignificant.

Don't take this idea of "buying" too literally. We use this term literally to speak of dollars and cents; we also use it metaphorically to speak of credibility. Credibility is built primarily through – here is where the other shoe drops – *telling stories*. Indeed, to reach the mass of people, the number-laden results of quantitative research must be translated into narrative or "story" form. It is through narrative that people become convinced to study the field, create laws that support it, fund research for it, and become acupuncture patients.

Thus, the telling of stories – if they are built upon a base of properly collected and well-analyzed data – is at the core of all communication about oriental medicine.

9.6
Closing Remarks

Qualitative research is a powerful method – indeed the only method – for gathering the "stories" of people's lives and assembling information on the assumptions and beliefs that reveal motivations and explain people's behaviors. When we know what has meaning for others, we can put this information to work to solve daily problems from the local (e.g., how to design clinics to enhance patient recovery, how to minimize student dropout in acupuncture schools) to the general (how the theory of Chinese medicine translates into the American setting, why patients find oriental medical care satisfying).

Qualitative research lends itself to use by practitioners in their offices. However, to use the techniques described, clinicians must clearly distinguish their research task from their medical task and develop systematic designs for data collection. This chapter has introduced some basic techniques, warned about pitfalls, and proposed ideas for needed qualitative research in the field of Chinese medicine. I hope that readers will pursue some of the ideas proposed in this chapter and develop their own ideas putting qualitative methods to work.

References

1. Bernard HR (1993) Research methods in cultural anthropology. Second edn. Sage Publications, Thousand Oaks
2. Bernard HR (1998) Handbook of methods in cultural anthropology. Altamira Press, Thousand Oaks
3. Brink PJ, Wood MJ (1988) Basic steps in planning nursing research, from question to proposal. Third edn. Jones and Bartlett Publ, Boston

4. Cassidy C (1995) Social science methods in alternative medicine research. J Altern Compl Med 1:19–42
5. Cassidy CM (1994) Unraveling the ball of string: Reality, paradigms, and the study of alternative medicine. Advances. J Mind-Body Med 10:5–31
6. Cassidy CM (1998) Chinese medicine users in the United States, Parts 1 and 2. J Altern Compl Med 4:17–27, 189–202
7. Creswell J (1994) Research design, qualitative and quantitative approaches. Sage Publications, Thousand Oaks
8. Denzin NK, Lincoln YS (1994) Handbook of Qualitative Research. Sage Publications, Thousand Oaks
9. Emad M (1994) Does acupuncture hurt? Cultural shifts in experience of pain. Proc Soc Acupunct Res 2:129–140
10. Emad M (1998) Feeling the qi: Emergent bodies and disclosive fields in American appropriations of acupuncture. Dissertation available from Univ Michigan Microfilms, Ann Arbor
11. Feldman MS (1995) Strategies for interpreting qualitative data. Sage Publications, Thousand Oaks
12. Fontana A, Frey J (1994) Interviewing, the art of science. In: Denzin NK, Lincoln YS (eds) Handbook of qualitative research. Sage Publications, Thousand Oaks, pp.361–376
13. Hare M (1992) East-Asian medicine among non-Asian New Yorkers: A study in transformation and translation. Dissertation available from Univ Michigan Microfilms, Ann Arbor
14. Hare M (1993) The emergence of an urban U. S. Chinese medicine. Med Anthropol Quart 7:30–49
15. Kirk J, Miller ML (1986) Reliability and validity in qualitative research. Sage Publications, Thousand Oaks
16. Marshall C, Rossman GB (1989) Designing qualitative research. Sage Publications, Thousand Oaks
17. McCracken G (1988) The long interview. Qualitative research methods, Vol 13, Sage Publications, Newbury Park
18. MacPherson H, Kaptchuk T (1997) Acupuncture in practice, case history insights from the west. Churchill Livingstone, Edinburgh
19. Miles MB, Huberman AM (1994) Qualitative data analysis. Second edn. Sage Publications, Thousand Oaks
20. Morse J, Field PA (1995) Qualitative research methods for health professionals. Second edn. Sage Publications, Thousand Oaks
21. Schlusser G (1992) Coping strategies and individual meanings of illness. Soc Sci Med 34:427–432
22. Yin R (1994) Case study research, design and methods. Second edn. Applied Social Research Methods Series, Vol. 5. Sage Publications, Thousand Oaks

Recommended Reading

Brody H (1987) Stories of sickness. Yale Univ Press, New Haven
Carmines EG, Zeller RA (1979) Reliability and validity assessment. Quantitative applications in the social sciences. Sage Publications, Thousand Oaks
Gephart R (1988) Ethnostatistics: Qualitative foundations for quantitative research. Sage Qualitative Methods, Vol 12. Sage Publications, Thousand Oaks
Lee ES, Forthofer R, Lorimor R (1989) Analyzing complex survey data. Quantitative Applications in the Social Sciences. Sage Publications, Thousand Oaks
McDowell I, Newell C (1996) Measuring health, a guide to rating scales and questionnaires. Oxford Univ Press, Oxford
Ogles BM, Lambert MJ, Masters KS (1996) Assessing outcome in clinical practice. Allyn and Bacon, Boston
Reissman C (1993) Narrative analysis. Qualitative research methods, Vol 30. Sage Publications, Newbury Park
Schuman H, Presser S (1996) Questions and answers in attitude surveys. Sage Publications, Thousand Oaks
Stewart AL, Ware JE (1992) Measuring functioning and well-being, the Medical Outcomes Study Approach. Duke Univ Press, Durham
Streiner DL, Norman GR (1989) Health measurement scales: A practical guide to their development and use. Oxford Univ Press, Oxford

CHAPTER 10

Proposed Standards of Acupuncture Treatment for Clinical Studies

G. Stux · S. Birch

10.1
Introduction

The quality of clinical trials of acupuncture conducted since the early 1970s is often poor. General reviews and formal evaluations of the literature are uniform in this finding [22, 23, 26, 27, 30, 32, 34, 37–39, 43, 51, 53, 55, 59, 66, 67, 70–74]. While the literature evaluating these clinical trials continues to grow, it has focused largely on the methodological quality of the study designs and the soundness of their results, but there has been little discussion of the adequacy of the acupuncture treatment itself. A few authors have suggested that the quality or adequacy of the acupuncture in these clinical trials may be problematic [17, 32, 57, 63], and some have discussed guidelines to suggest what constitutes adequate treatment [4, 64]. There is generally a paucity of systematic analysis of the adequacy of the acupuncture tested in these clinical trials. One review team merely assessed whether the treatment was reported or not [34, 66, 67]. Another team attempted to develop criteria for such an evaluation but experienced difficulties with the method selected [39]. This essay will outline criteria for evaluating the adequacy of treatment in acupuncture studies, present evaluations of the adequacy of a number of clinical trials, and describe a systematic method for ensuring adequacy in future studies. Preliminary versions of some of these methods and data have been presented in previous research conferences and publications [4–6, 23, 64].

10.2
Acupuncture Treatment – What Is Involved?

When acupuncture is administered, several decisions are made as the basis for selecting the optimal treatment:
1. What are the most appropriate sites of treatment for a patient?
2. What is the optimal number of treated sites?
3. What is the optimal number of treatment sessions?
4. What is the optimal frequency of treatment?
5. What techniques of treatment should be applied at each treated site and what tools are best used to do this?
6. Is acupuncture to be used alone or as a complement to standard therapy?

Prior to asking these questions, two more questions are usually raised: who shall administer the acupuncture treatment and what are that person's training requirements?

The treatment is usually selected based on answers to all these questions. However, many of the questions are not explicitly addressed or answered in the acupuncture literature and hence in practice. Most texts describe how one should apply the prescribed treatment once the diagnosis is selected, with certain pluses and minuses according to the patient. But this process is not always an explicit one and, as happens in many areas, the decisions and issues are constantly evolving. Take for example the treatment of drug addiction using acupuncture. Addiction is a complex health problem for which acupuncture has been applied over the last 25 years. The treatment was initially applied by needling the auricles with additional electrical stimulation of the needles [75]. Then, as it became more widely used, needles started being used alone, at set points that practitioners had noticed seemed to be most helpful [12]. These treatments were added into existing treatment programs where group and individual counseling is the standard treatment [13]. Many using this approach stated that the counseling was an essential part of therapy and that the acupuncture should be used principally as an adjunctive treatment. It was also recommended that the acupuncture be applied daily if possible, at least for the detoxification stage of treatment, and then as needed. Clinical trials testing the auricular needling then started being conducted. However, a close examination of them reveals a certain heterogeneity in the approach. Some used three, some four, some five auricle points, and some used additional body acupoints [14, 48]. Most used the acupuncture adjunctively to the standard counseling therapy, but some used it alone without concurrent counseling [40]. Frequency of treatment also varied. Reviewers examining the clinical trial literature of acupuncture in the treatment of addictions have expressed their frustration with the variability of approaches, noting the need for a more standardized approach [51].

The variation in this area of acupuncture practice and trial literature is not unique. In general, we can say that acupuncture is not a homogenous method, unvarying in its applications in the different countries and cultures where it is used [9]. There are many different models of acupuncture practice and many different methods and techniques that may be used [7]. Thus, the answers to the above series of questions are usually tailored to the training and background of the acupuncturist asking them. For example, the traditional Chinese medicine (TCM) acupuncturist is trained to identify the "zheng," or pattern giving rise to the patient's complaint, and to treat this while also applying treatment to relieve the symptoms. In the TCM model, there are hundreds of possible zheng [76]. The practitioner of the Japanese Keiraku Chiryo style is trained to identify one of only four patterns, or "sho", and apply treatment to correct this and relieve the symptoms [61]. Some styles of acupuncture do not apply any particular assessment methods to determine a sho or zheng, but rather they apply treatment simply to relieve the symptoms [19]. As a consequence of this diversity, we must recognize the following if we are to proceed with an examination of the standards for acupuncture treatment in clinical studies of acupuncture:

1. To test a particular style or method of practice, care must be taken to ensure that relevant methods are used. Thus, in answer to the series of questions above, it is important that each answer is congruent with that style or method of practice. If

testing the TCM style of acupuncture, the characteristic "de qi" sensation should be obtained at each site of insertion as is prescribed by the literature [16] and, similarly, the zheng should be determined to be able to administer optimal treatment [11].

2. Additionally, the conclusions of the study should discuss that style of acupuncture rather than acupuncture itself, as such generalizing may be misleading. For example, it would be misleading to discuss how acupuncture can treat addictions, since the treatment is principally of the auricles. It would be more precise to discuss the effects of auricular acupuncture.

3. If one wants to test acupuncture itself and be able to start generalizing across the entire field, it is necessary to take the diversity of practice approaches into account. This requires a systematic method of examining the literature to find appropriate answers to the above series of questions. These questions and issues related to the diversity of practice approaches have not been addressed in most clinical trials, creating many problems in their interpretation.

10.3
A Systematic Analysis of the Adequacy of Treatment in Acupuncture Studies

In an effort to understand the scope of the problem of adequacy of treatment in acupuncture studies, Birch conducted a review of the literature describing acupuncture treatment of chronic headache and low back or neck pain. Twenty-six Japanese, Chinese, and English texts were examined. This review found that a conservative minimum treatment for each condition involves ten treatment loci for a course of ten treatment sessions [4, 6]. (See below for details and examples.) Based on this review, 34 controlled clinical trials were examined to see if treatments approximated what was found in the literature review. Table 1 shows the results from applying these criteria to those 34 studies [6].

Applying these basic criteria in the three chronic pain conditions, none of the 34 studies clearly administered adequate treatment. Some may have, but because of inadequate reporting of the treatment methods, it is not possible to determine this one way or the other [5]. When these minimum adequate criteria were relaxed, it was found that half the studies administered approximately adequate treatment (Table 1).

Berman and colleagues conducted a formal review of 47 pain studies incorporating the above criteria for adequate and approximately adequate minimum treatment [23]. Using logistic regression analyses to examine the adequacy of treatment as a variable in outcome, they found that both the adequate and approximately adequate minimum treatments were significantly associated with a positive outcome when controlling for study quality [23]. This finding suggests that conservative minimum treatments derived from the literature reviews are valid.

Table 1. Adequacy of treatment in 34 controlled studies of acupuncture for head, neck and back pain

N administered adequate treatments (10 loci, 10 sessions)	0
N administered approximately adequate treatments (6 loci, 6 sessions)	17
N administered clearly inadequate treatments	8
N about which we cannot say if adequate treatment was administered	9

A further examination of the clinical acupuncture trial literature found other related problems. Some reviewers found that the actual treatments are not described at all in some studies and that there is no source referencing of the applied treatments, thereby hindering determination of what treatments were actually applied [5, 32, 34, 66, 67]. In an analysis of 86 controlled studies, Kersken found that no description of therapy was given in 18 studies (21 %) and that no description of the number of treatment sessions or other important parameters were given in 19 (22 %), [32]. Kersken found additionally that, while adequate descriptions were made of treatment principles in 15 of the 86 studies, 34 (40 %) did not [32]. It is hard to imagine a study of an analgesic drug where the actual drug and doses used are not described nor references given so that one can check elsewhere what was done; but the equivalent problem can be found in acupuncture studies [17, 18, 20].

In his analysis of the acupuncture quality in 86 studies, Kersken found that only 33 % describe obtaining a de qi response [32]. Pomeranz also noted that in many studies recommending the specific needle technique, elicitation of the de qi response (obtaining the qi) was not applied and that thus many studies did not adequately apply treatment [56]. While de qi is a very common method of needling and characteristic of some but not all forms of acupuncture [7], it is important that the study utilizes this technique when testing those models in which it is normally indicated.

Some have also argued that the optimal use of acupuncture includes traditional diagnostic methods to individualize treatment appropriately for patients in clinical studies [17, 44]. While this is not necessarily a valid claim, given the diversity of practice approaches [6, 8], it is important to individualize treatments when testing models that usually employ these assessments. However, these methods require prior testing to establish their reliability [5, 69]. To date, very few studies of traditional diagnostic assessment methods have been conducted [69]. While evidence of the reliability of those assessments is slowly growing [8], it is still essential to incorporate reliability studies into future prospective trials that wish to use them.

The training of the person administering the treatments can be an additional issue. In their three reviews, Ter Riet et al. addressed whether the training was mentioned in the 86 studies they reviewed [34, 66, 67], finding that "good quality of the acupuncturist" was mentioned in only 30 studies. Hammerschlag and Morris examined 23 studies to find that the acupuncturist's qualifications were mentioned in only one [27], a much smaller percentage than when all studies were pooled by Ter Riet and colleagues. However, mentioning the skill of the acupuncturist or simply stating his qualifications are clearly not enough, since training in acupuncture is not the same as real qualification to administer the treatment in a clinical study. For example, how much experience do they have?

Obviously, more needs to be specified. Here we find a very contentious issue, as training requirements for acupuncturists vary considerably around the world [3]. There are places where physicians may practice with no training and others where practice is unregulated and anyone can practice. However, many countries and states within those countries have come up with some minimum training standards, but these vary tremendously from place to place. One of the principle variables has to do with whether the acupuncturist is also a physician. Typically, physicians study acupuncture in shorter programs than nonphysicians. Training programs for physicians can run from 1 or more weekends to several hundred hours; a review in Australia found programs that ranged from 50 to 390 hours [3]. The recommended length of training programs for physicians in Germany is proposed to be 350 hours, 50 % theoretical and 50 % practical. The World Federation of Acupuncture and Moxibustion Societies (WFAS) recommends a minimum of 200 hours' training for physicians wishing to practice acupuncture [28]. Training for nonphysicians is usually at least 400 hours and can be substantially more [9]. For example, in Australia, training programs run from 1562 to 3824 hours [3], with the number of acupuncture- and TCM-specific training hours ranging from 906 to 2936 hours [3]. In the U.S., accredited programs contain a minimum of 2175 hours, with the average program lasting 450 hours more than this [21]. It is difficult to ascertain a clear minimum standard of training for acupuncturists in studies of acupuncture, but at the least a minimum needs to be established in the context of the country of study. Ideally, an approved course of study should have been completed. We would feel uncomfortable with a physician not experienced in a particular medical procedure to administer that procedure in a clinical trial.

While we cannot generalize for all trials from these reviews, it does appear that there is a significant problem in how acupuncture treatments are tested in clinical trials. Putting aside questions about what some proponents believe are the correct styles of treatment [2, 17, 44], in simple numerical terms (number of points treated and number of treatment sessions), it appears that many clinical trials did not apply sufficient treatment. This is akin to testing a drug in a controlled clinical trial at inadequate doses for an inadequate length of time. If the results of such a trial were positive for the drug, many might consider it to be very effective and capable of working at lower doses than expected. Were the results of the drug trial negative, few would argue that it had been properly tested. However, knowledge of this issue has not yet been adequately incorporated into reviews of the acupuncture clinical trial literature. In the absence of such analyses, many reviewers assumed that the treatments were adequate and, upon finding little robust data or other problems with study design, concluded that acupuncture does not appear to be very effective [34, 66, 67, 71]. Were analyses of the adequacy of treatment incorporated into such reviews, it could be that many authors would need to change their conclusions.

In the following, we outline methods for determining what might constitute minimum adequate treatment in a clinical trial of acupuncture. These methods and their results can be used both in reassessment of the published literature and by researchers planning prospective studies. Based on the minimum adequate treatment, we then describe what might be the optimal treatment, or that expected to produce optimal results for a patient or group of patients.

10.4
Proposed Method for Review of the Literature

Birch pointed out previously that one of the principal reasons for finding treatment inadequate was that many research teams appear to have read little of the available acupuncture literature, as evidenced by the lack or inadequate citation of sources in published studies [5], some even citing no acupuncture literature at all [17]. The solution to this problem is obviously that more acupuncture literature needs to be read before researchers embark on clinical trials. But here there are still a number of issues that will need to be dealt with:

1. There are often problems with the literature itself [5]
2. There are problems stemming from the nature of the question to be addressed and the related issue of generalizability of results [5, 11]
3. There is a problem with variability in the literature [6, 12]. We propose a systematic and extensive literature review to address these issues in each relevant area.

Table 2 illustrates how the literature review process is applied. It shows the findings from a review of 18 texts describing the treatment of low back pain by acupuncture. The recommended treatments in each text are compiled to show the ranges and averages of recommended numbers of treatment points and sessions. The review included a variety of texts from different approaches, so that when averaging the recommended numbers of points and sessions, we can increase the generalizability of results. The points recommended by each text for low back pain and the various subcategories of low back pain are recorded. By examining the specific points, the total number of discrete sites to be treated could be extrapolated. If the text indicated the number of treatment sessions necessary, this is also recorded.

According to these sources, low back pain is treated with 2–14 points, or 3–28 needles, at an average range of 5.1–7.8 points and 9.5–13.8 discrete sites per treatment. Further, at least ten treatments need to be given, which matches clinical experience [64]. It thus appears that at least ten discrete sites treated for at least ten sessions can be considered the minimum adequate treatment for chronic low back pain. Hence, treatment should involve these parameters in a clinical trial for chronic low back pain.

Acupuncture texts rarely discuss the number of sessions and frequency of treatment. As shown in Table 2, only three of 18 texts discussed the recommended number

Table 2. Recommended treatment outlines for low back pain

Source	Recommended number of treatment points
Kwok et al. 1991	4/6/7/5/5/5/6 (7–14)
Manaka 1970	6/3/2 (3–10)
Shanghai Institute of TCM, n.d.	8–10/8–10/8–11/8–10/8–13 (16–26)
O'Connor, Bensky 1981	6–10 (10–18) [10 or more sessions]
Anon 1980	3/6/3 (5–10)
Cheng 1987	5/5/5/3 (5–9)
Feit, Zmiewski 1990	6/6/6 (10–11)
Liu 1988	5/5/5/3 (6–10)
Qiu, Su 1985	8/4/5/5 (7–15)
Chen, Wang 1988	6 (12) (actual cases) [15 sessions]
So 1987	5 (9) [over 10 sessions for chronic pain]
Mann 1974	6 (12)
Tianjin Chinese Med Coll 1988	6/4 (7–10)
Stux, Pomeranz 1988	5+3–4 (10–14)
Nagahama et al 1983	Up to 14 depending on pressure pain (probably 10–16)
Kinoshita 1983	7/6/8/up to 5 (10–14)
Ikeda 1985	10–14/8–12/6/10–13/12 (12–28)
Lee, Cheung 1978	6/5 (10–11)

The entry "6/6/5" indicates three alternative treatments (including treatments according to differential diagnostic patterns) with six, six, and five points listed, respectively. The entry "(10–11)" indicates that from 10 to 11 discrete sites are treated
N.d., no year given.

Table 3. Summary of low back pain treatments in TCM related acupuncture texts [12]

Source	N patterns	N points
1. Kwok et al 1991	7	Mean 5.7 points (10.3–10.5 discrete sites)
2. Manaka 1970	3	Mean 3.7 points (6.3 discrete sites)
3. Shanghai Institute of TCM, n.d.	5	Mean 8.2 points (14.6 discrete sites)
4. O'Connor, Bensky 1981	3	Mean 6 points (11–12 discrete sites)
5. Anon 1980	3	Mean 4.7 points (7.7 discrete sites)
6. Chang 1987	4	Mean 5 points (8.3–8.5 discrete sites)
7. Feit, Zmiewski 1990	4	Mean 6 points (10.3–10.5 discrete sites)
8. Liu 1988	4	Mean 3.8 points (6.3–7.3 discrete sites)
9. Qiu, Su 1985	3	Mean 4 points (6.7–7.3 discrete sites)
10. Wiseman, Feng 1998	19	Mean 7.6 points (12.9–13.8 discrete sites)
11. Ying, De 1997	4	Mean 5 points (9.3–9.5 discrete sites)
12. Liu 1996	4	Mean 9.5 points (17–17.5 discrete sites)
13. Geng, Su 1991	3	Mean 5.7 points (9.3–10.3 discrete sites)
14. Maciocia 1994	3	Mean 12 points (15–19 discrete sites)
15. Zheng 1990	3	Mean 6 points (11–11.3 discrete sites)
16. Wu, Fischer 1997	5	Mean 6.2 points (10.6–10.8 discrete sites)

N.d., no year given.

of treatments, and frequency is recommended even less often. Since this is a common problem, it will be necessary to use additional methods to determine the appropriate number and frequency of treatments. Since the literature is not forthcoming on this, it would be useful to conduct practitioner surveys to ascertain actual practice habits and augment this with expert panel reviews.

It is possible to use the same overall process to examine the recommended treatments within a specific style or tradition, such as zhong yi or TCM. Table 3 summarizes the findings from a review of 16 different TCM acupuncture-related texts [11]. Quite a wide range of diagnostic patterns were found (3–19 patterns, median 3.5).

Four TCM diagnostic patterns of chronic low back pain were commonly discussed. The recommended numbers of points and discrete sites of treatment are [11]:

1. Cold damp: mean 6.6 points (range 3–12), mean 9.6–11.5 discrete sites (range 5–21)
2. Kidney yang vacuity: mean 6.4 points (range 5–9), mean 10.3–10.4 discrete sites (range 8–14)
3. Kidney yin vacuity: mean 6.3 points (range 5–8), mean 11.7–11.9 discrete sites (range 9–15)
4. Blood stasis: mean 6.4 points (range 2–11), mean 11.2–11.8 discrete sites (range 3–20)

Thus, in a study testing TCM acupuncture for low back pain, the considerable variation in the literature makes selecting the treatment somewhat complicated. However, these four TCM diagnostic categories could be used, with the conservative minimum treatment for each category given as ten sessions each with treatment of 10, 10, 12, and 11 discrete sites, respectively [11].

The literature review methods described above can be used between or within traditions of practice to examine what might constitute an adequate treatment in any

Table 4. Summary of neck pain, headache, and asthma treatment recommendations

Condition	N sources consulted	N points recommended	N sessions recommended	Minimal adequate treatment
Neck pain	12 Chinese, Japanese, and English	4–11 points, mean 6–7.5 points, 7–20 discrete sites; mean 10.5–13.8 sites	At least 10	At least 11 sites in each of at least 10 sessions
Headache	15 Chinese, Japanese, and English	4–21 points, mean 7.3–11.4 points; 5–24 discrete sites, mean 10.8–14.5 sites	At least 10	At least 11 sites in each of at least 10 sessions
Asthma (long-term treatment, not relief of acute attack)	22 Chinese, Japanese, and English	4–17 points, mean 8.3–8.9 points; 5–30 discrete sites, mean 12.2–16.8 sites	At least 10 and probably more than 20	At least 12 sites each in more than 10 sessions

condition for which acupuncture is used. Table 4 summarizes results of similar reviews on the acupuncture treatment of neck pain, headaches, and asthma.

One review of acupuncture treatment of osteoarthritis showed that this literature review method can encounter difficulties. These difficulties arise in part because of considerable inconsistencies in the acupuncture literature, in part from difficulties with terms, and in part because this condition has many manifestations, some of which are described separately. In a review of 34 texts from the world literature, only 15 had any actual description of the treatment of arthritis, including osteoarthritis. In these texts, a range of 3–16 sites of treatment were recommended, depending upon location of the arthritis and text reviewed.

These difficulties with the osteoarthritis literature suggest that it may be possible to use the number of treatment sessions only as the cutoff point for determining adequacy of treatment in each trial examined, since the selection of treatment points is quite varied. However, were there an effort to incorporate an analysis of the extent of treatment into each session, then it may also be advisable to use the above recommendations as tentative guidelines for discussion by a group of carefully selected experts. It would be better if this group had broad representation of the major traditions of practice so that its considerations could be more generalizable.

It should be noted that the methods cited in Tables 2–4 yield a range of number of acupoints and discrete sites to be treated for each condition. We assumed that the lower end of that range should constitute the minimum adequate treatment for the given condition. In their review of pain studies, Berman and colleagues found that the cutoff point for minimum adequate treatment was a significant predictor of treatment outcome [23]. It thus appears that this guideline is useful in analyses of published studies. However, when designing prospective studies, it is advisable to define adequate treatment in more positive terms such as "optimal," so there can be no doubt that the treatment tested was a fair test of acupuncture.

Defining this optimal treatment can be somewhat difficult. It is possible to use the higher ranges of average numbers of acupoints and discrete sites of treatment as optimal. For example, the data in Tables 3 and 4 would therefore suggest using 14, 14, 15, and 17 sites for the treatment of low back pain, neck pain, headache, and asthma, respectively. It may also be necessary to process these data with surveys of practitioners and expert panels to achieve a greater level of agreement on the optimal treatment in a particular condition.

10.5
Proposals for Systematizing the Selection of Acupuncture in Clinical Trials

Since many clinical trials of acupuncture use so-called sham or irrelevant acupuncture as the control treatment, the method used for selecting the appropriate and adequate acupuncture treatment could also be used to select the control treatment [4, 5]. A systematic method of ensuring that an appropriate control treatment is selected can be just as important for selecting the test treatment. The following proposal provides a method for selecting both types of treatment.

In addition to selecting the test and control treatments, it may be possible to tackle the problem of generalizability of results. To date, this problem has not been well-addressed. Is it possible to generalize the results from one study of acupuncture to other studies or acupuncture as a whole? What must we to do to ensure or enhance the generalizability of results? The broad range of therapeutic techniques and approaches in the field [7, 9, 22] can be problematic in this sense. However, it may be possible to develop a method allowing generalization of results across methods or at least increased generalizability without repeating logical errors.

A reproducible method for selecting both test and control treatments is needed. The Birch relevant and irrelevant treatment selection (BRITS) method is offered as a solution to this problem. Essentially, it seeks to establish treatment validity and improve generalizability of results through extensive literature reviews. Developed in early 1993 and named by one of the authors, this method was first presented at the Second Symposium of the Society for Acupuncture Research in September, 1994 [4] and has since been adopted in major clinical acupuncture trials in the U. S. These include trials for chronic neck pain at Harvard Medical School [10] and cocaine dependence at Yale University School of Medicine [49], and a large multicenter trial for cocaine dependence through Columbia University including the substance abuse treatment centers at the Universities of Yale, Minnesota, Miami, Washington, and California at Los Angeles and San Francisco [50]. Other, smaller studies in the U. S. have also utilized this method.

10.6
The BRITS Method

10.6.1
Purposes

In brief, the BRITS method aims to develop:
1. An easily applied standardizable approach to selecting and validating relevant acupoints for the test treatment in needle controlled acupuncture studies, thereby helping ensure appropriateness and adequacy of the test treatment.
2. An easily applied standardizable approach to selecting and validating irrelevant acupoints for the control treatment.

3. A pool of standardized irrelevant acupoints for specific conditions that can be used in future needle-controlled studies.
4. A method that allows for a broad generalization of the results of controlled acupuncture studies using that method.
5. Aid in formulating assessment criteria used to evaluate the quality and quantity of the test and control acupuncture treatments in published clinical trials.

10.6.2
Selecting and Validating Test (Relevant) Treatment Points

The BRITS methodology for determining relevant treatment points uses the following guidelines:
1. Review treatment texts or papers directly related to the method or tradition of practice being tested. Confirm that all acupoints to be treated are recommended for the condition in a minimum number of sources, e.g., at least six.
2. Review other treatment texts to confirm that the treatment points are generally indicated in these other texts for the condition at hand. This step enhances the potential generalizability of the results and is optional, but preferred.
3. Test the treatment in a pilot study before going to a full-scale study. Data from the pilot study can help fine-tune the design and size of the larger follow-up studies. This step is preferable but not always necessary.

10.6.3
Selecting and Validating Control (Irrelevant) Treatment Points

To determine control treatment points, the BRITS method uses the following steps:
1. Review the same treatment texts and papers used to validate the test acupoints and pick out the same number of inappropriate points as test points.
2. The selection criteria for these points should be:
   A. They are hardly or not at all mentioned as being good for the condition or related conditions being treated in the study.
   B. They are in similar regions of the body. The credibility of the control treatment will likely decrease if the treatment is perceived as being ridiculous or unrelated to the pain. Needling in the proximity of the pain will tend to appear more credible.
   C. *Always* test the control treatment in a pilot study before going to a full-scale study. This will allow estimates of relative effectiveness of the control treatment to be made. These can then be used to determine the appropriateness of the control and make sample size calculations for larger scale studies [4, 6]. If the control treatment appears almost as effective as the test treatment, it may be an inappropriate control treatment. Additional steps may be required to investigate this further [49, 50].

This method provides a greater guarantee of validity of selected "active" and "control" treatment sites than previous methods and, by including a broad range of literature from diverse sources, it increases the generalizability of results. The more agreement there is about a particular concept or method across varied traditions of practice, the greater the generalizability of that concept or method to the whole field.

If the literature review yields unclear results, as was found with the osteoarthritis review discussed above, it should be augmented by practitioner surveys and a panel of experts. These experts could use the review findings as a starting point for their considerations. Once a majority or consensus opinion develops, this can be used to outline treatment protocols in a particular study.

The following example illustrates how the BRITS method can be used. In their study of acupuncture in the treatment of chronic neck pain, Birch and Jamison reviewed 24 classical Chinese, modern Chinese (including English language texts), and modern Japanese texts to determine the most commonly referenced local points for the treatment of neck pain and validate the selection of nonlocal points [6, 10]. The same texts were also reviewed to select points that were never cited in the treatment of neck pain; these were used as the control or irrelevant treatment points. Reviewing these texts allowed for the derivation of treatment protocols that were supportable by a significant body of modern and historical literature. In addition, the protocols had broad generalizability because of the selection of treatment points from a variety of schools and traditions. The review also justified the selection of the specific treatment techniques used.

Coupled with the broader literature reviews discussed above, this method allows one not only to ascertain the minimum adequate treatment (numbers of discrete sites and number of treatment sessions) for the condition studied, but also the choice of specific acupoints themselves. It is also possible to use this method for focusing on the specific techniques to be tested.

Extending this concept of minimum adequate treatment, we can derive an optimal treatment, one we think will produce optimal results. The BRITS method allows for precise selection of treatment points and associated methods. However, as we saw above, the literature usually specifies little about numbers of treatment sessions needed. In 1995, Stux addressed this issue. For example, he recommended that at least 16 treatments be administered for headache and migraine [64]. Generally, it is poor research practice for a study to discover after the fact that an inadequate treatment or dose of treatment had been administered. To compensate for this, we feel justified in recommending to guarantee optimal treatment. Our recommendations for optimal treatments in clinical trials of acupuncture are as follows:

1. Since the reviews of the treatment of head, low back, and neck pain found a minimum of 10–11 and a maximum of 14–17 treatment sites (Tables 2, 4), we feel it is better to use an average of 15 sites per treatment. Variations on this should be based on an extensive literature review and, if necessary, practitioner surveys complemented by expert panel reviews. However, if the goal of a particular study is to look only at palliative care, the reviews for chronic pain suggest that six sites of stimulation in each of six treatment sessions appears to be a good cutoff point for minimum adequate treatment [23]. In the treatment of asthma, our review suggests that the optimal treatment should involve 17 sites (Table 4).

2. There has been little discussion of numbers of treatment sessions needed. However, our reviews suggest that for the treatment of chronic pain, a minimum of ten sessions is needed (Tables 2, 4). Thus, for optimal treatment, we feel it better to err on the side of too much, so at least 15 treatment sessions should be administered (except as mentioned for palliative care). In treating asthma, optimal treatment probably should involve more than 15 and possibly as many as 20 treatment sessions (Table 4).

3. Frequency of treatment is discussed even less often than number of treatment sessions. However, we feel again that it is better to err on the side of the optimal treatment and that treatment should be at least twice per week (more, for example, with addiction), and cut back to once a week or less, based on some algorithm.

4. Treatment techniques should match the practice model being tested. If a TCM acupuncture model is being used, de qi should be elicited at all points. If electrostimulation treatment is being tested, it is important to specify the machine, intensity and frequency of stimulation, wave form used, etc. Each technique should be justified through an appropriate literature review. The type and gauge of needles and depths of insertion should all be recorded, as well.

5. Inserted needles are usually retained for some minimum length of time. This length is not always specified. However, we feel it most appropriate to retain them for at least 15–20 minutes and longer, as necessary. Since our approach is to recommend in favor of optimal treatment, we feel that if the study is to retain needles for less than 15 minutes, it should justify this through an appropriate literature review.

6. An important issue barely raised in the literature is the adequacy of training of the person administering the acupuncture. It is not enough merely to state that the person had some training. Perhaps the safest standard is that the person administering the treatments should have completed an approved course. It is clearly not appropriate for a so-called surgeon from China to administer the acupuncture, nor is the completion of a single weekend of training sufficient. We discussed above the variation in training programs. Further work is necessary to establish an international standard for the training of acupuncturists in clinical trials but, at least for now, ensuring that the acupuncturist satisfies the standards in the country of practice should be sufficient. Additionally, it is probably advisable that the acupuncturist have a minimum number of years of experience.

7. Finally, it is evident that the methodology of most acupuncture studies has been poor. It is therefore recommended as a matter of course that any proposed study bring in the services of at least three different experts: an acupuncture expert (separate from the person administering the treatment), an expert in methodology, and a statistical expert. With appropriate advice, it is hoped that the methodology in future studies of acupuncture will improve.

10.7
Conclusions

It is apparent from the above discussions that there is considerable variety in how acupuncture textbooks describe the treatment for a particular condition. This variety exists even among texts purportedly describing the same tradition of practice. It is also apparent that the adequacy of treatment in clinical trials of acupuncture has been poor, raising yet more questions about how to interpret such trials. Further, with inadequate reporting of treatments and their origins, it is likely that idiosyncratic treatments have been tested, raising still more questions about the generalizability of results. There is clearly a need for a method that helps guarantee adequacy of treatment in future studies and helps resolve contradictions in the acupuncture literature itself.

References

1. Anonymous (1980) Essentials of Chinese acupuncture. Foreign Languages Press, Beijing
2. Bensoussan A (1991) The vital meridian. Churchill Livingstone, Edinburgh
3. Bensoussan A, Myers SP (1996) Towards a safer choice: The practice of traditional Chinese medicine in Australia. Faculty of Health, University of Western Sydney MacArthur, Sydney
4. Berman BM, Ezzo J, Lao L, Singh BB, Jadad A (1997) Penetrating the methodological issues in randomized controlled trials of acupuncture and chronic pain: A systematic review. In submission
5. Birch S (1995) Testing the clinical specificity of needle sites in controlled clinical trials of acupuncture. Proceedings of the Second Annual Meeting. Society for Acupuncture Research, Georgetown, pp 274–294
6. Birch S (1997) Issues to consider in determining an adequate treatment in a clinical trial of acupuncture. Compl Ther Med 5:8–12
7. Birch S (1997) An exploration with proposed solutions of the problems and issues in conducting clinical research in acupuncture [Doctoral thesis]. University of Exeter
8. Birch S (1998) Diversity and acupuncture: Acupuncture is not a coherent or historically stable tradition.. In Vickers AJ (ed) Examining complementary medicine: The sceptical holist. Stanley Thomas, Cheltenham
9. Birch S (1999) Preliminary investigations of the inter-rater reliability of traditionally based acupuncture diagnostic assessments. In submission
10. Birch S, Felt R (1999) Understanding acupuncture. Churchill Livingstone, Edinburgh
11. Birch S, Jamison RN (1998) A controlled trial of Japanese acupuncture for chronic myofascial neck pain: Assessment of specific and nonspecific effects of treatment. Clin J Pain 14:248–255
12. Birch S, Sherman K (1999) Zhong yi acupuncture and low back pain: Traditional Chinese medical acupuncture differential diagnoses and treatments for chronic lumbar pain. J Alt Compl Med 5:415–425
13. Brumbaugh A (1993) Acupuncture: New perspectives in chemical dependency treatment. J Subst Abuse Treat 10:35–43
14. Brumbaugh A (1994) Transformation and recovery: A guide to the design and development of acupuncture-based chemical dependency treatment programs. Stillpoint Press, Santa Barbara
15. Bullock ML, Culliton PD, Olander RT (1989) Controlled trial of acupuncture for severe recidivist alcoholism. Lancet 1:1435–1439
16. Chen J, Wang N (1988) Acupuncture case histories from China. Eastland Press, Seattle
17. Cheng XN (1987) Chinese acupuncture and moxibustion. Foreign Languages Press, Beijing
18. Coan R, Wong G, Ku SL, Chan YC, Wang L, Ozer FT, Coan PL (1980) The acupuncture treatment of low back pain: A randomized controlled treatment. Amer J Chin Med 8:181–189
19. Coan R, Wong G, Coan PL (1982) The acupuncture treatment of neck pain: a randomized controlled study. Amer J Chin Med 9:326–332
20. Debata A (1986) Diagnosis and treatment of knee joint pain for the private practitioner acupuncturist [Japanese]. Ido no Nippon Sha, Yokosuka
21. Emery P, Lythgoe S (1986) The effect of acupuncture on ankylosing spondylitis. Brit J Rheum 25:132–133
22. Ergil KV (1997) Acupuncture licensure, training, and certification in the United States. NIH Consensus Development Conference on Acupuncture: Panels and abstracts. NIH, Bethesda
23. Ernst E, White AR (1997) A review of problems in clinical acupuncture research. Amer J Chin Med 25:3–11
24. Feit R, Zmiewski P (1990) Acumoxa therapy – treatment of disease; vol II. Paradigm Publications, Brookline
25. Geng JY, Su ZH (1991) Practical traditional Chinese medicine and pharmacology. Acupuncture and moxibustion. New World Press, Beijing
26. Hammerschlag R (1998) Methodological and ethical issues in clinical trials of acupuncture. J Alt Compl Med 4:159–171
27. Hammerschlag R, Morris MM (1997) Clinical trials comparing acupuncture with biomedical standard care: A criteria-based evaluation of research design and reporting. Compl Ther Med 5:133–140
28. Helms JM (1996) Educational and licensing requirements for medical practitioners. J Alt Compl Med 2:39
29. Ikeda M (1985) Acupuncture and moxibustion treatment of lumbago. Shinkyu Chiryo Shitsu; vol 3. Ido no Nippon Company, Yokosuka, pp 16–19
30. Jobst KA (1995) A critical analysis of acupuncture in pulmonary disease: Efficacy and safety of the acupuncture needle. J Alt Compl Med 1:57–85

31. Jobst K, Chen JH, McPherson K, Arrowsmith J, Brown V, Efthimiou J, Fletcher HJ, Maciocia G, Mole P, Shifrin K, Lane DJ (1986) Controlled trial of acupuncture for disabling breathlessness. Lancet 2:1416–1419
32. Kersken T (1993) Teil II: Einschätzung der handwerklichen Qualität durchgeführter Akupunkturtherapien in 86 Studien. In: Buhring M, Kemper FM (eds) Naturheilverfahren – Grundlagen, Methoden, Nachweissituationen. Springer-Verlag, Berlin
33. Kinoshita H (1983) In: Nagahama Y, Kinoshita H, Nakamura R (eds) Shinkyu Chiryo no Shin Kenkyu, third edn. Sogensha, Osaka
34. Kleijnen J, Ter Riet G, Knipschild P (1991) Acupuncture and asthma; a review of controlled trials. Thorax 46:799–802
35. Kwok CY, Wang PZ, Wong R, Yang LG, Zhang DZ (1991) Applying mathematical models to traditional Chinese medicine for the diagnosis and treatment of low back pain. Amer J Acup 19:129–135
36. Lee JF, Cheung CS (1978) Current Acupuncture Therapy. Medical Book Publications, Hong Kong
37. Lewith GT, Machin D (1983) On the evaluation of the clinical effects of acupuncture. Pain 16:111–127
38. Lewith G, Vincent C (1996) On the evaluation of the clinical effects of acupuncture: A problem reassessed and a framework for future research. J Alt Compl Med 2:79–90
39. Linde K, Worku F, Stor W, Wiesner-Zechmeister M, Pothmann R, Weinschutz T, Melchart D (1996) Randomized clinical trials of acupuncture for asthma – a systematic review. Forsch Kompl 3:148–155
40. Lipton DS, Brewington V, Smith M (1994) Acupuncture for crack cocaine detoxification: Experimental evaluation of efficacy. J Subst Abuse Treat 11:205–215
41. Liu GW (1996) Clinical acupuncture and moxibustion. Tianjin Science and Technology Translations and Publishing Corp, Tianjin
42. Liu YC (1988) The essential book of traditional Chinese medicine. Columbia University Press, New York
43. Lytle CD (1993) An overview of acupuncture; U. S. Department of Health and Human Services, Public Health Service, Food and Drug Administration, Center for Devices and Radiological Health
44. Maciocia G (1993) Letter to the editor. Compl Ther Med 1:221–222
45. Maciocia G (1994) Practice of Chinese medicine. Churchill Livingstone, New York
46. Manaka Y (1970) Clinical dictionary of acupuncture and moxibustion [Japanese]. Ido no Nippon Sha, Yokosuka
47. Mann F (1974) Treatment of disease by acupuncture. William Heinemann Medical Books Ltd, London
48. Margolin A, Avants SK, Chang P, Kosten TR (1993) Auricular acupuncture for the treatment of cocaine dependence in methadone-maintained patients. Amer J Addict 2:194–200
49. Margolin A, Avants SK, Chang P, Birch S (1995) A single blind investigation of four needle puncture conditions. Amer J Chin Med 23:105–114
50. Margolin A, Avants SK, Birch S, Falk CX, Kleber HD (1997) Methodological investigations for a multisite trial of auricular acupuncture for cocaine addiction. A study of active and control auricular zones. J Subst Abuse Treat 13:471–481
51. McLellan AT, Grossman DS, Blain JD, Haverkos HW (1993) Acupuncture treatment for drug abuse: A technical review. J Subst Abuse Treat 10:569–576
52. Nagahama Y, Kinoshita H, Nakamura R (1983) Shinkyu Chiryo no Shin Kenkyu; third edn. Sogensha, Osaka
53. National Institutes of Health (1998) NIH consensus conference: Acupuncture JAMA 280:1518–1524
54. O'Connor J, Bensky D (1981) Acupuncture. A comprehensive text. Eastland Press, Seattle
55. Patel M, Gutzwiller F, Paccaud F, Marazzi A (1989) A meta-analysis of acupuncture for chronic pain. Intl J Epid 18:900–906
56. Pomeranz B (1997) Scientific bases of acupuncture. In: Stux G, Pomeranz B (eds) Basics of acupuncture, fourth edn. Springer-Verlag, Berlin, pp 6–72
57. Prance SE, Dresser A, Wood C, Fleming J, Aldridge D, Pietroni PC (1988) Research on traditional Chinese acupuncture – science or myth: A review. J Royal Soc Med 81:588–590
58. Qiu ML, Su XM (1985) NanJing Seminar Transcripts. Journal of Chinese Medicine, London
59. Richardson PH, Vincent CA (1986) Acupuncture for the treatment of pain: A review of evaluative research. Pain 24:15–40
60. Shanghai Institute of TCM (nd) Zhen Jiu Zhi Liao Xue, Acu-moxa therapy treatment studies. Shao Hua Cultural Service Publishing Company, Hong Kong

61. Shudo D (1990) Japanese classical acupuncture: Introduction to meridian therapy. Seattle, East-land Press
62. So JTY (1987) Treatment of disease with acupuncture. Paradigm Publications, Brookline
63. Stux G (1990) Migraine treatment with acupuncture and moxibustion. Acup Sci Intl J 1:16–18
64. Stux G (1995) Qualitatskriterien fur die Akupunktur bei klinischen Studien. In: G. Stux. Einfuhrung in die Akupunktur, fourth edn. Springer-Verlag, Berlin
65. Stux G, Pomeranz B (1988) Acupuncture: Textbook and atlas. Springer-Verlag, Berlin
66. Ter Riet G, Kleijnen J, Knipschild P (1990) Acupuncture and chronic pain: A criteria-based meta-analysis. J Clin Epid 43:1191–1199
67. Ter Riet G, Kleijnen J, Knipschild P (1990) A meta-analysis of studies into the effect of acupuncture on addiction. Brit J Gen Prac 40:379–382
68. Tianjin Chinese Medical College; translated by Ikegami S (1988) Shinkyu Rinsho no Riron to Jisai. Kokusho Publishing Association, Tokyo
69. Tsutani K, Birch S (in press) Evaluating complementary and alternative diagnostics. In: Jonas W, Leyin JS (eds.) Textbook of complementary, alternative and unconventional medicine. Williams and Wilkins, Baltimore
70. Vickers A (1996) Can acupuncture have specific effects on health? A systematic review of acupuncture antiemesis trials. J Royal Soc Med 89:303–311
71. Vincent CA (1993) Acupuncture as a treatment for chronic pain. In: Lewith GT, Aldridge D (eds) Clinical research methodology for complementary therapies. Hodder and Stoughton, London, pp 289–308
72. Vincent C, Lewith G (1995) Placebo controls for acupuncture studies. J Royal Soc Med, 88: 199–202
73. Vincent CA, Richardson PH (1986) The evaluation of therapeutic acupuncture: Concepts and methods. Pain 24:1–13
74. Vincent CA, Richardson PH (1987) Acupuncture for some common disorders: A review of evaluative research. J Royal Coll Gen Prac 37:77–81
75. Wen HL, Cheung SYC (1973) Treatment of drug addiction by acupuncture and electrical stimulation. Amer J Acup 1:71–75
76. Wiseman N, Ellis A (1985) Fundamentals of Chinese medicine. Paradigm Publications, Brookline
77. Wiseman N, Feng Y (1998) A practical dictionary of Chinese medicine. Paradigm Publications, Brookline
78. Wu Y, Fischer W (1997) Practical therapeutics of traditional chinese medicine. Paradigm Publications, Brookline
79. Ying ZZ, De JH (1997) Clinical manual of Chinese herbal medicine and acupuncture. Churchill Livingstone, New York
80. Zheng EQ (ed) (1990) Chinese acupuncture and moxibustion. Publishing House of Shanghai College of TCM, Shanghai

Assessing Clinical Efficacy of Acupuncture: Considerations for Designing Future Acupuncture Trials

L. Lao · J. Ezzo · B. M. Berman · R. Hammerschlag

11.1
Introduction

The recent interest in acupuncture has led to an unprecedented amount of research funding in this area. This chapter presents a systematic, stepwise approach to research. It proposes investigating the efficacy of acupuncture by adapting the U. S. Food and Drug Administration (FDA) approach to clinical trials (Table 1). Two examples, one for chronic osteoarthritic (OA) pain [1, 2] and one for acute postextraction dental pain [3–5] are used to demonstrate how this method can be applied to acupuncture research. The final section discusses ways to integrate Western medicine more closely with traditional Chinese medicine (TCM) in research.

11.2
Phase I

According to the FDA description, phase I trials are small, typically do not have a control group, and are designed to establish basic parameters of dose and safety (Table 1). The phase I OA trial [2], for example, consisted of 12 patients with no control group. Although acupuncture has already been recognized as generally safe, establishing an adequate dose (i.e., a specific acupuncture protocol) in a phase I trial is a major challenge. This has seldom been done in past trials. Consequently, a number of randomized controlled trials (RCTs) of acupuncture have administered acupuncture treatments not based on preliminary data. The following key items should be considered in a phase I acupuncture trial: dose, primary and secondary outcomes, follow-up time, and safety.

Table 1. Features and types of clinical trials according to FDA nomenclature

Type	Key features
Phase I	Initial human studies; provides preliminary information on safety, appropriate dose, and chemical action; typically does not include a control group
Phase II	Larger than phase I but still generally small numbers of patients; provides preliminary information on efficacy; provides additional information on dose and safety; usually includes a control group; may randomize
Phase III	Large sample size based on phase II results; assesses dose effects; evaluates term safety and efficacy; always controlled and randomized; treatment must demonstrate favorable risk/benefit ratio

11.2.1
Establishing an Adequate Dose

Establishing an adequate treatment/dose of acupuncture is one of the fundamental first steps of a trial. In the past, many acupuncture treatments used in trials have been shown to be inadequate according to minimal criteria [6 and see Chapt. 10]. The fundamental decisions a researcher must make when establishing an adequate acupuncture treatment pertain to:
1. Type of acupuncture treatment (e.g., TCM, Japanese, five-element)
2. Formulaic vs. individualized treatments
3. Qualifications/experience of the acupuncturist
4. Point selection
5. Depth and techniques of needle manipulation, i.e., manual (reinforced or reducing technique) or electrical stimulation (frequency and intensity)
6. Whether de qi will be pursued
7. Duration of each treatment
8. Number of treatments per week and spacing between treatments
9. Total number of treatments.

11.2.2
Formulaic vs. Individualized Acupuncture

The ongoing debate about whether to use formulaic or individualized acupuncture revolves around two points of view. Those who argue for individualized treatment suggest that this approach reflects clinical reality whereas formulaic approaches do not. Those who argue for formulaic approaches suggest that individualized approaches may compromise methodological rigor and that a standardized treatment is less likely to create unintended confounders or noise in the study. There is no golden key that fits all the locks. Both methods are useful if the design is appropriate. Part of the decision depends on the condition being treated. Homogeneous populations are more conducive to formulaic acupuncture than are heterogeneous populations. For example, formulaic acupuncture was used in the postextraction dental pain study [3–5]. All the patients shared the same Western medicinal diagnosis (postoperative acute pain) and the same traditional Chinese medicinal diagnosis (excess heat condition with qi and blood stagnation), making this group an exceptionally homogeneous patient population. Heterogeneous populations in whom multiple signs and symptoms are treated, e.g., quality of life, pain, function, and mental status, may require individualized treatments.

Deciding on formulaic vs. individualized acupuncture can also be an integrated rather than either/or approach. For example, both can be considered in a stepwise approach, progressing from the more rigorously controlled (formulaic) to the more practical (individualized). If results are positive using a formulaic approach, then research can progress into individualized treatments based on TCM diagnoses. Another integrated approach is to select comprehensive formula points which cover multiple TCM diagnoses. For example, the formulaic treatment used in the osteoarthritis study [1] covered most of the TCM points that would have been used, had individual syndromes been treated. Yet another option is to include at least one point from every TCM diagnosis. An additional compromise between formulaic and individualized protocols is to stratify patients by TCM subgroup diagnosis and treat patients at subgroup-specific acupoints (see discussion of double screen design later in this chapter).

11.2.3
Training/Experience of the Acupuncturist

How skilled and experienced the acupuncturist should be in clinical trials is another common question. Proficiency requirements of the acupuncturist may differ, based on whether formulaic or individualized treatments are used. Obviously, when individualized treatments are given, the acupuncturist must be very experienced in both diagnosing and treating the condition under investigation in order to make treatment decisions based on TCM diagnoses. However, when formulaic treatments are given, it may suffice for the acupuncturist to demonstrate proficiency and replicability of the needling technique being used.

11.2.4
Selection of Points

Birch has observed [7] that there is no consensus among acupuncture textbooks on the points to use for a given condition. The absence of standardized treatments makes it important to base the selected points both on the literature and personal clinical observations of effectiveness.

11.2.5
Total Number of Treatments

The sufficient total number of treatments to administer in a trial, especially for chronic conditions, is largely unknown and seldom specified in the literature. Phase I presents a low-cost opportunity to establish both total number of treatments and the frequency of treatments for the investigated condition. In establishing these parameters, outcomes need to be measured frequently to determine when improvement begins and whether additional improvements occur with more treatments. For example, in the osteoarthritis study, both clinical experience and prior RCTs in the literature suggested that treatments twice weekly for three weeks were probably not adequate [8–10]. Phase I results showed substantial improvements at 4 weeks and continued improvements at 8 weeks. Therefore, treatment twice weekly for 8 weeks was selected as the treatment modality for phase II.

11.2.6
Selecting Outcomes

Phase I provides an opportunity to select appropriate outcomes to be tested. The outcomes should be measurable according to validated instruments. A validated instrument means that it has been demonstrated through prior research that it is measuring what it says it is measuring. Examples of well-validated general health assessment tools include the Sickness Impact Profile (SIP) [11] and the SF-36 [12]. Because these measurement tools have been validated using the whole instrument, it is a good idea when using these instruments to use them intact; using pieces of an instrument can jeopardize the validity of a trial. Instruments can be generic (measuring overall health status) or disease-specific (measuring clinically important changes pertinent to that specific disease) [13]. Frequently, studies include both. It is helpful to look at the recent literature pertaining to the disease under investigation in order to decide which instruments to use. Excellent, user-friendly guides on measurement selection exist [14].

Another important decision to be made is which will be the primary and which the secondary outcomes. Primary outcomes, designated by investigators as the most important outcomes, should be limited to one or two, clearly defined, and used for calculating sample size in subsequent trial phases. Secondary outcomes can represent other symptoms of interest, quality of life, sleep patterns, appetite, bowel movements, and mental status. However, it is important to remember that because sample size is not based on secondary outcomes, significant changes between groups might not be observed in all of these secondary outcomes. For example, in the dental pain study [5], the primary outcome was pain-free time after surgery, and sample size calculation was based on that. A secondary outcome was pain relief after the first acupuncture treatment. Results showed a significant difference between groups in the primary but not the secondary outcome. One possibility for this finding is that, in reality, there is no significant difference in pain relief in real vs. placebo acupuncture once the pain has reached moderate intensity. However, another possibility is that the sample size may have been too small to detect a difference between groups in the secondary outcome. Similar situations have occurred in other acupuncture trials [15].

11.2.7
Choosing a Follow-up Time

Selecting the appropriate follow-up time depends on the condition being tested and can be investigated in the early phases of a trial because, especially in chronic conditions, this may influence the final treatment protocol to be used in subsequent phases. For acute conditions such as dental pain [3–5], a week may be adequate to determine whether the treatment is effective. By contrast, for chronic conditions such as OA, a follow-up of 3, 6, or 12 months may be more appropriate [1, 2]. Long-term follow-up is important to determine long-term efficacy with acupuncture. If efficacy is not sustained, investigators can examine ways to sustain it.

Follow-up data can provide useful information for designing future trial phases. For example, long-term follow-up data from two previous OA studies guided the formulation of the acupuncture protocol in the large, randomized OA trial. Firstly, long-term follow-up data by Christensen and colleagues [9] in a group of OA patients showed that improvements could be sustained for a year using monthly acupuncture after treatments twice a week had stopped. However, it was not evident from this study whether improvement would be sustained without booster treatments. Then, long-term follow-up data from Berman and colleagues [1] showed that, without booster treatments, pain scores returned to pretreatment baselines by 24 weeks. As a result of these follow-up data, the decision was made in a large OA trial to give monthly booster acupuncture treatments after patients had completed the 8-week treatment regimen.

11.2.8
Measuring Safety

Unlike phase I trials for a new drug, which must closely examine safety, acupuncture is already considered safe. However, it is important as part of any clinical assessment to document adverse events. Confusion arises when a paper mentions that no adverse effects were observed. Frequently, it is not clear whether adverse effects did not occur or simply were not measured. Therefore, it is advisable to have an explicit and systematic methodology such as a symptoms checklist for documenting side effects. Phase I provides the opportunity to refine the checklist based on the condition being investigated.

11.2.9
Comment

The major advantage of a phase I trial is that it enables investigators to generate preliminary information on dose and safety in a cost-effective way. If no benefit is observed during phase I, it may be because the selected acupuncture protocol (dose) is not appropriate and/or because the condition under investigation is not responsive to acupuncture. In such a circumstance, the researcher might alter the acupuncture protocol or inclusion/exclusion criteria and conduct another phase I trial. If patients do not respond, then the researcher knows early on that the research question may not be worth pursuing in a larger, more costly, randomized controlled trial.

However, if benefit is observed in phase I, it cannot be assumed to be due to the acupuncture protocol. This is because phase I trials have no control group and are not efficacy trials. There are three explanations for why patients may experience benefit during an intervention: (1) treatment effects, (2) nonspecific effects, and (3) disease remissions [16]. To be able to attribute improvements to treatment effects, the investigator must first rule out disease remissions and nonspecific effects. "Nonspecific effects" is frequently used to describe all of the nontreatment effects which result from the milieu in which the treatment occurs, including the physical environment, the caring staff, and beliefs and expectations of the patients. Confusion arises in acupuncture trials because the term "nonspecific effects" is often used to describe physiological effects due to needling stimulation, such as diffuse noxious inhibitory control (DNIC). For clarity, this term will be used to describe nontreatment-related effects, and "nonspecific physiological effects of needling" will be used to describe the effects of acupuncture that result from needle stimulation but are not acupuncture point-specific. Ruling out improvements due to nonspecific effects and spontaneous remissions requires the use of a control group, which is commonly introduced in phase II.

11.3
Phase II

Phase II trials build on the information gained in phase I. Phase II trials generally have a control group and generate additional information on dosing and safety as well as preliminary information on efficacy (Table 1). Comparison groups can concern different doses of the same treatment, different treatment, or placebo groups. Randomization is frequently done in phase II, although the numbers are generally small.

11.3.1
Selecting an Appropriate Control Group

Unlike pharmaceutical research, in which a placebo is easy to design and double blinding is easily achieved, it is difficult to design an appropriate control group for acupuncture, because acupuncture is an invasive, physical modality. No single control group can answer all the research questions. Therefore, many types of control groups, each with its own advantages and disadvantages, have been used, depending on the specific question being asked (Table 2) [17]. In choosing an appropriate control group, it is important to consider what current treatments are available for the condition being investigated. If a condition already has an effective standard medical treatment, then it makes no ethical or financial sense to examine sham vs. real acupuncture. It is more logical to examine acupuncture effectiveness compared to standard care. In addition to overall effectiveness, it can also be noted whether acupuncture has a quicker onset, lasts longer, or has a milder side effect profile than standard care. It is also logical to examine whether additional benefit to standard care can be derived by adding acupuncture treatments.

11.3.2
Waiting Lists

Waiting lists can track the natural history of a disease and assess for spontaneous remissions. Therefore, the value of a waiting list over not using a control group is that waiting lists provide a way to estimate remissions due to disease variation rather than treatment effectiveness. For example, in the OA trial [1], a waiting list control group was used. Both patient groups were instructed to continue using whatever medications they were already using. Acupuncture was administered immediately to one group and delayed in the other group. There were several advantages to the choice of this control group. It controlled for spontaneous remissions, provided clinically useful information on acupuncture as an adjunct to treatments already being used and offered an ethical design for the control group to receive the experimental acupuncture treatment. Obviously, the limitation to this group was that it could not control for placebo effects.

The importance of controlling for disease remissions using a waiting list group was underscored in an acupuncture trial in which 30 % in the waiting list group experienced remissions in pain [18].

Table 2. Control groups in acupuncture trials

Type of control	Questions asked	Advantages	Disadvantages
Waiting list (delayed treatment)	Is acupuncture more effective than no treatment?	Controls for disease remissions; all patients receive treatment	Does not control for placebo effects
Nonacupuncture inert controls (sham TENS, sugar pills)	Is acupuncture more effective than a placebo?	Controls for some placebo effects	Does not resemble acupuncture; cannot blind patients
Placebo acupuncture (noninserted needle)	Is acupuncture more effective than placebo?	Resembles real acupuncture; patients can be blinded; eliminates the possibility of nonspecific needling effects	Difficult to implement in long-term studies; may be effective only for acupuncture-naïve patients; does not test for specificity of acupoints
Sham acupuncture (inserted needle)	Is real acupuncture more effective than sham acupuncture? Does real acupuncture have point-specific effects on the condition under investigation?	Resembles real acupuncture; patients can be blinded	Likely to produce nonspecific physiological effects of needling
Combined controls (e.g., placebo acupuncture plus sham acupuncture)	What is the magnitude of placebo acupuncture (no treatment vs. placebo)? What is the magnitude of nonspecific effects (placebo vs sham)?	The two treatments resemble each other, so patients can be blinded; can minimize nonspecific needling effects of sham	If placebo acupuncture is used, it may be difficult to implement in long-term studies
Positive controls (standard medical care)	Is acupuncture equivalent/ superior to standard medical care or is it, when combined with standard care, more effective than standard care alone?	Compares the effectiveness of acupuncture as replacment or adjunctive care; has practical value, since cost effectiveness, adverse effects, and efficacy can be compared	Cannot blind patients or practitioners; may risk a type II error (where the two treatments are believed to be equivalent but, in reality, one is better)

11.3.3
Nonacupuncture Inert Controls

A placebo is a physiologically inert intervention. Sham transcutaneous electrical nerve stimulation (TENS) has been used in acupuncture trials to estimate placebo effects because it provides a control intervention that is undoubtedly physiologically inert and has been demonstrated to be a credible treatment [19]. Unlike patients in the waiting list control, patients in the sham TENS group receive amounts of practitioner time and attention similar to those for patients in the acupuncture group. Therefore, the sham TENS group controls for some nonspecific effects, such as those resulting from patient-practitioner relationship. However, the placebo effect of acupuncture cannot be measured, because sham TENS does not resemble acupuncture. Patients cannot be blinded in a sham TENS vs. acupuncture trial. In other words, patients know whether they received acupuncture or not.

Sugar pills, another type of nonacupuncture inert control, have also been used [20]. However, sugar pills bear even less resemblance to acupuncture and cannot control for the nonspecific effects resulting from the patient-practitioner relationship, because the practitioner time and attention is not comparable in patients receiving acupuncture relative to those receiving sugar pills.

11.3.4
Placebo Acupuncture

Placebo acupuncture is a true control for the acupuncture treatment because it is not only physiologically inert but also resembles real acupuncture. In placebo acupuncture, the blunt end of the needle [21], acupuncture needles, or objects resembling needles such as toothpicks [22], needling guiding tubes [3–5], or specifically designed noninsertion needling devices [23, 24] create the appearance of insertion but are not actually inserted.

In order to enhance the success of patient blinding in placebo acupuncture, some investigators [3–5] exclude patients who have previously received real acupuncture. Patient blinding might also be improved by creating the expectation that acupuncture is painless, such as by showing placebo patients that the diameter (≤ 0.2 mm) of the commonly used acupuncture needle is much thinner than hollow hypodermic needles. Placebo acupuncture may be especially useful in short-term, acute intervention trials. A possible disadvantage is that in conditions requiring long-term treatment, maintaining patient blinding may be difficult. This is because curiosity of the patients to discover the type of treatment they have been receiving may lead to unblinding (e.g., patients may talk to each other, read about acupuncture, or go to another acupuncturist). A few investigators [3–5, 22, 32] have checked the blinding credibility after the placebo intervention by administering a questionnaire asking patients which treatment they believe they have received. This procedure is important in order to validate whether blinding has succeeded.

11.3.5
Sham Acupuncture

11.3.5.1
Sham Acupuncture for Measuring Nonspecific Effects of Needling

Unlike placebo acupuncture that involves noninvasive procedures, sham acupuncture involves actual needling but at sites inappropriate to the condition being examined [8,11, 25–28]. Like placebo acupuncture, the advantage in sham acupuncture is its resemblance to real acupuncture so that patients can be blinded to treatment group assignment. However, since sham needling mimics both the nonspecific effects and the nonspecific physiological effects of needling, the difference between real and sham groups may be slight, especially in pain trials. Such nonspecific physiological effects of needling may include local alteration in circulation and immune function [29] and triggering of neural pathways such as those resulting in diffuse noxious inhibitory control (DNIC) of pain [30].

In order to minimize the nonspecific physiological effects of needling, the sham procedure may use distal points, minimal needling depth, and minimal needle stimulation rather than local points, standard depth, and needle stimulation [31]. Avoiding de qi in the sham group is also important. Because of the magnitude of these nonspecific needling effects, careful consideration is needed to calculate an adequate sample size. As in placebo acupuncture, it is important to confirm patient blinding by providing a questionnaire asking patients which treatment they believe they have received [32].

In addition to producing nonspecific needling effects, another disadvantage of sham acupuncture is that there is no general agreement as to how it should be designed [17]. For example, sham acupuncture may be applied by needling nonpoints adjacent to real points [26], nonpoints distal to real points [27], or real acupuncture points not specific for the condition to be treated [33]. Needling techniques in sham acupuncture can be applied at various depths, e.g., superficial or standard, with various types of stimulation, e.g., manual or electrostimulation, using various needle manipulation techniques, e.g., reinforcing, reducing, and changes in needling angles and directions, and retaining needles for various times, e.g., for similar or shorter duration than in treatment groups. These variations in the way sham acupuncture is applied make it difficult even to compare the results of two sham acupuncture trials investigating the same condition. For example, in an OA RCT, Takeda and Wessel [10] noticed that de qi was sometimes inadvertently elicited in the sham group and sometimes not elicited in the real acupuncture group. Although results showed no significant differences between groups, de qi was a predictor for significant improvement in both the *Western Ontario and McMaster Universities Osteoarthritis* Pain Index and the pressure threshold scores in both groups. Clearly, comparing the results of this sham acupuncture trial may not be comparable with the results of another trial which avoids de qi in the sham group.

11.3.5.2
Sham Acupuncture for Measuring Acupuncture Specificity

Sham acupuncture is also the appropriate control for examining the validity of TCM claims for acupuncture point specificity. It can be used to test point specificity by comparing the physiological effects of needling a precisely located real acupoint to an adjacent nonpoint according to standard TCM textbooks. It can also test specificity by comparing the effects of needling a group of real points prescribed for a condition according to TCM theory to a group of inappropriate points. And it is useful for testing specific physiological effects of various needling techniques such as reinforced or reducing technique, or techniques that elicit de qi.

When sham acupuncture is devised to investigate acupuncture specificity, different design issues need to be considered than when sham is devised to measure placebo effects. In the latter case, the goal is to minimize nonspecific physiological effects of needling and, therefore, several features of the sham procedure may differ from procedures with the real acupuncture group, including points selected, depth of insertion, and amount of stimulation applied to the needle. In contrast, when sham acupuncture is used in the former case as a control to examine acupuncture specificity, i.e., to test whether stimulation of a real point has greater physiological effects than a nonpoint, then all the features of the sham treatment should be identical to the real treatment except for the feature under investigation, i.e., point locations.

11.3.6
Combined Controls

Combining various controls within the same study is a creative way to minimize the limitations of each type of control. It is apparent that a major challenge in acupuncture research is the ability successfully to blind patients to their treatment group assignment, because when the comparison group's treatment does not resemble acupuncture, blinding is impossible. One innovative approach is to combine various placebo interventions within the same study to make the treatments in the two groups appear comparable. For example, in comparing medication to acupuncture for migraine, Hesse et al. [21] gave real medication plus placebo acupuncture to one group and real acupuncture plus placebo medication to the other. This innovative approach enabled them to blind patients to treatment group assignment.

Another challenge in acupuncture research is to develop placebos that resemble acupuncture while minimizing nonspecific needling effects. A rarely used, innovative approach is to combine both sham acupuncture (inserted needles) and placebo acupuncture (noninserted needles) in the same design. For example, in a recently funded dental study, the real treatment consisted of real acupuncture at points St.6 and 7, SJ.17, and LI.4. The placebo treatment consisted of placebo acupuncture (noninserted needles) administered to these same points. However, in order to improve blinding in the placebo group, a sham acupuncture (inserted needle) point was added to the leg 1 inch posterior to Liv.8, thereby ensuring that the placebo group experiences the sensation of needle insertion. Then, to make the two groups comparable in appearance, placebo acupuncture (noninserted needle) was added to the same leg point in the real acupuncture group. Combined controls such as these have two advantages: (1) blinding in both groups is enhanced because the two treatments are comparable in appearance, and (2) blinding in the real acupuncture group is further enhanced because the placebo leg point may make the real treatment appear less real.

11.3.7
Positive Controls

The question asked in the type of research design that uses a positive (active) control group [34] is different from those asked with any of the above control groups: is acupuncture at least as effective as standard medical care such as medication, physiotherapy, or occlusal splint? This design is useful for conditions in which side effects of medications are problematic, since it allows for side by side comparisons of adverse outcomes [21, 35]. Acupuncture can also be added to standard care to determine if it can increase the effectiveness of other treatment [36] or even reduce the required dose [37]. Designs which assess acupuncture compared or added to standard care also provide an opportunity for cost effectiveness comparisons [36]. When planning a trial using positive controls, it is important to ensure adequate power, because otherwise nonsignificant results are difficult to interpret. It cannot be assumed that acupuncture has performed as well as standard care unless a type II error can be ruled out. A type II error occurs when there actually is a difference between the two treatments but the sample size is too small to detect it. Such results are not significant, but a larger sample size would have found a significant difference between the two treatments.

11.3.8
Selecting the Study Design: Parallel or Crossover

A final consideration for phase II trials is which type of study design to select. Several acupuncture trials have used crossover designs, mostly for the sake of convenience, because crossover designs increase statistical power without increasing patient enrollment. Three assumptions must apply for crossover designs to be an appropriate experimental design: (1) the disease must be stable throughout the study, (2) there is no reason to believe that the treatments interact with each other, and (3) the effects of the proposed intervention cease soon after discontinuing the intervention[38].

The latter point calls into question the appropriateness of crossover designs for acupuncture trials. Evidence of long-term effects of acupuncture have been observed in controlled clinical trials in which significant pain relief achieved after 6 weeks of treatment for migraine [26] or 3 months of treatment for dysmenorrhea [27] was maintained at 1-year follow-up. Not surprisingly, carryover effects (treatment effects which persist long after treatment ceases) have been documented in crossover trials of acupuncture [39]. The presence of carryover effects in acupuncture studies suggests that crossover designs are an inappropriate design choice, except in trials with very long washout periods.

Furthermore, in crossover studies comparing real versus sham acupuncture, it is questionable whether patients can maintain blindness to treatment groups once they have experienced both real and sham acupuncture treatments. For these reasons, parallel rather than crossover designs are preferred for acupuncture efficacy trials.

11.3.9
Summary and Example

There are several advantages to conducting a phase II trial before plunging into a large, definitive phase III randomized controlled trial (RCT): it (1) allows for the hypothesis to be tested on a small, cost effective scale, (2) provides the data needed to do the power calculation for a larger trial, (3) assesses the feasibility of the research setting, including staffing availability, and (4) provides a forum where unforeseen problems can arise and be resolved so that a solid study protocol can be developed for the larger phase III randomized trial.

For example, phase II of the dental pain trial [4] provided an excellent opportunity to refine the timing of activities within the trial. Prior to phase II, the treatment protocol had been based on a previous trial in the literature which administered acupuncture when patients experienced moderate pain [25]. However, during phase II, the investigators observed that acupuncture given pre-emptively was a more effective analgesic, so the protocol was modified accordingly.

Another example was that phase II provided an opportunity to assess whether the timing of administering the blinding questionnaire was appropriate. Prior to phase II, it was determined that patients would be asked before they left the clinic which treatment they believed they had received. The investigators learned during phase II that, by that time, patients' guesses were based on their level of pain relief and were fairly accurate. However, when the question was asked immediately after the first treatment, prior to the experience of breakthrough pain, guesses were based on characteristics of the treatment, and the placebo acupuncture procedure was found to be credible.

11.4
Phase III

Phase III trials are the definitive efficacy trials. They are large and often conducted at multiple locations. In the OA study, the phase III trial consists of a three-arm parallel design (n = 570) comparing real and sham acupuncture vs. an attention control group. The systematic reviews discussed in chapter 7 provide excellent commentaries on the methodological quality of acupuncture efficacy trials. This section proposes guidelines for strengthening acupuncture efficacy trials based on those commentaries. Obviously, many of these guidelines apply to both phase II and III trials.

11.4.1
Select Biologically Meaningful Inclusion/Exclusion Criteria

One must be explicit about the biological rationale for the inclusion/exclusion criteria. For example, there are advantages and disadvantages to including heterogeneous study populations. An advantage of heterogeneous study populations is that the study results may be generalized to a broader group of people. Furthermore, as has been mentioned previously, it is unlikely that formulaic acupuncture can ever be devised for a very heterogeneous study population. The disadvantage is that heterogeneity may dilute treatment effects. In either case, the most important consideration is that the inclusion criteria make biological sense based on knowledge of the disease and of acupuncture.

11.4.2
Ensure Adequate Power

The most universal observation made in systematic reviews of acupuncture trials is that, with few exceptions, the numbers of patients were notably small. This makes acupuncture trials difficult to interpret because they can be prone to type II errors. Type II errors occur when a study obtains a nonsignificant result although a significant difference between groups exists in reality [40]. Unfortunately, there is no way to tell whether nonsignificant results reflect reality or result from type II errors due to inadequate statistical power. To reduce the possibility of type II errors, it is important to base sample size estimates a priori on a statistical formula [40], estimate expected differences from studies which used a control group comparable to the one intended for the planned study and, when possible, base sample size estimates on pilot data. It is best to recruit the skills of a biostatistician when addressing these statistical issues throughout the trial.

Trials comparing real vs. sham acupuncture for the treatment of pain may be especially prone to type II errors because they have larger sample size requirements than trials comparing real acupuncture to inert placebos for the treatment of pain. This is because sham (invasive) needling induces nonspecific physiological effects that include partial pain modulation [17]. A systematic review of acupuncture [41] for chronic pain demonstrated that the proportions of patients responding to sham acupuncture were significantly higher than the proportions responding to inert placebos.

11.4.3
Minimize Selection Bias Through Adequate Randomization

One of the most important potential biases can result from the way that patients are allocated to treatment groups. Known as selection bias, this is a systematic difference in the baseline characteristics of comparison groups [42]. Randomization offers the best way to balance known and unknown prognostic factors equally between groups. There are two distinctly important features in group allocation, both of which must be present in order to reduce the chances of selection bias: the first is that a true randomization procedure needs to be implemented (i.e., using a table of random numbers or a computer-generated randomizing scheme). The second, to be discussed in Section 11.4.4, is that the allocation procedure needs to be tamperproof.

Small studies are prone to selection bias because they are unlikely to achieve balance on important prognostic factors. If imbalances in group allocation result in less severely impaired patients being allocated to the treatment group and more severely impaired patients to the control group, then selection bias can lead to an artificially high response rate in the treatment group. Small trials are often thought to be problematic only because insufficient power may lead to findings of no treatment effect. However, they can truly be problematic due to selection bias and actually overestimate treatment effects by as much as 30 % [43]. The importance of baseline comparability has led Linde et al. [44] to include a question in their quality checklist which asks whether groups were comparable at baseline. It is always a good idea to report baseline comparisons of the two groups in any of the study publications. The difficulty of how to interpret results of a trial when groups are not comparable in baseline characteristics was recently evidenced in an RCT for headache [22]. The results of this methodologically rigorous pilot study, which scored a perfect score on the Jadad scale, were deemed impossible to interpret [45] due to a baseline difference in the weekly headache index. More severe headache index scores clustered in the real acupuncture group, thus giving placebo acupuncture an unfair advantage.

One way to assist the balance between groups is to stratify before randomizing. Generally, one or two factors known to be associated with the outcome of interest, such as CD4 counts in an AIDS study, are selected for the strata. Randomization is then done within each stratum.

11.4.4
Minimize Selection Bias Through Allocation Concealment

Allocation concealment is a term used to describe the method by which foreknowledge of treatment assignment is prevented and the allocation procedure is kept tamperproof [42]. Each patient's eligibility for the trial should be determined before he is randomly given a group assignment. Once assignment has been made, both the treatment group assignment and the eligibility decision should be unalterable. Obviously, allocation concealment is more likely to succeed if the person responsible for allocation is not the same one responsible for recruiting subjects or assessing eligibility.

Lack of adequate allocation concealment is more strongly associated with bias than how the randomization sequence is generated [42]. Lack of adequate allocation concealment can exaggerate treatment effects by as much as 41 % [46]. Obviously, transparent allocation systems such as alternate assignment, open lists, allocation by date of birth, or pulling numbers from a hat are not sufficient. Systems which sufficiently conceal allocation can include calling a central office for the next allocation assignment or an in-house computer file which yields the allocation only after the study identification number of the eligible person is entered.

11.4.5
Minimize Performance Bias by Blinding Patients and Practitioners

Performance bias is a systematic difference in the way patients or practitioners behave as a result of knowing the treatment group assignment [42]. Performance bias in unblinded patients, for example, can result in patients' reporting more symptoms.

Performance bias in unblinded practitioners can occur if the practitioner inadvertently treats the patients in treatment and control groups differently, such as being more caring or encouraging with those in the treatment group. Because practitioners can seldom be blinded in acupuncture trials, care must be taken to minimize practitioner performance bias. For example, the protocol might require that practitioners minimize verbal communication with the patient or use only standardized answers. It has also been suggested that videotaping treatment sessions could provide a way of detecting differences in practitioner behaviors so that they may be corrected while the trial is in progress [47].

Clearly, the optimal way to prevent performance bias is to blind those providing and receiving care to treatment group assignment (called double blinding). If a trial is not double blind, effects can be overestimated [43]. Double blinding is seldom possible in acupuncture trials because blinding those who are receiving the treatment is not possible if the two treatments do not resemble each other, as in sham TENS vs. acupuncture. Therefore, investigators must anticipate how performance bias might be influencing results and find ways to minimize it.

11.4.6
Minimize Detection Bias by Blinding the Outcome Assessors

Even when patients and practitioners cannot be blinded, the outcome assessor always can and should be blinded. Avoid detection bias by blinding outcome assessors. Detection bias is a systematic difference in the way outcomes are assessed due to lack of unblinded outcome assessors [42]. Put another way, unblinded outcome assessors may see what they want to see. This is particularly problematic in outcomes such as x-rays or global estimates of improvement that require a level of subjective judgment. It is less problematic in outcomes that require no subjective judgment, such as death. In acupuncture trials, unblinded outcome assessors who believe that acupuncture is beneficial may tend to find more global improvements or less disease progression in the real acupuncture group. It is important to note that some investigators use the term "double blinding" to mean that the outcome assessor is also blinded [48]. Therefore, it is important to ascertain exactly who is being blinded when "double blinding" is used.

11.4.7
Control for Cointerventions

Cointerventions, those treatments other than the experimental treatment that the patient may use while enrolled in the trial, must be accounted for in order to ascertain if benefit can be attributed to the experimental treatment [49]. Cointerventions can include medications, massage, physiotherapy, meditation practice, or lifestyle changes such as diet and exercise.

For example, one scenario might be that the control group does not experience benefit from the control treatment so that they turn to cointervention for relief. If cointerventions are not accounted for, then the two groups could appear to have equally effective treatments. This potential problem often leads trialists to ask patients to refrain from using cointerventions during the study period. When this is neither practical nor ethical, providing patients a way to document the use of cointerventions, such as recording in a daily diary, will provide a way to control for cointerventions in the statistical analysis.

11.4.8
Avoid Attrition Bias by Performing Intention-to-Treat Analysis

Even if selection bias has been successfully prevented during the allocation stage of a trial, it can still occur during the follow-up trial if only completers are counted. Selection bias during the follow-up period due to dropouts and withdrawals is called attrition bias. Attrition bias, therefore, results from a systematic difference in withdrawals [42]. Intention-to-treat analysis, which treats dropouts as nonresponders, is the preferred statistical approach to preventing attrition bias. Examples of intention-to-treat analysis are a relatively recent occurrence in the acupuncture literature [1, 50].

The rationale behind intention-to-treat analysis is to preserve the randomization scheme, thus preserving the balance in prognostic factors achieved during allocation to treatment group. Therefore, intention-to-treat analysis counts everyone who was randomized, including those who dropped out before ever receiving treatment, those who stopped coming for treatment, and those who were lost to follow-up. Although treating all dropouts and withdrawals as nonresponders may downplay the true effect of a treatment, it will not bias results.

11.4.9
Avoid Reporting Bias by Reporting on all Prespecified Outcomes

Reporting bias, the systematic difference in how outcomes are reported, can occur during writeup [42]. Because some consider positive findings more interesting than nonsignificant findings, investigators might be inclined to report only those outcomes which yield positive findings. The best way to prevent reporting bias is to specify in the planning stage of the study which outcomes will be measured and then to report on all of them, regardless of whether they yield positive or nonsignificant results.

11.4.10
Report *p* values, Relative Risk, and Confidence Intervals

Randomized controlled trials typically report between group differences in *p* values. By convention, differences are considered significant if $p < 0.05$, which means a less than 5 % chance that treatment A is the same as treatment B. When *p* values are presented with the relative risks and confidence intervals are presented near the relative risk, then a great deal more information about the results is provided. *P* values alone cannot estimate the magnitude of the treatment effect or indicate the precision of that magnitude estimate. Relative risk (RR), on the other hand, is the ratio of the incidence of the outcome in the treated group to the incidence of the outcome in the control group. The 95 % confidence intervals are generally presented with the RR and used to estimate its precision. A 95 % confidence interval indicates a 95 % chance that the difference between groups actually lies within that interval.

As a case in point, consider the recent RCT assessing the efficacy of acupuncture for dental pain. [5] Using *p* values alone, it was reported that after the first acupuncture treatment, subjects treated with real acupuncture compared to placebo acupuncture reported a longer time to moderate pain ($p = 0.008$). Then, by using RRs and confidence intervals, the investigators presented additional information that could not be provided by *p* values alone. The magnitude of effect was depicted as an RR of 0.40, which indicated that those in the real acupuncture group were 60 % less likely to experience moderate pain after third molar extraction than those in the placebo group. The precision of this estimate was depicted in the 95 % confidence interval (0.19–0.84), which showed that, although the RR estimated that the real acupuncture group was 60 % less likely to experience moderate pain, the real estimate may be as high as 81 % or as low as 16 %. That the confidence interval did not exceed these limits indicates that the true effect is likely to be statistically significant.

11.4.11
Summary

The three phases of clinical trials have been discussed in this chapter. By outlining the major goals in each phase of research, these FDA descriptions offer a model for acupuncture research that provides information valuable in every phase. This method enables acupuncture research to be simultaneously comprehensive and cost effective.

11.5
Toward an Integrated Research Model of Western and Traditional Chinese Medicine

With acupuncture seeking acceptance in the West, it is understandable that the large majority of clinical efficacy trials have been framed by biomedical symptoms and designed according to the placebo-controlled model. Yet adapting the Western biomedical model to assess TCM has been likened to measuring Chinese distances with a Western ruler. The fundamental question becomes: what more can be learned from the tradition behind acupuncture and how can that knowledge be applied to optimize the potential health benefits? To answer this question means integrating Western biomedical and TCM diagnoses and treatments into the same conceptual framework. Once the paradigms of these two medical traditions are brought into the same clinical trial framework, the scope of questions that can be asked is broadened and the potential gain of information becomes apparent. It is a fair test of any medicine that clinical trials should be informed by and mirror clinical practice to the greatest extent possible. The remainder of this chapter proposes ways to integrate the two systems so that future research is better informed and reflects acupuncture as it is practiced.

11.5.1
Can Integrating Western and TCM Diagnoses in the Same Trial Improve Efficacy?

As has been mentioned, a controversy exists in research concerning whether to use formulaic acupuncture in trials (which satisfies Western methodological rigor) or individualized treatments (which more closely approximates how acupuncture is practiced). Traditional Chinese medicine practitioners express concern that, by following only Western methodology, TCM loses its original meaning and its potentially greatest contribution to medicine – a unique way of diagnosing and individualizing treatments commonly referred to as TCM differentiation. According to the Western point of view, the same disease with the same symptoms presents the same diagnostic criteria; but according to the TCM point of view, it may constitute two or more TCM differentiations. For example, the Western treatment for chronic diarrhea may be universal, but the TCM treatment would be based upon the differentiation (Table 3).

The double screen technique proposed in this section is designed to accommodate both Western and TCM diagnoses in the same clinical trial. It is applied when eligibility is being determined prior to randomization. During eligibility assessment, both Western and TCM diagnostic criteria apply. Firstly, the person is deemed eligible according to conventional medicine diagnosis, in this case chronic diarrhea. Next, he is deemed eligible according to TCM diagnosis made by a TCM practitioner. Because there may be several TCM differentiations, it is more appropriate to choose the most

Table 3. Example of TCM differentiation of chronic diarrhea

Presenting symptoms	Likely TCM diagnosis	Likely TCM treatment
Diarrhea plus poor appetite	Spleen qi deficiency	Enhance spleen qi
Diarrhea plus anxiety	Liver overacting on spleen	Soothe liver qi
Diarrhea plus cold limbs	Spleen and kidney yang deficiency	Warm spleen and kidney yang
Turbid (loose, not clear), sluggish (foul smelling) diarrhea	Heat and dampness in the large intestine	Eliminate heat and dampness
Diarrhea plus hot flashes and night sweats	Yin deficiency	Enhance yin

common ones (e.g., for chronic diarrhea, kidney yang deficiency, and spleen qi deficiency) for the practical reason that selecting a common TCM diagnosis will increase the likelihood of enrolling an adequate number of participants for the trial. Once eligibility is confirmed by both conventional and TCM diagnoses, the patient is entered into the trial and randomly assigned to either a treatment group with formulaic acupuncture based on that TCM diagnosis or a placebo control group. If herbs are being used as part of the treatment, placebo herbs can be easily formulated for the control group. The double screen design is highly rigorous and likely to be acceptable by Western clinical trial standards and more satisfactory from the TCM point of view than trials applying one acupuncture formula to multiple TCM diagnoses.

A variation of the double screen design is to admit into the study all those who meet the Western eligibility criteria and then subdivide participants according to their TCM diagnoses prior to randomization. Within each TCM diagnostic category, patients would be randomized to receive either a formulaic treatment devised for that TCM diagnosis or a control treatment. The formulaic treatment would consist of a core set of points that are common to all categories, with additional formulaic points for that particular diagnostic category.

Yet another variation of the double screen design permits changing the formulaic treatment within the same patient during the course of the trial. In this application, a variety of formulaic treatments based on the possible TCM diagnoses is developed ahead of time. Then, as the TCM diagnosis of the person changes during the study, the acupuncturist administers a different formulaic treatment that is appropriate for the new TCM diagnosis. This approach moves closer to satisfying the TCM philosophy, which recognizes that there can be variations in the same patient at different time points and not just variations between patients.

11.5.2
Can the Modulatory Effects of Acupuncture Prevent Disease?

Cassidy [51] found that one of the primary reasons people seek acupuncture is for wellness maintenance – a kind of physiological tune-up. Indeed, one of the most appealing principles of TCM is that health is preserved by restoring a state of balance through keeping meridians open and the qi moving freely. It is postulated that TCM can detect minor, subclinical imbalances before they manifest as overt signs and symptoms. Consequently, according to this philosophy, a person is wise not to wait until illness occurs but rather to use acupuncture as preventive care. If this aspect of TCM can be validated, it may be the strongest contribution that this medicine has to offer: health maintenance with enhanced quality of life, well-being, and the absence of disease. The basic question is: can the TCM assertion be validated that subclinical symptoms are detectable and correctable which, if left unchecked, would lead to predictable biomedical symptomology?

Several studies with animals and humans now document that physiological processes can be normalized by acupuncture (e.g., cardiovascular [52–53], immunological [54], and gastrointestinal [55]). For example, Ballegaard et al. [53] demonstrated that acupuncture has a modulatory effect on cardiovascular indicators including skin blood flow, heart rate, and product of blood pressure and heart rate (increasing low normal values while decreasing high normal values) and concluded there may be value in healthy people using acupuncture to maintain cardiovascular homeostasis. Lao et al. [5] found that postoperative dental patients demonstrated fewer surgical side effects such as swelling and inflammation after acupuncture, also suggesting an anti-inflammatory modulatory effect.

To assess whether acupuncture can prevent chronic conditions requires costly, longitudinal, long-term epidemiological studies. However, a starting point for examining the effects of acupuncture on prevention can focus on acute conditions. For example, does Chinese medicine given preventively during the flu season lessen the incidence and severity of illness? Does it reduce the incidence of illness in at-risk populations such as the elderly?

11.5.3
Can Acupuncture plus Chinese Herbs Improve Efficacy?

In contrast to several styles of acupuncture that use needling without herbal therapy notably the Worsely-originated Five Element school, the French energetic style favored by most M. D. acupuncturists, and several systems of Japanese acupuncture the predominant style taught at U. S. acupuncture colleges, practiced by most licensed acupuncturists and known as TCM, fully integrates Chinese herbal therapy into its treatments. However, virtually no clinical trials have assessed the efficacy of acupuncture plus herbs.

Most Western trials of Chinese herbal therapy have tested either single herbs or isolated components rather than the herbal formulas characteristic in clinical practice. It is ironic that the increasing interest in "complementary" and "integrative" approaches to medicine has resulted in trials of acupuncture [36, 56] or herbs [57–58] as adjunctive to biomedical care but not led to trials of acupuncture *plus* herbs.

One expanded research design would randomize patients to groups receiving acupuncture plus herbs or acupuncture plus placebo herbs. When an herbal formula is prepared in tablet form, it is relatively straightforward also to prepare an innocuous placebo, with both sets of tablets having a similar shape, color, and bland coating [59]. Alternatively, an herbal preparation can be prepared in a standardized manner as a decoction (tea), while a similar weight of herbs with no known benefit for the test condition but a smell and taste similar to those of the active herbs can be used for a placebo decoction [60]. Such testing of herbal therapy as adjunctive to acupuncture allows for the possibility of a dose-response curve, a component of pharmaceutical trials rarely attempted in herbal trials.

11.5.4
Can Acupuncture plus Conventional Care Improve Efficacy?

A second research design involving an active control would compare actual practices of Chinese medicine (either acupuncture alone or acupuncture plus herbs) and biomedicine. Patients selected according to strict inclusion and exclusion criteria would be randomly assigned to receive one or the other type of care. If a condition chosen for study were treatable by biomedicine within a known time course, then such a study would reveal if Chinese medicine is as effective in a similar time period. Additional endpoints, including adverse side effects and cost effectiveness, could be compared for the two types of treatment.

11.5.5
Additional Applications

11.5.5.1
Evaluating Acupuncture Within Its Own Paradigm

Few trials have asked whether acupuncture is effective for conditions within its own medical paradigm, and few have explored how much additional information can be gained by including Chinese medicine diagnoses as endpoint measures. Among the questions future trials could ask are:

- Can acupuncture be shown in randomized controlled designs to correct Chinese medicine diagnoses? Can it relieve liver qi stagnation, correct kidney yin deficiency, or balance a condition of "too much fire?"
- Do Chinese medicine symptoms improve at the same rate as biomedical symptoms? (For example, does tongue coloration return to normal prior to, at the same time as, or after serum enzyme markers return to normative values?)
- Do patients who respond well or poorly to a biomedical treatment tend to fall preferentially into particular Chinese medicine subgroups?

11.5.5.2
Controlling for Individual Variation in Response to Acupuncture

In designing and interpreting clinical trials of acupuncture, little attention has been given to the potentially confounding problem of individual variations in responsiveness to treatment. The need to consider this phenomenon has become especially clear in studies of acupuncture analgesia. In animal studies, good responders and poor responders are often identified on the basis of prescreening tests and treated separately when examining the mechanisms of acupuncture analgesia [61–62]. Such studies have shown that individual variations in acupuncture analgesia are closely paralleled by variations in morphine-induced analgesia and analgesia induced by stimulation of the periaqueductal gray (PAG), a midbrain region that plays a key role in the processing of pain signals [63–65]. Further, animals identified as poor responders not only show high levels of cholecystokinin (CCK-8, an endogenous antiopioid neuropeptide) in their PAG but also can be converted to good responders by decreasing their brain levels of CCK-8 [66]. In humans, the existence of responders and nonresponders to morphine analgesia has long been recognized and is often taken into account in the research design of clinical trials [67–68].

The consequences of individual variations for clinical trials of acupuncture lie in the importance of assessing, for example, whether patients with headaches unresponsive to acupuncture have a vascular or musculoskeletal condition subtype that does not respond well to the treatment and/or have a biochemical makeup that prevents acupuncture from effectively stimulating their endogenous pain regulating mechanisms. In this light, the outcome of a clinical trial may well be a composite of independently varying responses to acupuncture and, as such, can confound interpretation of results. One approach to lessening the impact of individual variation would be to stratify for good or poor responders to acupuncture analgesia prior to randomizing patients into treatment groups. By relying on the high correlation in individual responses to acupuncture and morphine analgesia, patients enrolled in clinical trials of acupuncture efficacy for pain could be classified as good or poor responders on the basis of plasma and urinary markers used to differentiate responders and nonresponders to morphine [69]. The recognition of individual variations should also prompt clinical trials of acupuncture to report individual responses in addition to mean values. With this information, as well as rigorously defined inclusion and exclusion criteria at the outset, the contribution of individual response variations to trial outcome can be more clearly assessed.

11.6
Conclusions

Future acupuncture research holds many promising possibilities as clinical trials are creatively designed to reflect acupuncture as it is actually practiced. Once the Western and Chinese medical paradigms are brought into the same clinical trial framework, the scope of questions that can be asked is broadened and the potential information gain becomes apparent.

Acknowledgement. We would like to express appreciation to Victoria Hadhazy for her kind assistance with this manuscript.

References

1. Berman BM, Singh BB, Lao L, Langenberg P, Li H, Hadhazy V, Bareta J, Hochberg M (1999) A randomized trial of acupuncture as an adjunctive therapy in osteoarthritis of the knee. Rheumatol 39:346–354
2. Berman B, Lao L, Greene M, Anderson R, Wong RH, Langenberg P, Hochberg M (1995) Efficacy of traditional Chinese acupuncture in the treatment of symptomatic knee osteoarthritis: A pilot study. Osteoarthritis Cartilage 3:139–142
3. Lao L, Bergman S, Anderson R, Langenberg, P, Wong RH, Berman B (1994) The effect of acupuncture on postoperative oral surgery pain: a pilot study. Acup Med 12:13–17
4. Lao L, Bergman S, Langenberg, P, Wong RH, Berman B (1995) Efficacy of Chinese acupuncture on postoperative oral surgery pain. Oral Surg Oral Med Oral Pathol Oral Radiol Endod 79:423–9
5. Lao L, Bergman S, Hamilton GR, Langenberg P, Berman B (1999) Evaluation of acupuncture for pain control after oral surgery: A placebo-controlled trial. Arch Otolaryngol Head Neck Surg 125:567–572
6. Molsberger A, Bowing G (1997) Acupuncture for pain in locomotive disorders. Critical analysis of clinical studies with respect to the quality of acupuncture in particular. Der Schmerz 11:24–29
7. Birch S (1997) An exploration with proposed solutions of the problems and issues in conducting clinical research in acupuncture. University of Exeter, Exeter
8. Gaw AC, Chang LW, Shaw LC (1975) Efficacy of acupuncture on osteoarthritic pain. A controlled, double blind study. N Engl J Med 293:375–378
9. Christiansen BV, Iuhl IU, Vilbek H, Bulow HH, Dreijer NC, Rasmussen HF (1992) Acupuncture treatment of severe knee osteoarthrosis. A long-term study. Acta Anaesthesiol Scand 36:519–525
10. Takeda W, Wessel J (1994) Acupuncture for the treatment of pain of osteoarthritic knees. Arth Care Res 7:118–122
11. Bergner M, Bobbit RA, Carter WB, Gilson BS (1981) The Sickness Impact Profile: Development and final revision of a health status measure. Med Care 19:787–805
12. Ware JE (1995) The status of health assessment 1994. Ann Rev Public Health 16:327–354
13. Patrick DL, Deyo RA (1989) Generic and disease-specific measures in assessing health status and quality of life. Med Care 27:S217–S232
14. Hulley SB, Cummings SR (1992) Planning the measurements. In: Hulley SB, Cummings SR (eds) Designing Clinical Research. Williams and Wilkins, Baltimore
15. Deluze C, Bosia L, Zirbs A, Chantraine A, Vischer TL (1992) Electroacupuncture in fibromyalgia: Results of a controlled trial. BMJ 305:1249–1252

16. Turner J, Deyo R, Loeser J, Von Korff M, Fordyce WE (1994) The importance of placebo effects in pain treatment and research. JAMA 271:1609–1614
17. Hammerschlag R (1998) Methodological and ethical issues in clinical trials of acupuncture. J Alt Compl Med 4:159–171
18. Coan RM, Wong G, Ku S (1980) The acupuncture treatment of low back pain: A randomized controlled study. Am J Chin Med 8:181–189
19. Petrie J, Hazleman B (1985) Credibility of placebo transcutaneous nerve stimulation and acupuncture. Clin Exp Rheumatol 3:151–153
20. Richter A, Herlitz J, Hjalmarson A (1991) Effect of acupuncture in patients with angina pectoris. Eur Heart J 12:175–178
21. Hesse J, Mogelvang B, Simonsen H (1994) Acupuncture versus metoprolol in migraine prophylaxis: A randomized trial of trigger point deactivation. J Intern Med 235:451–456
22. White AR, Eddleston C, Hardie R, Resch KL, Ernst E (1996) A pilot study of acupuncture tension headache using a novel placebo. Acup Med 14:11–15
23. Streitberger K, Kleinhenz J (1998) Introducing a placebo needle into acupuncture research. Lancet 352:364–365
24. Emery P, Lythgoe S (1986) The effect of acupuncture on ankylosing spondylitis. [Letter.] Br J Rheumatol 25:123–133
25. Sung YF, Kutner MH, Cerine FC, Frederickson E (1977) Comparison of the effects of acupuncture and codeine on postoperative dental pain. Anesth Analg 56:473–478
26. Vincent CA (1989) A controlled trial of the treatment of migraine by acupuncture. Clin J Pain 5:305–312
27. Helms JM (1987) Acupuncture for the management of primary dysmenorrhea. Obstet Gynecol 69:51–56
28. Blom M, Dawidson I, Angmar-Mansson B (1992) The effect of acupuncture on salivary flow rates in patients with xerostomia. Oral Surg Oral Med Oral Pathol Oral Radiol Endod 73:293–298
29. Kendall DE (1989) A scientific model for acupuncture. Am J Acupunct 7:251–268
30. LeBars D, Villanueva L, Willer JC, Bouhassira D (1991) Diffuse noxious inhibitory controls (DNIC) in animals and man. Acupunct Med 9:47–56
31. Lewith G, Vincent C (1995) Evaluation of the clinical effects of acupuncture: A problem reassessed and a framework for future research. Pain Forum 1–29
32. Vincent CA (1990) Credibility assessment in trials of acupuncture. Complement Med Res 4:8–11
33. Allen JJB, Schnyer R, Hitt Sk (1998) The efficacy of acupuncture in the treatment of major depression in women. Psychol Sci 9:397–440
34. Hammerschlag R, Morris MM (1997) Clinical trials comparing acupuncture with biomedical standard care: A criteria-based evaluation of research design and reporting. Complement Ther Med 5:133–140
35. Wang H-H, Chang Y-H, Liu DM (1992) A study in the effectiveness of acupuncture analgesia for colonoscopic examination compared wth conventional premedication. Am J Acupunct 20:217–221
36. Johansson K, Lindgren I, Widner H, Wiklund I, Johansson BB (1993) Can sensory stimulation improve the functional outcome in stroke patients? Neurology 43:2189–2192
37. Zhou G, Jin S-B, Zhang L-D (1997) Comparative clinical study on the treatment of schizophrenia with electroacupuncture and reduced doses of antipsychotic drugs. Am J Acupunct 25:25–31
38. Max M (1991) Neuropathic pain syndromes. Advances Pain Res Ther 18:193–219
39. Mendelson G, Selwood TS, Loh TS, Kidson MA, Scott DS (1983) Acupuncture treatment of chronic back pain: A double blind placebo-controlled trial. Am J Med 74:49–55
40. Browner WS, Newman TB, Cummings SR, Hulley SB (1988) Getting ready to estimate sample size: Hypotheses and underlying principles. In: Hulley SB, Cummings SR (eds) Designing clinical research. Williams and Wilkins, Baltimore
41. Ezzo J, Berman B, Hadhazy V, Jadad A, Lao L, Singh B (2000) Is acupuncture effective for the treatment of chronic pain? A systematic review. Pain 86:217–225
42. Mulrow CD, Oxman A (eds) (1997) Critical appraisal of studies. Cochrane Collaboration Handbook. [Updated September 1997]. In: The Cochrane Library database on disk and CD-ROM. Issue 4. The Cochrane Collaboration, Oxford
43. McQuay H, Moore A (1998) An evidence-based resource for pain relief. Oxford Medical Publications, Oxford, p 33
44. Linde K, Worku F, Stor W, Wiesner-Zechmeister M, Pothmann R, Weinschutz T, Melchart D (1996) Randomized clinical trials of acupuncture for asthma – a systematic review. Forsch Komplementarmed 3:148–155
45. Melchart K, Linde K, Fischer P, Berman B, White A, Vickers A, Allais G (1999) Acupuncture for recurrent headaches. Review. Issue 3. The Cochrane Library, Oxford

46. Schultz KF, Chalmers I, Hayes RJ, Altman DG (1995) Empirical evidence of bias: Dimensions of methodological quality associated with estimate of treatment effects in controlled trials. JAMA 273:408–12

47. Vincent CA, Richardson PH (1986) The evaluation of therapeutic acupuncture: Concepts and methods. Pain 24:1–13

48. Jadad AR, Moore RA, Carroll D, Jenkinson C, Reynolds DJM, Gavaghan DJ, McQuay HJ (1996) Assessing the quality of randomized clinical trials: Is blinding necessary? Controlled Clin Trials 17:1–12

49. Deyo R (1991) Nonoperative treatment for low back disorders. Differentiating useful from useless therapy. In: Frymoyer J (ed) The adult spine: Principles and practices. Raven Press, New York, pp 85–104

50. Molsberger A (1998) Acupuncture in chronic low back pain. Paper presented at the International Society for the Study of the Lumbar Spine June 9–13, Brussels

51. Cassidy CM (1998) Chinese medicine users in the United States. Part I: Utilization, satisfaction, medical plurality. J Altern Complement Med 4:17–27

52. Yao T (1993) Acupuncture and somatic nerve stimulation: Mechanisms underlying effects on cardiovascular and renal activities. Scand J Rehab Med [Suppl] 29:7–18

53. Ballegaard S, Muteki T, Harada H, Ueda N, Tsuda H, Tayama F (1993) Modulatory effect of acupuncture on the cardiovascular system: A crossover study. Acup Electro Ther Res 18:103–115

54. Yang MMP, Ng KKW, Zeng HL, Kwok JSL (1989) Effect of acupuncture on immunoglobulins of serum, saliva, and gingival sulcus fluids. Am J Chin Med 17:89–94

55. Iwa M, Sakita M (1994) Effects of acupuncture and moxibustion on intestinal motility in mice. Am J Chin Med22:119–125

56. Shen J, Wegner N, Glaspy J, Hays R, Elliot M, Choi C, Shekelle P (1997) Adjunct antiemesis electroacupuncture in stem cell transplantation. Proc Am Soc Clin Oncol 16:42a

57. Xu GZ, Cai WM, Qin DX, Yan JH, Wu XL, Zhang HX, Hu YH, Gu XZ (1989) Chinese herb "destagnation" series I. Combination of radiation with destagnation in the treatment of nasopharyngeal carcinoma (npc): A prospective randomized trial on 188 cases. Int J Radiation Oncol Biol Phys 16:297–300

58. Yu G, Ren D, Sun G (1993) Clinical and experimental studies of JPYS in reducing side effects of chemotherapy in late stage gastric cancer. J Trad Chin Med 13:31–37

59. Burack JH, Cohen MR, Hahn JA, Abrams DI (1992) Pilot randomized controlled trial of Chinese herbal treatment for HIV-associated symptoms. J AIDS Hum Retrovirol 12:386–393

60. Sheehan MP, Rustin MHA, Atherton DJ, Buckley C, Harris DJ, Brostoff J, Ostlere L, Dawson A (1992) Efficacy of traditional Chinese herbal therapy in adult atopic dermatitis. Lancet 340:13–17

61. Xu M, Aiuchu T, Nakaya K, Arakawa H, Maeda M, Tsuji A, Kato T, Takeshige C, Nakamura Y (1990) Effect of low frequency electric stimulation on in vivo release of cholecystokinin-like immunoreactivity in medial thalamus of conscious rat. Neurosci Lett 118:205–207

62. Takeshige C, Oka K, Mizuno T, Hisamitsu T, Luo C-P, Kobori M, Mera H, Fang T-Q (1993) The acupuncture point and its connecting central pathway for producing acupuncture analgesia. Brain Res Bull 30:53–67

63. Takeshige C, Murai M, Tanaka M, Hachisu M (1983) Parallel individual variations in effectiveness of acupuncture, morphine analgesia, and dorsal PAG-SPA and their abolition by D-phenylalanine. Adv Pain Res Ther 5:563–569

64. Huang Z, Qiu X, Han J (1985) The individual variation in acupuncture analgesia: A positive correlation between the effects of electroacupuncture analgesia and morphine analgesia in the rat. Acupunct Res 10:115–118

65. Liu SX, Luo F, Shen S et al (1999) Relationship between the analgesic effect of electroacupuncture and CCK-8 content in spinal perfusate in rats. Chin Sci Bull 44:240–243

66. Tang N-M, Dong H-W, Wang, X-M, Tsui Z-C, Han J-S (1997) Cholecystokinin antisense RNA increases the analgesic effect induced by electroacupuncture or low dose morphine: Conversion of low responder rats to high responders. Pain 71:71–80

67. Lorenzetti ME, Roberts-Thomson IC, Pannall PR, Taylor WB (1991) Placebo-controlled trial of dexamethasone for chronic biliary pain after cholecystectomy. Clin J Pain 7:318–322

68. Sorensen J, Kalman S, Tropp H, Bengtsson M (1996) Can a pharmacological pain analysis be used in the assessment of chronic lower back pain? Eur Spine J 5:236–242

69. Roberts-Thomson IC, Jonsson JR, Pannall PR, Frewin DB (1991) Morphine responders with unexplained pain after cholecystectomy may have sympathetic overactivity. Clin Autonom Res 1:59–62

CHAPTER 12

Future Directions for Research on the Physiology of Acupuncture

R. Hammerschlag · L. Lao

12.1
Overview

Clinical research provides a systematic approach for identifying conditions of disease and dysfunction that can be effectively treated by acupuncture; *physiological* research examines how acupuncture works. Several rationales support the need for these latter studies. Evidence of mechanism imparts credibility to clinical findings of acupuncture as a drug-free alternative for treating conditions involving pain, inflammation, and nausea. Understanding the mechanisms by which needling promotes healing enhances the acceptance of acupuncture in the West, particularly when changes are detected in cells or molecules related to neural, hormonal, immune, cardiovascular, gastrointestinal, and other biomedically defined systems. Biomedical correlates of acupuncture action, in turn, assist researchers in improving the design of trials testing the efficacy of acupuncture treatment.

It can be argued, however, that the question guiding most mechanism-directed research "What biochemical or physiological changes correlate with acupuncture effectiveness?" is useful but limiting. Equally needed are studies that ask the broader question "What can acupuncture tell us about how the body functions that Western medicine and physiology have not yet discovered?"

The present chapter examines three fruitful areas for physiological research in acupuncture with the potential for revealing additional biomedical correlates of acupuncture effectiveness and for shedding light on new ways to understand human health and disease. Firstly, we address the need to identify mechanisms of acupuncture analgesia for management of chronic pain. The need for this new direction arises from an anomaly: that acupuncture practitioners most commonly treat *chronic* pain whereas neurophysiological models of acupuncture analgesia are based mainly on studies of neurologically distinct *acute* pain. Secondly, we examine a range of techniques used to stimulate acupoints, from electroacupuncture to qigong, to assess the degree of confidence with which we can accept neurophysiologically based models as the predominant means of explaining acupuncture analgesia. Thirdly, we review the concept that, as a treatment system not restricted to pain modulation, acupuncture acts by exerting a normalizing or homeostatic effect on physiological parameters, up-regulating *hypo* conditions while down-regulating *hyper* conditions. In this context, we consider proposals that view acupuncture as acting on a self-regulatory system, one that may not be fully explainable in terms of currently accepted nervous, endocrine, and immune system functions.

12.2
Acupuncture and Chronic Pain: Models and Mechanisms

Acupuncture-produced analgesia (AA) is one of the most extensively investigated areas in the field of research directed at the physiology of acupuncture [27, 41, 50]. The most common animal behavioral models in AA research challenge acupuncture to lengthen the time that a normal (noninjured) animal will tolerate a transient noxious stimulus. Increased tolerance, measured as an increase in time before the test animal flicks its tail, jerks its head, avoids a hot plate, or vocalizes, is equated with increased analgesia [20, 30, 40]. Typically, heat or subcutaneous electrical stimulation is applied to the skin, tail, or nostril region, and the tail-flick latency or "latency to squeak" is measured before and after acupuncture or in needled vs. sham needled animals [20, 41]. It has been frequently demonstrated that electroacupuncture (EA) increases response latency to noxious stimuli in animals, indicating that it produces an analgesic effect. These studies have proven valuable in establishing that AA does, in fact, have a physiological basis and that acusignals underlying AA appear to follow neural pathways well-known to researchers who study the neurobiology of pain.

A major drawback of such studies, however, is their limited clinical relevance. Four lines of reasoning support this argument:

1. Analgesic effects of EA diminish rapidly after the termination of EA treatment, typically within 10–20 minutes [20]. This provides an inadequate model of common clinical observations of post-treatment effects of AA, at least temporally.
2. Behavioral tests employed as endpoints in AA studies often require restraining the animals, which in turn may inadvertently cause stress-induced analgesia that can confound the experimental results [39, 54].
3. The intensity of EA used has often been higher (up to 18 V) than that used in clinical practice [30, 42]. This is because the clinically effective use of low intensity electrical stimulation may not be able to increase the pain threshold dramatically in normal animals.
4. The normal animal model does not resemble the pathological chronic pain conditions that acupuncturists are most often called upon to treat clinically.

Thus, in spite of numerous AA studies that have revealed considerable details of the physiological bases of acupuncture, many questions regarding clinical applications of acupuncture cannot be answered by examining animal models of acute transitory pain, for example:

1. What is the "optimal dose" of acupuncture treatment as determined in dose-response studies (the most appropriate frequency of treatments, duration of a treatment session, and follow-up protocols after the initial concentrated treatments) for a given chronic pain condition?
2. What is the role of acupuncture in treating underlying conditions that produce pain, such as inflammation or tissue injuries?
3. How can stress-induced analgesia be minimized in acupuncture studies that involve animal behavioral endpoints?

To answer these questions, acupuncture needs to be evaluated in clinically relevant, chronic pathological conditions such as an animal model of persistent inflammatory pain.

Persistent inflammatory pain models have been developed in the rat using inflammatory agents such as yeast, carrageenan, and complete Freund's adjuvant (CFA), which can produce inflammation lasting for hours, days, or weeks [26, 29, 57]. This class of noxious stimuli has recently been employed to develop a rat behavioral model of chronic inflammatory pain for the study of AA [28]. Injection of CFA into the intraplantar surface of the rat's hindpaw produces an intense inflammation characterized by edema, redness, and hyperalgesia that is limited to the injected paw [23, 44, 45]. The hyperalgesia is assessed by exposing the hindpaw to a thermal or mechanical stimulus and monitoring the paw withdrawal latency or the intensity of the stimulus that produces withdrawal [25, 45]. This model provides sufficient time (up to 10 days) to evaluate the post-treatment effects of EA and minimizes stress-induced analgesia by its use of unrestrained animals. This is because, in pathological conditions, lower EA intensities – comparable to those used in clinical practice – can produce desired antihyperalgesic effects. This CFA-mediated persistent inflammatory pain model may also allow the analgesic, antihyperalgesic, and anti-inflammatory effects of acupuncture to be investigated separately, under clinically relevant pathogenic conditions [28].

Although studies have demonstrated that the mechanism of acupuncture-mediated analgesia (AA) is attributable to the release of opioids from the central nervous system, clinically effective local acupuncture points, adjacent to the painful area, are often crucial for the treatment of musculoskeletal pain conditions [11, 37]. The effectiveness of using local acupuncture points to treat musculoskeletal conditions such as osteoarthritis has also been demonstrated in clinical trials [5, 14]. One question arising from these studies concerns to what extent *peripheral* mechanisms underlie the effectiveness of acupuncture. Recent studies have revealed that, in addition to a central opioid system, a peripheral opioid system exists which is also involved in modulating pain, particularly localized inflammatory pain [43, 51]. Zhang et al. [62] recently reported that AA is partially blocked by local application of naloxone, suggesting that peripheral opioids are released following electroacupuncture treatment. Additional studies are needed in this new direction of AA research not only to investigate further the physiological mechanisms induced by the needling, but to provide information that can improve the clinical practice of acupuncture.

12.3
Invasive and Noninvasive Stimulation of Acupoints: Implications for Mechanisms

Clinical practice as well as clinical trials have demonstrated that acupoints can be stimulated by a wide range of procedures. These modes of stimulation include the minimally invasive techniques of electroacupuncture and manual needling as well as noninvasive techniques involving surface contact, as with transcutaneous electrical nerve stimulation (TENS) electrodes, and noncontact, as with the practice of external qigong. (Pressure and lasers are among an array of additional means that are not included in this discussion.) The most intense form of acupoint stimulation is usually achieved via electroacupuncture, involving the mechanical effects of needling augmented by electric current delivered through the needle. When delivered at the same frequencies as electroacupuncture, TENS can, under some conditions, produce comparable effects [13, 33]. Manual needling alone, whether with the deeper, intramuscular techniques favored by Chinese-style practitioners or the relatively shallow, subcutaneous needling preferred in the Japanese style, involves mechanical effects of the needle often enhanced by the practitioner's intent (*yi,* in Chinese medical terminology). A more subtle form of acupoint stimulation is achieved in *toyo hari* acupuncture, with the needle placed either just touching the acupoint at the skin surface or held directly above the acupoint without skin contact and with the practitioner sensing or projecting *qi* (*ki* in Japanese) through the needle [6, 18]. Finally, qigong practitioners typically stimulate acupoints by projecting their qi at a distance from the patient [24, 47].

Viewed in this manner, where the mode of acupoint stimulation varies from electrical current to mechanical activity to the undefined transmission of qi, several questions arise with regard to the neurobiology-based models of AA elegantly described in the earlier chapters of Han, Pomeranz, and Takeshige.

How well do these models, derived predominantly from studies employing strong electrostimulation techniques, hold up when manual needling is employed? With very few exceptions, e.g., the first demonstration in humans that naloxone partially inhibits acupuncture analgesia induced by manual needling [34], virtually all the evidence for the acupuncture-endorphin connection has been derived from studies using electroacupuncture. From a research perspective, electroacupuncture (as well as TENS) has an obvious advantage over manual acupuncture in that defining the frequency, amplitude, duration, and wave form of electrostimulation allows experiments to be reproduced with a greater degree of confidence than do descriptions of twirling, thrusting, and other traditional techniques of manual stimulation.

From a clinical perspective, electrostimulation parameters for acupuncture analgesia have been chosen for their effectiveness in reproducing therapeutic outcomes of different styles of manual needling. For example, high frequency (100 Hz) and low frequency (2 Hz) electroacupuncture are described as mimicking traditional needling techniques known as "dense" and "disperse," respectively [10]. However, systematic studies are needed to test whether disperse needling preferentially induces nervous system release of enkephalin and β-endorphin similar to that under 2–4 Hz electrostimulation (via needles or TENS) and whether dense needling preferentially releases dynorphin and serotonin similar to that with 100–200 Hz electrostimulation [12, 21, 22]

Does Japanese style shallow needling stimulating cutaneous afferent nerve endings release the same endogenous substances as Chinese style deep needling, which predominantly stimulates muscle afferents? While no clinical trial has been designed to compare these two types of needling performed by practitioners trained in the respective traditional medicine, several trials have inadvertently approximated this design by performing shallow needling on the "control group" at the same acupoints used for deep needling of the "acupuncture group" [19, 58]. It is clearly inappropriate to assess the magnitude of acupuncture efficacy relative to sham needling in a trial where, in fact, two different styles of acupuncture are compared. Clinical trials of deep vs. superficial needling would be of value if clinical effectiveness and corresponding release of endogenous opioids were compared. A related issue is to assess clinical effectiveness and patterns of neurochemical release under conditions where deep needling, which elicits patient reports of *de qi* sensations (often claimed by traditional Chinese acupuncture as essential to produce clinical results), is compared to Japanese style shallow needling, where practitioners treat with no attempt to elicit this sensation.

Do noninvasive toyo hari needling and external qigong also release endogenous opioids as they clinically suppress pain? Clinical reports of pain modulation resulting from nonpuncture and noncontact treatment at acupoints are not readily explainable within the framework of neurobiological models of acupuncture analgesia. In such models, electrical signaling along peripheral and central nerve pathways is initiated predominantly by *physical contact* between the acupuncture needle and mechanoreceptive nerve endings in skin and muscle. While these models can be expanded to include nonpuncture initiating stimuli such as pressure (acupressure) and electrical fields (TENS), there is no generally accepted understanding of what types of stimuli are generated during *toyo hari* noncontact needling and external qigong treatment, nor is there direct evidence that such practices stimulate the same neural pathways proposed for electro- and manual acupuncture. Of considerable interest, however, is that the propagating sensations along the meridians, reproducibly reported by sensitive subjects in response to manual needling at single points [59], has also been reported in response to noninvasive *toyo hari* needling [7] and external qigong [24].

Several types of research studies are needed to begin examining the phenomena of acupoint stimulation at a distance in relation to invasive needling techniques. Randomized clinical trials comparing electroacupuncture, manual acupuncture, *toyo hari* needling, and external qigong should be designed to assess (a) pain modulation, (b) endogenous opioid release, and (c) direct microelectrode recording from single nerve fibers [55]. These latter experiments in human subjects have demonstrated similar neural activity patterns in response to manual acupuncture with and without electrostimulation. Clearly, it is also important to identify the nature of the signal passing from the *toyo hari* or qigong practitioner to the acupoint. Preliminary studies suggest that electromagnetic [36, 49] and microwave [15] emissions detected from the palms of practitioners may be involved

12.4
Bidirectional Effects of Acupuncture

A clinically recognized but little-researched phenomenon of acupuncture is its ability to induce bidirectional effects such that needling at the same acupoint(s) can return a particular physiological parameter, e.g., heart rate, gastric acid secretion, or antibody levels from a hypo- or hypercondition to normative levels. For example, blood pressure and heart rate in strains of rats bred to be either congenitally hypotensive or hypertensive were "normalized" by acupuncture [61]. Pharmacological studies suggest that the pressor effects of acupuncture in hypotensive rats, being naloxone-insensitive but attenuated by scopolamine, involve central cholinergic mechanisms, whereas the depressor effects in the hypertensive animals, being inhibited by naloxone or parachlorophenylalanine, are mediated by the release of endogenous opioids and serotonin. Similar normalizing effects of acupuncture have been described in rats made hypotensive by withdrawing blood [52]and in dogs made hypertensive by intravenous infusion of epinephrine [31].

In light of the evidence supporting a homeostatic action of acupuncture, it is not surprising that studies on cardiovascular function in *normal* human subjects have shown only slight or nonsignificant effects on heart rate or blood pressure when the data was presented in mean values [35, 53]. However, a different picture emerges when the effects on *individual* subjects are analyzed. A trial involving electroacupuncture at LI.4 and LI.10 [1] revealed that individuals whose pretreatment heart rates were in the lowest third of the normal test group had their rates increased by acupuncture, whereas those with initial values in the highest third experienced a decrease. Similar bidirectional effects were observed for cutaneous blood flow and the product of blood pressure and heart rate. Had these sets of data been analyzed as mean effects, none of the results would have been statistically significant.

Indications of the normalizing or balancing effect of acupoint stimulation have also been detected in immune system responses. In healthy human subjects, the levels of IgA (the main class of salivary immunoglobulins) increased after 30 minutes of acupuncture (LI.4, St.7, endocrine ear point) and at 24 hours post-treatment in individuals whose initial levels were low and decreased in those whose initial levels were high [60]. While the effects of acupuncture have been examined on a wide range of other immune responses, including cell-mediated (white blood cell levels, macrophage phagocytic activity, T cell proliferation and transformation, and natural killer cell cytotoxic activity) and humoral immunity (competency of B-cells to engage in antibody production) [9, 16, 17, 48], only the IgA study cited above was designed to examine the bidirectional effects of acupuncture.

While the logic of biomedicine is to monitor specific cellular and molecular biomarkers in response to acupoint needling, this approach causes acupuncture to be regarded as a set of finely tuned procedures that, similar to pharmacologically designed drugs, selectively affect different cell populations. An arguably more useful physiological model is to consider acupuncture as facilitating the release and balancing the circulating levels of the same endogenous substances, e.g., cytokines and endogenous opioids, that immune system cells use to communicate with each other as well as with cells of the endocrine, nervous, and other regulatory systems [8, 38, 56]. In a body that has lost the ability to regulate one of its systems, biomedicine prescribes an agonist or antagonist drug that mimics or blocks the action of an inadequately functioning regulatory molecule. In contrast, acupuncture may stimulate a regulatory system in a manner that induces self-correction mechanisms.

What is needed are systematic studies of the bidirectional effects of acupuncture, with multiple measurements of regulatory or affector molecules, such as the cytokines, as well as affected cell and molecular markers. Only with this broader approach can questions be framed and answers sought as to how acupuncture regulates internal activities. As the data accumulates, it should become clearer whether the homeostatic actions of acupuncture are initiated directly via known neural and hormonal mechanisms, as occurs when a drug binding to its target receptor initiates a cascade of events. Alternately, it may also become clearer that acupuncture triggers homeostatic regulation by acting on an integrative system that is separate from but interfaces with the known autonomic and humoral systems [4, 32].

What clues do we have in the search for such an integrative system? If, as briefly discussed earlier in this chapter, the clinical effectiveness of *toyo hari* and external qigong treatments-at-a-distance are mediated by bioelectromagnetic (BEM) field effects, the question arises whether these fields, externally applied to acupoints, have informational content. It has long been recognized that electromagnetic fields of brain, muscle, and heart give rise to EEG, EMG, and EKG patterns that contain diagnostic information. Only recently has it also been observed that living organisms emit BEM radiation as biophotons that contribute to the regulation of a range of cell biological events from membrane transport to gene expression [46]. The question to be explored is whether "energy" practitioners have learned to transmit this form of BEM field as a therapeutic signal. The intriguing possibility is that practitioner-generated weak electromagnetic fields may entrain or "pattern-correct" abnormal BEM fields within the body [2].

There is promising evidence that such BEM fields arise from the direct current generated by cells that surround neurons [3]. The nature of this DC phenomenon, the possible role of acupoint stimulation in the maintenance of the BEM field integrity, and the manner in which the BEM field acts via stimulation of acupoints to regulate energetic, molecular, and cellular events are highly exciting directions for future research.

References

1. Ballegaard S, Muteki T, Harada H, Ueda N, Tsuda H, Tayama F, Ohishi K (1993) Modulatory effect of acupuncture on the cardiovascular system: A crossover study, Acupunct Electrother Res 18:103–115
2. Becker RO (1982) Electrical controls of regeneration. J Bioelectr 1:239
3. Becker RO, Marino AA (1982) Electromagnetism and life. State University Press, New York, Albany
4. Bensoussan A (1991) The vital meridian: A modern exploration of acupuncture. Churchill Livingstone, Melbourne, pp 127–132
5. Berman B, Singh B, Lao L, Hochberg M, Langenberg P, Li H, Hadhazy V (1999) A randomized trial of acupuncture as an adjunctive therapy in osteoarthritis of the knee. Br J Rheumatol 38:346–354
6. Birch S, Ida J (1997) A brief report on the 1996 U. S. Toyohari workshop, with reflections on the development of keiraku chiryo (Japanese meridian therapy) in America. Amer J Acu 25:71–74
7. Birch S (1999) Personal communication
8. Blalock JE (1989) A molecular basis for bidirectional communication between the immune and neuroendocrine systems. Physiol Rev 69:1–32
9. Bossy J (1994) Acupuncture and immunity: Basic and clinical aspects. Acupunct Med 12:60–62
10. Chen X, Guo S, Chang C, Han J (1992) Optimal conditions for eliciting maximal electroacupuncture analgesia with dense and disperse mode stimulation. Eur J Pharmacol 211:203–210
11. Cheng X (1987) Chinese acupuncture and moxibustion. Foreign Languages Press, Beijing
12. Cheng RSS. Pomeranz B (1981) Monoaminergic mechanism of electroacupuncture analgesia. Brain Res 215:77–92
13. Cheng RSS. Pomeranz B (1987) Electrotherapy of chronic musculoskeletal pain: Comparison of electroacupuncture and acupuncture-like transcutaneous electrical nerve stimulation. Clin J Pain 2:143–149
14. Christensen BV, Iuhl IV, Vilbeck H, Bulow HH, Dreijer NC, Rasmussen HF (1992) Acupuncture treatment of severe knee osteoarthritis: A long-term study. Acta Anaesthesiol Scand 36:518–525
15. Edrich J, Jobe WE, Cacek RK, Hende WR, et al (1980) Imaging thermograms at centimeter and millimeter wavelengths. Ann NY Acad Sci 335:456–476
16. Filshie J, White A (1998) The clinical use of and evidence for acupuncture in the medical systems. In: Filshie J, White A (eds) Medical acupuncture: A western scientific approach. Churchill Livingstone, Edinburgh
17. Fujiwara R, Tong ZG, Matsuoka H, Shibata H, Iwamoto M, Yokoyama MM (1991) Effects of acupuncture on immune response in mice. Intern J Neurosci 57:141–150
18. Fukushima K (1991) Meridian therapy: A hands-on text on traditional Japanese hari. Toyo Hari Medical Association, Tokyo
19. Haker E, Lundeberg T (1990) Acupuncture treatment in epicondylagia: A comparative study of two acupuncture techniques. Clin J Pain 6:221–226

20. Han JS (1987) The neurochemical basis of pain relief by acupuncture. Chinese Medical and Technology Press, Beijing, pp 21–76
21. Han JS (1993) Acupuncture and stimulation produced analgesia. Handbook Exp Pharmacol 104/II:105–125
22. Han JS, Chen XH, Sun SL, Xu XJ, Yuan Y, Yan SC, Hao JX, Terenius L (1991) Effect of low- and high-frequency TENS on met-enkephalin – Arg-Phe and dynorphin A immunoreactivity in human lumbar CSF. Pain 47:295–298
23. Hargreaves K, Dubner R, Brown F, Flores C, Joris J (1988) A new and sensitive method for measuring thermal nociception in cutaneous hyperalgesia. Pain 32:77–88
24. He Q, Zhou J, Yang B, Zhao G, Zhai T, Liu Y (1984) Research on the propagated sensation along meridians excited by qigong. Second National Symposium on Acupuncture and Moxibustion and Acupuncture Anesthesia, abstracts, pp 262–263
25. Hylden JLK, Nahin RL, Traub RJ, Dubner R (1989) Expansion of receptive fields of spinal lamina I projection neurons in rats with unilateral adjuvant-induced inflammation: The contribution of dorsal horn mechanisms. Pain 37:229–243
26. Kayser V, Guilbaud G (1987) Local and remote modifications of nociceptive sensitivity during carrageenin-induced inflammation in the rat. Pain 28:99–107
27. Kho HG, Robertson EN (1997) The mechanism of acupuncture analgesia: Review and update. Am J Acupunct 25:261–281
28. Lao L, Zhang G, Wei F, Berman B, Meszler RM, Ren K (1998) Electroacupuncture attenuates hyperalgesia and modulates FOS protein expression with unilateral persistent inflammation. Soc for Neurosci 24:884
29. Larson AA, Brown DR, El-Atrash S, Walser MM (1986) Pain threshold changes in adjuvant-induced inflammation: A possible model of chronic pain in the mouse. Pharmacol Biochem Behav 24:49–53
30. Lee JH, Beitz AJ (1993) The distribution of brainstem and spinal cord nuclei associated with different frequencies of electroacupuncture analgesia. Pain 52:11–28
31. Li P, Sun F-Y, Zhang A-Z (1983) The effect of acupuncture on blood pressure: The interrelation of sympathetic activity and endogenous opioid peptides. Acupunct Electrother Res 8:45–56
32. Manaka Y, Itaya K, Birch S (1995) Chasing the Dragon's Tail. Paradigm Publications, Brookline, pp 17–38
33. Martelete M, Fiori AMC (1985) Comparative study of the analgesic effect of transcutaneous nerve stimulation (TNS), electroacupuncture (EA), and meperidine in the treatment of postoperative pain, Acupunct Electrother Res 10:183–193
34. Mayer DJ, Price DD, Raffi A (1977) Antagonism of acupuncture analgesia in man by the narcotic antagonist naloxone. Brain Res 121:368–373
35. Nishijo K, Mori H, Yosikawa K, Yazawa K (1997) Decreased heart rate by acupuncture stimulation in humans via facilitation of cardiac vagal activity and suppression of cardiac sympathetic nerve. Neurosci Lett 227:165–168
36. Nordenström, BEW (1992) Hand movements above the unshielded tail of a shielded rat induces differences of voltage inside the animal. Amer J Acupunct 20:157–161
37. O'Connor J, Bensky D (eds) (1981) Acupuncture: a comprehensive text. Eastland Press, Chicago
38. Pert CB, Dreher HE, Ruff MR (1998) The psychosomatic network: Foundations of mind-body medicine. Altern Ther Health Med 4:30–41
39. Pomeranz B (1986) Relation of stress-induced analgesia to acupuncture analgesia. Ann NY Acad Sci 467:444–447
40. Pomeranz B, Stux G (1988) Scientific bases of acupuncture. Springer-Verlag, Berlin Heidelberg, pp 7–33
41. Pomeranz B (1994) Acupuncture in America, a commentary. APS Journal 3:96–100
42. Pomeranz B, Paley D (1979) Electroacupuncture hyperalgesia is mediated by afferent nerve impulses: An electrophysiological study in mice. Exp Neurol 66:398–402
43. Przewlocki R, Hassan AHS, Lason W, Epplen C, Herz A, Stein C (1992) Gene expression and localization of opioid peptides in immune cells of inflamed tissue: Functional role in antinociception. Neuroscience 48:491–500
44. Ren K, Ruda MA (1996) Descending modulation of Fos expression after persistent peripheral inflammation. NeuroRep 7:2186–2190
45. Ren K, Williams GM, Hylden JLK, Ruda MA, Dubner R (1992) The intrathecal administration of excitatory amino acid receptor antagonists – selectively attenuated carrageenan-induced behavioral hyperalgesia in rats Eur J Pharmacol 219:235–243
46. Rubik B, Becker RO, Hazlewood CF, Liboff AR, Walleczek J (1995) Electromagnetic applications in medicine. NIH-OAM Panel Report

47. Sancier KM, Hu BK (1991) Medical applications of qigong and emitted qi on humans, animals, cell cultures, and plants: Review of selected scientific research. Amer J Acupunct 19:367–377
48. Sato T, Yu Y, Guo SY, Kasahara T, Hisamitsu T (1996) Acupuncture stimulation enhances splenic natural killer cell cytotoxicity in rats. Japan J Physiol 46:131–136
49. Seto A, Kusaka C, Nakazato S, Huang WR, Sato R, Hisamitsu T, Takeshige C (1992) Detection of extraordinary large biomagnetic field strength from human hand during external qi emission. Acupunct Electrother Res 17:75–94
50. Sims J (1997) The mechanism of acupuncture analgesia: A review. Compl Ther Med 5:102–111
51. Stein C, Millan MJ, Yassouridis A, Herz A (1988) Antinociceptive effects of mu- and kappa-agonists in inflammation are enhanced by a peripheral opioid receptor-specific mechanism of action. Eur J Pharmacol 155:255–64
52. Sun X-Y, Yu J, Yao T (1983) Pressor effect produced by stimulation of somatic nerve on hemorrhagic hypotension in conscious rats. Acta Physiol Sin 35:264–270
53. Tayama F, Muteki T, Bekki S, Yamashita T et al (1984) Cardiovascular effect of electroacupuncture. Kurume Med J 31:37–46
54. Terman GW, Shavit Y, Lewis JW, Cannon JT, Liebeskind JC (1984) Intrinsic mechanisms of pain inhibition: Activation by stress. Science 226:1270–1277
55. Wang K, Yao S, Xian Y, Hou Z (1985) A study on the receptive field of acupoints and the relationship between characteristics of needle sensation and groups of afferent fibers. Sci Sin 28:963–971
56. Weigent DA, Blalock JE (1995) Associations between the neuroendocrine and immune systems. J Leukoc Biol 58:137–150
57. Winter CA, Flataker L (1965) Reaction thresholds to pressure in edematous hindpaws of rats and responses to analgesic drugs. J Pharmacol Exp Ther 150:165–171
58. Wyon Y, Lindgren R, Lundeberg T, Hammar M (1995) Effects of acupuncture on climacteric vasomotor symptoms, quality of life, and urinary excretion of neuropeptides among postmenopausal women. Menopause 2:3–12
59. Xie Y, Li H, Xiao W (1996) Neurobiological mechanisms of the meridian and the propagation of needle feeling along the meridian pathway. Sci China C Life Sci 39:99–112
60. Yang MMP, Ng KKW, Zeng HL, Kwok JSL (1989) Effect of acupuncture on immunoglobulins of serum, saliva, and gingival sulcus fluid. Am J Chin Med 17:89–94
61. Yao T (1993) Acupuncture and somatic nerve stimulation: Mechanism underlying effects on cardiovascular and renal activities. Scand J Rehab Med Suppl 29:7–18
62. Zhang G, Graczyk Z, Ren K, Stein C, Berman B, Lao L (1999) Local naloxone blockade of acupuncture analgesia: Peripheral opioids implicated. Proc Soc Neurosci 29th Annual Meeting 25:688

Subject Index

A

Druck: Strauss Offsetdruck, Mörlenbach
Verarbeitung: Schäffer, Grünstadt

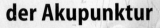
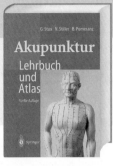
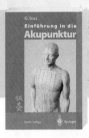
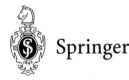

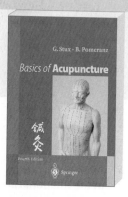
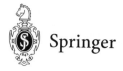